New Horizons in Medical Anthropology

New Horizons in Medical Anthropology is a cutting edge volume in honour of Charles Leslie, a highly respected medical anthropologist whose influential career has shaped this branch of anthropology as it is studied and theorized today. Written by former students and colleagues of Charles Leslie, this collection of papers deals with issues as diverse as AIDS and new medical technologies, therapy management and over-population with case studies from Africa and Asia.

The first section of the book reflects recent research by medical anthropologists working in Asia who have been inspired by Charles Leslie's earlier research on medical pluralism, the social relations of therapy management, the relationship between state and medical systems, and health discourse. The latter part of the volume then reflects the lesser known aspects of Leslie's work – his contribution as an editor and the role he played in carrying the field forward; his ethics as a medical anthropologist committed to humanism and sensitive to racism and eugenics; and the passion he inspired in his co-workers and students.

Charles Leslie is a remarkable and influential social scientist. *New Horizons in Medical Anthropology* is a fitting tribute to a sensitive man whose ethics, theories and codes of practice provide an essential guide to all future medical anthropologists.

Mark Nichter is Professor of Anthropology at the University of Arizona. **Margaret Lock** is Professor in the Department of Social Studies of Medicine and in the Department of Anthropology, McGill University.

Theory and Practice in Medical Anthropology and International Health
A series edited by *Susan M DiGiacomo*
University of Massachusetts, Amherst

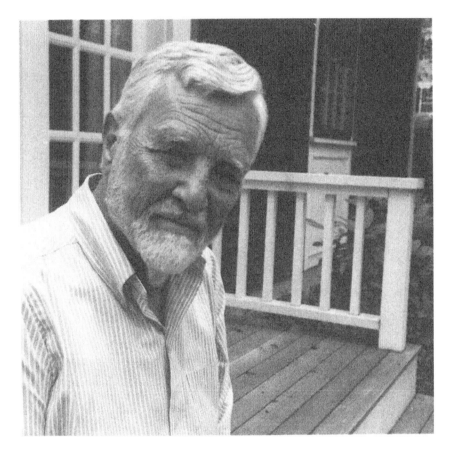

Charles Leslie

New Horizons in Medical Anthropology

Essays in Honour of Charles Leslie

Edited by Mark Nichter
and Margaret Lock

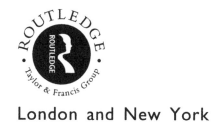

London and New York

First published 2002 by Routledge
2 Park Square, Milton Park, Abingdon, Oxon, OX14 4RN

Simultaneously published in the USA and Canada
by Routledge
270 Madison Ave, New York NY 10016

Routledge is an imprint of the Taylor & Francis Group

Transferred to Digital Printing 2005

Typeset in Times by Florence Production Ltd,
Stoodleigh, Devon

British Library Cataloguing in Publication Data
A catalogue record for this book is available from the British
Library

Library of Congress Cataloguing in Publication Data

A catalog record for this book has been requested

ISBN 0–415–27793–0 (hbk)
ISBN 0–415–27806–6 (pbk)

Printed and bound by Antony Rowe Ltd, Eastbourne

Contents

Contributors

Vincanne Adams is Associate Professor of Anthropology in the Department of Anthropology, History and Social Medicine at the University of California, San Francisco. Her research interests include contemporary resurrections of debates on ethnomedicine, postcoloniality and colonialism, globalized alternative medicine research, and the medical domains of Tibet, Nepal and the Himalayas. Her books include *Tigers of the Snow and Other Virtual Sherpas* (Princeton University Press) and *Doctors for Democracy* (Cambridge University Press).

Gilles Bibeau is Professor of Medical Anthropology in the Department of Anthropology at the Université de Montréal. In the 1960s and 1970s he carried out long-term fieldwork in Africa studying African healing modalities and religions in both rural and urban settings. During the past two decades his research activities have centered around four main topics: the international comparative studies of mental health problems (Brazil, India, Mali, Peru, Côte d'Ivoire, Italy); the culture of drug addicts and street gangs in Montreal; the adaptation of young African immigrants to Québec society; and sexuality and AIDS. He is currently chairing an international network of Latin American Schools of Public Health on the social determinants of health. His most recent books are: *Dérives Montréalaises* (Boréal Press, 1995) (a study of shooting galleries in Montreal); and *Juvenile Street-gangs* (Boréal Press, 2001).

Steve Ferzacca is Assistant Professor of Anthropology at the University of Lethbridge in Lethbridge, Alberta, Canada. A major focus of his ethnographic research is medical pluralism in Indonesia. His recent book, *Healing the Modern in a Central Javanese City* (Carolina Academic Press, 2001) is an interpretive and phenomenological exploration of the relationship between medical practice, the health of modernity, and Javanese structures of experience. Professor Ferzacca is presently finishing a project on the works and life of a Javanese healer. His current research examines Javanese articulations of self and emotivity and relationships among space, place, and health in and around the city of Yogyakarta.

Patricia Jeffery and **Roger Jeffery** are Professors of Sociology at the University of Edinburgh. Their common research interests focus on aspects of gender and communal politics in South Asia, including: women's seclusion, childbearing, reproductive health, fertility and population issues, and the interconnections between gender and communal politics among Muslims and Hindus in rural north India. Their joint publications include *Labour Pains and Labour Power: Women and Childbearing in Rural North India* (Zed, 1989); *Don't Marry me to a Plowman! Women's Everyday Lives in Rural North India* (Westview & Sage, 1996) and *Population, Gender and Politics: Demographic Change in Rural North India* (Cambridge University Press, 1997). In addition, Patricia Jeffery has co-edited (with Amrita Basu) *Appropriating Gender: Women's Activism and Politicized Religion in South Asia* (Routledge, 1998). A new edition of her *Frogs in a Well: Indian Women in Purdah* (originally published in 1979) has just been published (Manohar, 2000). Roger Jeffery is the author of *The Politics of Health in India* (University of California Press, 1988) and has co-edited (with Nandini Sundar) *A New Moral Economy for India's Forests?* (Sage, 1999). Patricia and Roger Jeffery are currently Visiting Fellows at the Institute of Economic Growth in Delhi, conducting research on the secondary schooling and the social reproduction of inequality and social exclusion in rural Uttar Pradesh.

Margaret Lock is Professor in the Department of Social Studies of Medicine and the Department of Anthropology at McGill University. She is the author of *East Asian Medicine in Urban Japan: Varieties of Medical Experience* (University of California Press, 1980) and *Encounters with Ageing: Mythologies of Menopause in Japan and North America* (University of California Press, 1993), which won the Eileen Basker Memorial Prize, the Canada-Japan Book Award, the Wellcome Medal of the Royal Anthropological Society, the Staley Prize of the School of American Reseach, the Berkeley Prize, and was a finalist for the Hiromi Arisawa Award. Her most recent book is *Twice Dead: Organ Transplants and the Reinvention of Death* (University of California Press, 2001). Lock has edited seven other books and written over 150 scholarly articles. She was the recipient of a Canada Council Izaak Killam Fellowship for 1993–1995, and is a Fellow of the Royal Society of Canada, a member of Canadian Institute of Advanced Research, Population Program, and was awarded the Prix Du Quebec, domaine Sciences Humaines in 1997. Lock is currently working on the social impact of the new genetics with particular emphasis on Alzheimer's disease.

Mark Nichter is Professor of Anthropology at the University of Arizona and Coordinator of the graduate program in medical anthropology. He has conducted long-term fieldwork in South India as well as research in the Philippines, Sri Lanka, and Thailand on issues related to ethnomedicine as well as the interface between anthropology, international health and development. The author of numerous articles and book chapters on medical anthropology, Mark is editor of the collection of essays, *An Anthropological Approach To Ethnomedicine* (Gordon & Breach, 1994), and co-author (with Mimi Nichter) of *Anthropology and International Health: Asian Case Studies* (Gordon & Breach, 1996). His current research focuses on health care transition and pharmaceutical practice in Asia; TB in India; women's reproductive health in Thailand; trajectories of tobacco use and dependence; and harm reduction as a response to perceptions of risk and environmental degradation

Duncan Pedersen is Director of the Psychosocial Research Division at the Douglas Hospital Research Centre and Associate Professor at the Department of Psychiatry, McGill University. He is also Lecturer at the Department of Social Medicine, Harvard Medical School and Senior Editor (Medical Anthropology) of Social Science and Medicine. He has done extensive field research in social epidemiology and medical anthropology in various countries in Latin America (Andean countries, the Amazon region and Northeast Brazil), working amongst indigenous peoples and the urban poor. More recently he has become involved in the field of trauma and social suffering and is focusing his research on the long-term impact and health outcomes of sociopolitical violence and wars.

Stacy Leigh Pigg is Associate Professor of Anthropology at Simon Fraser University and editor of Medical Anthropology. Her interests lie at the intersection of medical anthropology and the study of postcolonial cultural relations, especially those organized through international development activities. Her current work on the production of public knowledge about AIDS in Nepal focuses on the ways the internationalization of biomedicine is tied to the social production of cultural difference. She has published essays on these questions of development, identity, and knowledge in *Comparative Studies in Society and History*, *Cultural Anthropology*, and *Social Science and Medicine.*

Marina Roseman is Associate Professor and Clinical Research Coordinator at Pacifica Graduate Institute, California, and Research Associate on the faculty in the Department of Anthropology at Indiana University. Recipient of Fellowships from the Guggenheim Foundation, the National Endowment for the Humanities, Asian Cultural Council,

Social Science Research Council, Fulbright, Wenner-Gren, Rockefeller Foundation, and the National Science Foundation, she has conducted research on indigenous arts and medical practices in Indonesia, Malaysia, Vietnam, and among Asian and Hispanic populations in the United States. Medical and psychological anthropology join ethnomusicology and dance ethnology in her publications, which include *Healing Sounds from the Malaysian Rainforest: Temiar Music and Medicine* (University of California Press, 1991; Japanese translation by Shouwada Press, 2000), *The Performance of Healing* (Routledge, 1996), *Dream Songs and Healing Sounds: In the Rainforests of Malaysia* (Smithsonian-Folkways Recordings, 1995), and *Engaging the Spirits of Modernity* (University of California Press, 1991).

Margaret Trawick is Professor of Social Anthropology at Massey University in New Zealand. She has conducted long-term research with Tamil-speaking people in southern India and Sri Lanka. Her previous work has explored indigenous systems of medicine, Tamil poetry and song, culture and emotion, concepts of the body, untouchability, family, and religious devotion. Her present research focus is children's agency. Some of her recent publications relevant to this volume include *Writing the Body and Ruling the Land: Western Reflections on Chinese and Indian Medicine*, in *Knowledge and the Scholarly Medical Traditions*, edited by Don Bates (Cambridge University Press, 1995); *Notes on Love in a Tamil Family* (second edition, Oxford University Press, Delhi, 1996); *Reasons for Violence: A Preliminary Ethnographic Account of the LTTE* (*South Asia*, Vol. XX, 1997, pp. 153–180); and *On the Status of Child Combatants* (*Journal of Social Sciences*, Volume 4, Number 2, April 2000, pp. 1–18).

Allan Young is Professor of Anthropology at McGill University in the Departments of Social Studies of Medicine, Anthropology, and Psychiatry. His early anthropological research was in Ethiopia, where he studied medical practices and institutions indigenous to the Begemder region. For the last fifteen years, he has worked on psychiatric subjects with a focus on the history and ethnography of traumatic memory. He is co-editor, with Charles Leslie, of *Paths to Asian Medical Knowledge* (University of California Press, 1992) and is the author of *The Harmony of Illusions: Inventing Posttraumatic Stress Disorder* (Princeton University Press, 1995).

Acknowledgements

We would like to acknowledge Lorna Rhodes for her careful reading and constructive comments on an early version of the volume and Carol Gifford for her valuable editorial assistance.

Chapter 1

Introduction

From documenting medical pluralism to critical interpretations of globalized health knowledge, policies, and practices

Margaret Lock and Mark Nichter

Medical anthropology has a history that covers nearly four decades. Although Charles Leslie's career is much longer, this volume is devoted almost exclusively to recognition of his unsurpassed contribution to medical anthropology from the time of its formal inception in the late 1960s to the present day. The authors represented in this volume, three generations of social scientists, one or two themselves close to retirement, all acknowledge a debt to Charles for intellectual stimulation through interactions with him and reflections on his writings on Asian medical traditions. He has frequently influenced the course of our professional lives, facilitated many of our publications, and provided forums in various locations for an exchange of ideas, most of which have become central to medical anthropology.

Considering the range of age and experience of the authors, one might expect to find quite dramatic differences in the perspectives taken in these chapters. But a critical, and in some cases, activist approach to the subject matter unites them, one in which a sensitivity is evident to both globalized political and economic issues as well as to a situated meaning-centered approach to ethnography. Above all, everyone is alert to global pluralism in medical knowledge and practice, a lesson first disseminated by Charles Leslie many years ago and one that has proved to be indelibly robust.

Toward a comparative study of medical traditions

The obvious place to start when tracing Charles Leslie's contribution to medical anthropology is with the symposium funded by the Wenner Gren Foundation and held in 1971 at the gothic castle in Burg Wartenstein in Austria that the Foundation kept at that time for such gatherings. Out of that conference came the now classic *Asian Medical Systems: A Comparative Study* published in 1976 by the University of California Press. In the introduction Charles set out the project that would occupy him for many years and become a source of inspiration for numerous others. This book was the first collection of essays to undertake a study of the professional, literary, medical traditions of Asia, highlighting characteristics in the production, organization, and communication of medical knowledge. The styles of thought used in these traditions are explicitly compared with those characteristic of medicine in the West.

It was of particular interest to Charles to show the historical processes that have mediated the relationship of these medical systems to modern science and technology. The integrity of each of the "great medical traditions" is stressed, but at the same time it is argued that Galenic/Arabic, Indian, and Chinese medicine exhibit epistemologies and features of social organization permitting general comparisons with each other as well as with "cosmopolitan medicine." Charles favored this latter term (first coined by Fred Dunn in 1976) to "Western medicine" because it drew attention to the manner in which biomedicine and other forms of medicine were adopted in and adapted to cosmopolitan lifeworlds, thereby contributing to lifestyles concordant with capitalist expansion. Charles Leslie challenges the dualism commonly made at that time between "traditional" and "modern" medicine and insists that all bodies of medical knowledge are dynamic and change as the result of political and social factors as well as the diffusion of knowledge and technological innovations.

Warning against the reification of "traditional medicine," Charles argues that no medical traditions are inherently conservative. Similarly he challenges the use of "scientific" medicine to describe biomedicine alone and argues forcefully for acknowledgement of the scientific and rational principles present in Ayurvedic, Unani, and Chinese medicine. In a later paper (Leslie 1995), where Charles revisits his reflections on comparative medical systems, he calls for recognition of the power of aesthetics associated with medical systems. Reacting to the tendency to dismiss those aspects of medical systems that cannot be assessed scientifically as having any value, Charles' observations suggest that we consider not only symbolic and performative dimensions of healing but aesthetic dimensions as well. The work of such medical anthropologists as Briggs 1994; Csordas 1996; Desjarlais 1992, 1995; Farquhar 1994a, 1994b; Roseman 1988, 1991; and You 1994 (to name a few) lend support to this position.

Even though Charles's vision of a medical system has always been of an entity that is open and infinitely malleable, nevertheless a certain amount of conflict arose among the contributors to *Asian Medicine* as to how best to delineate the idea of a medical "system." Some authors emphasized historical continuities whereas others stressed discontinuities. But one theme that emerged vividly across many of the essays was that of revivalism. Several authors made it clear that not only had the "great tradition" retained a firm foothold in the face of modernization and the spread of biomedicine, but the politics of nationalism was in many instances giving the indigenous literate medical traditions a powerful boost, assuring continued legitimization and even expansion.

A second ground-breaking conference was organized in Washington DC by Charles in 1977, sponsored jointly by the National Science Foundation and the Wenner Gren Foundation. Allan Young and Gilles Bibeau both participated, as did several well-known specialists in Asian medicine, including Francis Zimmerman, Paul Unschuld, and Arthur Kleinman. Theories of medical pluralism were central to this conference, and the majority of the papers were published in a special edition of *Social Science and Medicine* in 1978 entitled "Theoretical Foundations for the Comparative Study of Medical Systems." During the course of developing this Festschrift, Francis Zimmerman reminded us of Charles' important role in fostering dialogue between scholars engaged in classical and philological studies of Asian medical traditions and anthropologists studying contemporary medical practices. Charles more than anyone else attempted to analyze what was at stake in such an exchange. In particular, the different emphasis given to continuity and change, theory and practice, notably textual knowledge and contemporary clinical practice, and the knowledge and interests of healers as opposed to patients, were flashpoints for disagreement, as was the interest of many anthropologists in the political dimensions and applied aspects of health care. Zimmerman notes with sadness that today the close ties forged by Charles between scholars of classical medical texts and of contemporary medical practices have dissipated, although ensuing generations of scholars, including Vincanne Adams, Lawrence Cohen, Judith Farquhar, and others have been busy building new bridges.

In 1980 Charles Leslie edited a special issue of *Social Science and Medicine* entitled "Medical Pluralism in World Perspective." In the introduction Charles sets out his vision of Asia medical traditions as part of the globalized world. He revisits the notion of a medical "system," arguing that the very idea is a product of ordering and systematization integral to modernization and the emergence of so-called scientific medicine. The result is that all other forms of medicine are marginalized and the assumption is that they will shortly die out, although the goal in many Asian countries is to create a standardized medical system into which some aspects of local medical practices are incorporated. Charles notes that health care planners have often assumed that these national medical systems will eventually become part of a worldwide "cosmopolitan" medicine. Modern science will be used benevolently and rationally in the relief of human suffering and distress. Charles points out that nowhere has such a vision been realized, and that in reality pluralism and complementarity are the norm. Economic necessity has, of course, been a driving force in sustaining this situation.

This 1980 special issue explicitly questions the entrenched habit of judging medical practices everywhere in terms of measures of efficacy based on proscribed scientific (biomedical) standards. Critical medical anthropologists today question the alleged neutrality of such standards and recognize them as an instrument of governmentality (Foucault 1979). One way governmentality is exercised is through codification – be this the establishment of a system of weights and measures that govern trade and commerce (Appadurai 1996b), professional accreditation (for example, of medical practitioners) that determines legitimacy to practice, or an "evidence-based approach" to evaluating the efficacy of healing modalities through proscribed methods such as double blind trials. At issue in the case of efficacy is who gets to define what constitutes evidence, what sources of information and forms of knowledge are privileged as well as overlooked, and who determines the way "disease categories" are classified as well as samples of subjects selected (Kleinman 1980; Nichter 1992a).

This issue of *Social Science and Medicine* also highlights how patients are, almost without exception, pragmatic, and see nothing inconsistent about liberally combining different forms of therapy in their quest for restored health. These observations, commonplace today, were conceptualized clearly among relatively few medical anthropologists of the time (see also Janzen 1978; Kleinman 1980; Lock 1980; Nichter 1978).

A third conference organized by Charles Leslie in 1985 was also held in Washington DC. Like the Burg Wartenstein Symposium, it limited its sights to Asian medicine and was entitled "Permanence and Change in Asian Health Care Traditions." This, too, was sponsored by the Wenner Gren Foundation, with the support of the Department of Anthropology at the National Museum of Natural History, the Smithsonian Institute. The meeting was held in concert with the American Anthropological Association meetings at which 48 papers related to this theme were presented. Selected papers from the conference were published in a special edition of *Social Science and Medicine* edited by Beatrix Pfleiderer bearing the same name as the conference (1988, Vol. 12, no. 2B) and in a book published in 1992 by the University of California Press entitled *Paths to Asian Medical Knowledge*, co-edited by Charles Leslie and Allan Young. The presumption of so many intellectuals and medical professionals throughout the second half of the last century that, with "modernization" and "westernization," a scientific medicine would fully emerge, one that is, in effect, epistemologically free and corresponds closely with reality, is rigorously challenged in this book (see also Lock and Gordon 1988; Wright and Treacher 1982). Similarly, the idea that people everywhere, once exposed to modernization and a modicum of scientific knowledge, would rescind on "tradition" and resort only to "modern" medicine is refuted. For example, in a chapter examining local responses to an emergent disease in South India associated with deforestation (Kyasanur Forest Disease), Nichter presents a political ecological analysis that examines how the disease was interpreted within the local cosmology. Although ticks infected with arbovirus came to be recognized as an instrumental cause of the disease, the reason particular communities were affected was linked to such things as neglect for the shrines of patron deities associated with land reform. Scarce resources were expended on rituals and government hospitals set up to take care of the emergency were avoided by some as places of a bad death. A good death emerged as a primary health concern in a cosmology where disposition of one's spirit after death was taken seriously (Nichter 1992b).

The editors of *Paths to Asian Medical Knowledge* remind their readers that the medical systems of contemporary Asia are intellectually coherent, embedded in distinct cultural premises, but cannot be fully understood outside of the stream of history as they are intrinsically dynamic and continually evolving. They note that by the early 1990s these observations were not particularly remarkable, but nevertheless they need repeating for the benefit of some readers, including many anthropologists. The editors acknowledge the remarkable contribution of several historians and philologists, the majority of them European, to the study of Asian medicine. Given the vast corpus of written texts associated with the Asian medical traditions, the prodigious and patient work of these scholars, including Joseph Needham, Nathan Sivin, Paul Unschuld, Francis Zimmerman, Laurence Conrad, and Dominik Wujastyk, among others, provides invaluable insights that complement the work of social scientists studying change and continuity in healing traditions.

The shared perspective of *Paths to Asian Medical Knowledge* is epistemological. The authors each ask in their own way:

> How do patients and practitioners know what they know? What are their various rules of evidence, what kinds and categories of information do they find persuasive, and under what circumstances? How do they know when a medical judgment is wrong or correct? What do "wrong" and "correct" mean to patients, to village practitioners, and to experts trained in the great tradition? What sorts of inductive logic and analogy are at work here? Under what circumstances are these people inclined to accept or ignore novel medical ideas and practices?
>
> (Leslie and Young 1992: 14)

Responding to such theorists as Horton (1967) who argue that "traditional" thought systems are past oriented and therefore relatively closed to other possibilities and options, authors in this volume (for example, Obeyesekere; see also Trawick 1987) illustrate how multiple streams of reasoning guide the development and practice of major medical traditions such as Ayurveda. Although medical traditions like Ayurveda and the Chinese tradition are past oriented, they are also open to new sources of knowledge and empirical observation. They are dynamic and not static, capable of creative syntheses, not just a mere encompassment of ideas and resources. Case studies in *Paths to Asian Medical Knowledge* illustrate how practitioners base their diagnosis and treatment on both abstract principles as well as embodied knowledge and guided sensibility and on ad hoc experimentation as well as the formulations found in texts. The production of knowledge within great scholarly traditions of medicine both past and present is further examined by Judith Farquhar, Peggy Trawick, Francis Zimmerman and colleagues in a volume edited by the historian Don Bates (1995) and dedicated to Charles Leslie and the historian Owsei Temkin. In this book, the epistemology of medical traditions is expicitly examined and the question is posed: just how do practitioners of such medical systems convince others that they have privileged knowledge?

In addition to the organization of conferences and publication of books and special issues of *Social Science and Medicine*, Charles Leslie has carried out several other distinguished services for the medical anthropology community and for specialists in East Asian medicine over the years. He founded and was the General Editor between 1971 and 1985 of a book series in medical anthropology entitled "Comparative Studies of Health Systems and Medical Care," published by the University of California Press, and then was an editorial board member of the series until 1995. During his time as general editor, 21 volumes were published, including many books that have become classics in the sub-discipline of medical anthropology. The series acted as a catalyst for new scholarship as the critical mass of case studies published raised awareness about this domain of multidisciplinary scholarship, encouraging younger scholars to pursue research around new lines of research being modeled.

Charles has contributed to the field in yet other important ways. Between 1977 and 1989 Charles was the Senior Editor of the Medical Anthropology section of the journal *Social Science and Medicine* and a regular participant in the bi-annual conferences, usually held in Europe, under the auspices of the journal. In this capacity, Charles was able to encourage and shape the publication of medical anthropological articles that would be read by numerous social scientists from a range of disciplines. He actively encouraged contributions from scholars worldwide, making the journal truly international and opening up exchanges between south and north, east and west. Charles did not teach graduate students directly in his capacity as professor at the University of Delaware, but he helped scores of young scholars from all over the world publish their first articles and establish their careers.

Charles was also Secretary-General of the International Association for the Study of Traditional Asian Medicine (IASTAM) from its founding by A. L. Basham in 1984 until 1990, an organization that is still in existence. He has been deeply involved in the organization of the conferences held every five years under the auspices of IASTAM in Australia, Indonesia, India, Japan, Germany, and elsewhere. These conferences have been forums where historians, social scientists, and other intellectuals have made presentations together with practitioners of East Asian medicine. Several of the contributors to this volume (Adams, Ferzacca, Lock and Nichter) have served as office bearers in this organization nationally or internationally.

Medical pluralism and medical revivalism

Charles Leslie's own work on medical pluralism focused primarily on Ayurvedic practitioners and the conflict and accommodation that were apparent as they were increasingly confronted with cosmopolitan medicine. He was able to show conclusively how self-conscious attempts at revivalism of an "authentic" Ayurvedic tradition were closely associated with nationalism and were in large part responses to perceived threats by forces for modernization and, by implication, "westernization," emanating from both inside and outside India. This is a topic that is of ongoing importance to scholars of Asia and elsewhere. For example, Prakash (1999) points out that in India many Western-educated intellectuals and scientists found themselves in an acute dilemma: on the one hand they assumed that an embrace of Western science was a sign of modernity and progress, while on the other they were keen to identify evidence of scientific thought in indigenous knowledge and thus advance its claim to universalism. This dilemma is particularly fraught in India because to claim that a scientific tradition existed in India long before colonialism runs contrary to the assumptions of many Indians, namely, that what makes India unique are distinct rationalities juxtaposed to those of modernity and colonial power in which spiritual and practical interventions are blended. Indeed, Chatterjee (1993) argues that in India "anticolonial nationalism" emerged at a time when Western superiority in the domain of the material was recognized in large part through the conscious efforts made to preserve the distinctiveness of spiritual culture. Medicine was one of many spaces where "fragmented resistances" to the hegemonic project of modernity occurred and freedom of imagination was exercised (see also Nandy 1994).

The struggle to be modern and economically developed without being Western is an issue addressed by Steve Ferzacca in his examination of medical pluralism in Indonesia. Ferzacca notes that the Indonesian government has used a commitment to *pembangunan* (development) as an ideological apparatus to govern the daily lives of its citizens. At the same time traditional values are lauded as essential to the state's vision of reflexive and unique modernization. The modernity envisioned for Indonesia (and by other countries) looks backward to find something recoverable – something felt to be lost in the present – but it does so for the sake of a better future (Adams 2001).

Ferzacca draws on Foucault's concept of governmentality to explore medical pluralism as a form of state rule. In Indonesia, only forms of medicine that articulate the ideal of development or refined cultural citizenship are permitted. At a time when political and ethnic factionalism threaten national identity, hybrid forms of medical (or religious) eclecticism are not permitted. Sanctioned are healers and healing modalities that represent traditional Javanese culture and express principles of self-mastery and control, virtues that serve the state. Only those mixes of post-traditional medicine are deemed legitimate that fit the nation-state project of reflexive modernity. We clearly see in this essay the manner in which the state uses both biomedicine, public health, and traditional medical systems as instruments of governance. The research of medical historians and philologists have shown us that state projects have long influenced medical doctrine and that governance has long involved the privileging of particular health ideologies and healing practices over others. An excellent example is Unschuld's description of how Confucian ideology was propagated through everyday practices, including health and medical practices, as a way of reunifying the nation (Unschuld 1985; see also Sivin 1995). Farquhar (1995) has provided us with a more recent example of Maoist and post Maoist readings of medicine in line with state ideology.

Public health and the state

The tension between traditional values that define national identity and the forces of modernization and globalization is present in many of the papers in this volume. It is clear that although people may seek out certain medical technologies, they respond with ambivalence to other technologies (as well as to forms of medical and public health knowledge) when these are perceived as promulgating ideologies that threaten the moral order. This is well illustrated by Stacy Pigg in her essay on an HIV education hotline in Nepal. While AIDS prevention is welcomed by the State when in the form of warnings about disease that reinforce "proper" conduct within traditional social hierarchies, it nevertheless becomes a threat to the state's moral identity when sexual health is addressed more broadly and openly. More is at stake than a discussion of sexual practices: claims about norms and values draw social boundaries that are connected to important issues of national identity and social citizenship. To imagine that the difficulties in implementing a sexual health program merely involve getting the right balance of "cultural sensitivity" is to miss the social dynamics involved. States pursue their objectives through the everyday projects of regulation of bodies and spaces that they devise, in discursive battles over the boundaries and categories of social life and institutions, and in struggles over the power to represent what is deemed to be in the best interest of citizens. If educating consent is achieved through educating desire (Stoler and Cooper 1997), then discourse about sex touches at the very nerve of governance within the body politic.

Pigg investigates the complicated ways international public health priorities intersect with and contribute to local identity politics that in turn are informed by claims about local norms and values. Growing links between local and transnational NGOs having a progressive liberal democratic agenda create new spaces where the moral tenants of "national identities" may be revisited and challenged in the context of discourse on health and development. Diseases like AIDS force moral debates not only about sexual behavior, but about what kind of development a nation is pursuing. Pigg's (1992: 512) research on development encounters between foreign consultants/NGOs, Nepali health and development workers, and Nepali citizens hailing from different social classes encourages us to consider the project of modernization in Nepal as not simply a matter of western influence, but a matter of simultaneous Nepalization and globalization. Viewed in light of contestations, appropriations, and transformations occurring in multiple domains of life (reproduction, agriculture, health, and so on) development is best seen as an encounter resulting in hybridity (Vasavi 1994). It is by paying attention to the myriad ways in which encounters with development strategies have reconstituted and reworked modernity from within, producing multiple, alternative, fragmented, or hybrid modernities (Gupta 1998; Arce and Long 2000) while at the same time reassembling tradition, that we can better understand the effects and "side-effects of development" (Pigg 1997).

There is a great need for ethnographies that document the role of NGOs in both ushering in and resisting new moral orders propagated in the name of development (empowerment, emancipation, nationalism, internationalism, individualism, and so on), as well as studies of how the agendas of NGOs are co-opted by development agencies while advancing their own agendas by means of funding and workshops where local participants are resocialized and given new vocabularies with which to guide their thinking and constitute a form of symbolic capital (Fisher 1997; Farrington et al. 1995; Mencher 1999). As Pigg notes, struggles over the regulation of sexuality evident in the reactions to the HIV Hotline are inseparable from dependency on donor aid, the influence of international mass-media, and the formation of a middle class increasingly defined through its consumption practices.

In an era when international "development" is the order of the day, and health care is promoted under the banners of social welfare and human rights, it is no longer sufficient for medical anthropologists to focus on medical traditions (their respective knowledge and practices) and to document patterns of resort – the way in which patients move from one type of practitioner to another. Following Charles' advice that we consider contemporary medical pluralism in the context of cosmopolitanism we now need to reconsider medical cosmopolitanism from the vantage point of both local and global relationships, a topic of vital interest to anthropologists today. At this juncture, it is important to critically examine global public health agendas and how health and development agencies influence national health policies everywhere in the name of health care reform, "rationalizing" choices through the use of "evidence"-based criteria, homogenizing practice in the name of efficiency, and so on (Ginsberg and Rapp 1995; Lock and Kaufert 1998).

This transformation takes place in several different ways. Nationalistic competitiveness is fostered by the widely disseminated World Health Organization rankings of statistics on infant mortality rates, life expectancy rates, and so on. The concept of risk, and the "making up of people" (Hacking 1986) in terms of categories of risk, so central to the work of epidemiologists and public health practitioners is, of course, one of the principle ways in which biopower is put into practice globally.[1] It is one thing to know that you are poor, hungry, and often sick. It is another thing altogether to think of oneself as underdeveloped or a member of a risk group. One comes to understand how to be a "development category" (Pigg 1997: 267).

International organizations exert pressure on national bodies to follow global guidelines in the name of science if not expediency. It is worth considering, for example, how the World Health Organization has exerted pressure on the former Soviet Union to abide by its TB control policy of DOTS (direct-observation treatment plan with a fixed regimen). Several local medical scientists have argued against this policy, viewing it as more appropriate for Africa than their own context where medical standards are high, doctors numerous (and unemployed), and drug resistance to standard TB treatment high. DOTS has been imposed as a condition for receiving resources, although many doctors have expressed the opinion that DOTS is not sufficient to control the epidemic of multidrug-resistant TB (MDRTB) facing the region (Bukhman 2001; Farmer and Kim 2000; Perelman 2000). From their vantage-point, the imposition of TB policy from outside constitutes a form of neocolonialism. In this case, the colonial power is a global institution that threatens the nation's sovereignty and informed scientific judgment. In a likewise manner, it is worth examining the way in which the World Bank's Structural Adjustment and economic incentive policies have impacted negatively on primary health care, as well as fostered growth of the private health care sector in a country such as India (Nichter and Van Sickle 2002). Critics have argued that external assistance has guided the thinking behind the country's Ninth Plan, which cuts back on support to primary health care, draws heavily on external support for vertical programs, and implicitly fosters privatization (Nayar 2000; Qadeer 2000).

Risk, prevention, and harm reduction as features of biomedicine

Medical anthropologists no longer limit their analyses to the well-debated triad of disease, illness, and sickness (Young 1982). As social theorists including Beck (1992), Giddens (1991) and Hacking (1990) have argued, thinking in terms of risk is fundamental to modernity. Our lives are increasingly organized around managing risks. Nowhere is this more apparent than in the health field where attention is increasingly being directed to the calculation of risk as a means of targeting preventive health interventions. It is important to investigate how the public, health practitioners, and local leaders respond to risk talk and its representation as a form of biopower, as well as a call to action. Once individuals have been informed about risk, they are expected to act accordingly, a dynamic that sets in motion a politics of responsibility that is soon transformed into a social obligation (Lock 1993; Peterson and Lupton 1996). And yet exposure to information about risk does not always result in governments or individuals taking those actions advocated by health experts. Responses to risk discourse are complicated and dynamic, as well as politically and socially motivated. The degree of trust in the bearer of information is often implicated, as is a needed confidence in the data that are authoritatively presented.[2]

Anthropologists such as Stacy Pigg and Cris Lyttleton (who writes about HIV representation and education programs in Thailand, see Lyttleton 2000) lead us to question the politics underlying courses of action by governments (whether actually taken, postponed, or rejected) when they are confronted with decision-making in connection with supposed risks to individual bodies as well as to the body politic. Other anthropologists have drawn attention to the impact "risk awareness" and representations of a "dangerous other" have on social relations within the community and the manner in which risk discourse feeds into representations of gender, class, and ethnic difference. Reductionistic correlations of risk (such as correlations between ethnicity and HIV that do not take into account such confounding factors as economic status or environment) provide those who are so inclined with a seemingly "objective" and scientific substitute for other forms of prejudice (Nguyen 2001; Nichter 1999). As noted by Charles Leslie in his critique of Rushton and Bogaert's writing on ethnicity and HIV (discussed shortly), it is all too easy to misconstrue rates of a disease as traits of a people, and when this happens victim blaming usually follows. It is also important to bear in mind that being labeled at risk can place an individual or a group at further risk (Hahn 1997; Nichter 1999). This may occur when overwhelming risk contributes to a form of fatalism, or when others write off a people as "naturally" predisposed to particular types of problems and therefore not worth the investment of particular kinds of resources.

International health agencies are presently encouraging Ministries of Health and local NGOs to dedicate more time and resources to the three arms of prevention. Primary or "upstream prevention" entails not only preventing illnesses through the use of technical fixes such as vaccinations, but preventing the uptake of risky behaviors. Information about groups at risk, environments of risk, and high-risk behaviors are made public, and become the focus of intervention efforts. Secondary prevention involves locating problems early before they spread among the population. Early diagnosis enables not only early treatment, but also public health efforts to control endemic disease and swiftly respond to epidemics. Toward this end, community based sentinel surveillance systems have been set up for diseases like malaria, dengue fever, HIV, and TB as well as community-based screening programs for diseases such as cervical cancer. Tertiary or "downstream prevention" involves reversing and managing health problems once they progress. Given a middle health transition scenario (Gutierrex and Kendall 2000) in which longevity increases and late onset chronic diseases such as diabetes and hypertension become increasingly important public health problems, issues arise as to the roles of the household and state in providing curative care toward the end of tertiary prevention. Given the cost of such care, and population preferences for types of treatment, state interest in indigenous medicines, if not medical systems, is likely to increase.

Each of these strategies for preventive health demands investigation by social scientists. How are local communities responding to "risk talk" and the growing number of preventive health interventions promoted by international health agencies, governments, and NGOs? How do they relate to surveillance systems and screening programs for diseases that are both familiar and unfamiliar to local populations? How does the way in which an illness is interpreted influence when and if people seek diagnostic tests and consent to being screened? What are their expectations about diagnostic tests and what latent health and social concerns are triggered by community-based screening programs (Boonmongkon et al. 1999; Kavanagh and Broom 1998; Kaufert 2000; Wood et al. 1997). And what happens when indigenous medicines are commercialized and appropriated by cosmopolitan practitioners for use in chronic disease management (Lock 1984, 1990; Janes 1999)?

Since the birth of the discipline in the 1970s, medical anthropologists have been asked to investigate "cultural barriers" to health programs that represent "progress and modernity." Over the years anthropologists have come to better appreciate how stakeholders use the language of "culture barriers" to deflect attention from program failures or justify reasons for not investing in particular programs due to an assumption that they would not be culturally acceptable. The essays by Pigg, the Jefferys, and Nichter (as well as Leslie 1989b) invite us to further examine the extent to which public response to state health interventions is a feature of how a program has been implemented and the social relations of program management, identity politics, and public trust.

Another issue, not limited of course to developing countries, is how increasing risk consciousness influences the health consumption behavior of the public. Ministries of health, the media, and the health care industry routinely alert the public to health risks in the course of promoting beneficial health behavior and health related products. The reality is that many recommended health practices are unfeasible or untenable to various sectors of the population, given the availability of resources, their lifestyle, and the existing gender and power relations (Bujra 2000). In need of investigation are what forms of harm reduction both local populations and practitioners employ in lieu of recommended courses of action (Nichter 1996 a, 2001a).[3] The pharmaceutical industry is heavily invested in playing off the health anxieties of populations by providing a wide array of ready-made harm reduction and health promotion resources (Nichter 1996b; Nichter and Vuckovic 1993; Vuckovic and Nichter 1994). These range from curative biomedicines cleverly marketed as a means to prevent serious illness (Nichter 1994; Boonmongkon et al. 2001), to traditional medicines marketed as antidotes for the long term side effects of strong modern medicines (such as antibiotics), to medicines which are remedies for the ill effects of modernity itself (Miles 1998a,b; Nichter and Vuckovic 1993).

This trend was well recognized by Charles Leslie (1989), who considered harm reduction and medicalization important expressions as well as drivers of cosmopolitan medicine in all of its forms. (Nichter: personal communication). Leslie recognized that the revival of interest in indigenous pharmaceuticals was driven by the marketing of medicines made to appear traditional yet modern, appealing to the middle-class consumer who wanted the best of both worlds (Leslie 1989; Nichter 1996a). As van der Geest and Whyte have noted, one of the "charms" of such medicines is the metonymic relationship set up between their form, labeling, and packaging, the power and prestige of western technology, and traditional wisdom and nostalgic values associated with a simpler purer past (van der Geest and White 1989).

Given the well recognized global health and health care transition that is under way, limiting observation to what takes place between healers and their patients, while of great interest, is too narrow a research frame. Ethnographic accounts of health care related behaviors (prevention, promotion, harm reduction, cure) clearly need to take into account the political economics fostering and inhibiting particular care modalities; the impact of globalization, the media (local and international), and identity politics, among other factors. Such an approach should be attentive to the active rivalries as well as cooperative partnerships and exchanges among different types of healers and health care professionals as they respond to broader national and global interests.

Therapy management: the contribution of circumstantial ethnography

Ethnographies attentive to circumstance and the nested contexts within which people live out their daily lives provide us with valuable lessons about how social obligations and personal interests are balanced and prioritized, how identity is managed and reflected upon, and when and how agency is expressed. In his essay on the social relations of therapy management, Nichter contributes to both medical anthropology and an anthropology of self that challenges simplistic notions of sociocentric (collectivist) versus individualist selves. He examines when social obligations determine behavior toward the ill, as well as when illness leads individuals to re-examine their relations with kin in light of pressing problems; when illness serves to mobilize therapy management groups and when it places a strain on social relations in contexts of poverty. At the core of his research is an appreciation for "the politics of responsibility" as they are played out in multiple contexts: the household, the larger kin network, the local health care setting, and the national health care system.

Nichter pays special attention to the harsh economic realities in which health care decisions are and are not made. He examines entitlement to resources during illness as an issue that leads the ill to reject treatment options that would take scarce resources from others, and also as prompting reflection about one's relationship to others who may prove to be of little or no assistance in time of need. Research topics such as these beg further exploration. When is noncompliance with medical treatment actually self-sacrifice and a means of reserving resources for others? How have reciprocal exchange and mutual assistance survival strategies changed as a result of increased poverty, social transformation, or structural adjustment policies, and so on? And how has the diminished integrity of local safety nets influenced health care seeking? There are relatively few ethnographic studies (Oths 1994 is a notable exception) that address how changing economic conditions influence health care behavior. Far more attention should be focused on the relative importance of economics and cultural predispositions in determining the health care seeking behavior of various people. Equally important is to examine where people seek out care and under what circumstances, and how quickly they are able to act on options once they recognize the need to do so (Nichter and Kendall 1991).

A second theme explored by Nichter is how illness, even the possibility of illness, provides a space in which one's priorities may be (re)established while conflicting social relationships are sorted out. In one case, potential illness suggested by diagnostic tests provides the patient refuge from the pressing demands of kin. A sick role (in this case a risk role) enables him to make decisions that are beneficial to him and his wife without going against kin expectations. Assuming a sick role on the basis of diagnostic tests constitutes a form of self-medicalization (Nichter 1998) enabling the patient to mobilize and manipulate a therapy management group organized around support. This case leads us to appreciate one social dimension to the growing popularity of diagnostic tests in developing countries, a dimension fostered by medical entrepreneurs. As Nichter notes, by accommodating to consumer demand and market forces, such practitioners have unintentionally provided new barometers of well-being as well as new means of communicating distress, care, and concern. Tests are not just instruments of surveillance in the sense of Foucault's writings on biopower, they also provide a space within which social relations and agency may be articulated in a relatively self-conscious manner.

Confronting the shock of modernity

Research into medical pluralism not only reveals the endurance and stability of an enormous range of medical practices, but provides a lens through which to see how indigenous medical systems have confronted the forces of modernity. Writing about the Senoi Temiar in Malaysia, Marina Roseman considers how ritual healing not only deals with the distress of individuals, but also mitigates the effects of colonialism and postcolonialism experienced by Temiars as a whole. In her essay in this volume (see also Roseman 1996, 2001), Roseman analyzes the way healing rituals are employed as a therapeutic means of mediating traumatic cultural change secondary to encounters with deforestation, Islamic religious evangelism, and economic transformation. In recent times, the Temiar have experienced a shift from semi-nomadic mobility and rainforest symbiosis to a sedentary, restricted lifeway based on an alien market economy. As a means of coping, the Temiar perform rituals that attempt to conjoin the strands of their life as rainforest dwellers to the lifeworld of contemporary Malaysia. Ritual becomes a means for re-establishing cultural integrity and resolving new types of illness/soul loss associated with disruption and dislocation.

For the Temair, illness is understood as dislocation, a condition where one has lost one's way, but songs provide paths that lead to known places. The Temiar have begun to incorporate representations of varying spirit-entities associated with modernization into their cosmology. Potentially disruptive social, political, and ecological forces are configured into spirit-entity-song-pathways. By positioning "foreign" illness agents and new concepts, like statehood, within repetitive rhythms conjoining forest and body, past and present, the Temiar cope with adversity by encompassing it and reorienting the self in a changing social and environmental order.

Like Nichter's research on Kyasanur forest disease (Nichter 1992b), Roseman's research among the Temiar provide us with a powerful illustration of a political ecological analysis that goes far beyond a consideration of the impact of political economy on the physical environment. At stake is the Temiar's entire cosmos and sense of self derived from their relationship to this cosmology. Both these cases point to ways in which environmental and medical anthropology overlap and are informed by a consideration of the spiritual dimension of land-human relationships, and the way in which disorders of the land and the human body are read both as signs and symptoms.

Roseman provides us with a detailed analysis of the coping strategies employed by the Temiar when confronted by global forces that stretch the horizons of their local cosmology. How do other groups whose sense of well-being is tied to sacred landscapes cope with such challenges (see, for example, Adelson 2001)? How is displacement handled by these groups when they are forced to relocate (Cassey 1993)? How are emergent epidemics (of infectious or chronic disease) interpreted in relation to the violation of sacred landscapes? And when such is the case, how are attempts to heal bodies and control epidemics associated with attempts to pacify both old and new powers, purify the land, reaffirm sacred trusts, and so on? We might also ask if there are parallels in the way the Temiar encompass forces of social disruption and the way we medicalize and thereby locate social disorders in our conceptual system? How do we use medicines and support groups to reorient populations to new temporal and spatial, environmental, and occupational orders? It is also worth examining the extent to which rituals and healing modalities have been used as spaces for experimental practice and transformational action where possible modernities and selves are imagined (Comaroff and Comoroff 1993; Geschiere 1998).

Science as the arbiter of truth

In 1990 Charles Leslie published a paper in *Social Science and Medicine* that created quite a stir. This paper was a passionate response to one published the previous year in the same journal by two psychologists, J. Philippe Rushton and Anthony F. Bogaert. This paper created such controversy in Charles' opinion that the paper should have been rejected out of hand for publication through the usual mechanism of a competent peer review. In brief, the argument put out by Rushton and Bogaert is that the AIDS virus infects Negroid populations more than Caucasoids, and Caucasoids more than Mongoloids. It is argued that this variation in incidence can be explained by "racial" differences in anatomy, temperament, and in sexual behavior that arose during the course of human evolution. The thesis of these psychologists was dismissed out of hand in Social

Science and Medicine not only by Charles Leslie, but also by the biological anthropologist Owen Lovejoy on whose theories Rushton and Bogeart draw. Lovejoy describes their tenets as "virtual nonsense" dressed up in a language of pseudoscience (Lovejoy 1990: 909).

Charles' response to this paper opened up a breech between himself and the then editor of Social Science and Medicine, which led in large part to Charles' resignation as the editor of the section of that journal devoted to medical anthropology. It is of note that Philippe Rushton (1999) continues to publish this same thesis, elaborating on the same flawed data. His latest book is entitled *Race, Evolution, and Behavior: A Life History Perspective* and includes statements such as the following: "In Black Africa and the Black Caribbean, as in the American underclass ghetto, groups of pre-teens and teenagers are left quite free of adult supervision" with major consequences, the author claims, for "promiscuous sexual behavior" and "out-of-wedlock" births (Leslie 1999: 35). This slim volume, with supportive blurbs by Charles Murray, Arthur Jensen, and Hans J. Eysenck, was sent unsolicited by Philippe Rushton to academics across Canada (Margaret Lock received a copy) and perhaps to academics in other countries as well.

Gilles Bibeau and Duncan Pederson take up some of the issues raised by Charles in his rebuttal, notably why scientists involved in the peer review program failed to recognize the inherently racist premises so evident in the Rushton and Bogaert paper. Bibeau and Pederson focus on the way in which scientific explanations are so often flawed by an unexamined "ideological substratum," and they explicitly deconstruct the commentary on African sexual practices made by Philippe Rushton and, from a very different vantage point, by two demographers, John and Pat Caldwell. Bibeau and Pederson take exception to many facets of the writings of these authors. Above all they are critical because postulated biological structures and neuro-endocrinal mechanisms are given more explanatory power than are historical, social, political, or economic arguments, resulting in a crude genetic determinism buttressed by methodologies that are blatantly biased.[4] Bibeau and Peterson conclude that images of an "invented" Africa permit this kind of bias to persist and, following Mudimbe (1988), they argue that such images not only perpetuate dangerous distortions about daily life in Africa, but also have a negative effect on Africans as they in turn partially re-invent themselves in light of powerful discourses supposedly grounded in science that emanate from the West.[5]

Patricia and Roger Jeffery take up similar themes with respect to Indian Muslims among whom they have carried out ethnographic work for several decades. They depict the way in which global discourse about "populations out of control" is mobilized by the so-called Hindu Right in order to generate essentialized arguments about Muslims who are portrayed as taking over politically through the continued practice of polygamy with resultant high fertility rates (see also Jeffery and Jeffery 2000). The Jefferys present a nuanced analysis of historical and contemporary data to show how this discourse, with its emphasis on "excessive" reproduction, is demonstrably false. They then critique the macro-level data compiled by local demographers to show how their findings mask the fine-grained reality that accounts for fertility differentials. In common with the majority of sociologists and anthropologists who use the ethnographic method, the Jefferys argue forcibly that "situated accounts" have greater explanatory potential than does survey research. Only through recognition of the value of qualitative findings might the position of the Hindu Right be undermined – although the Jefferys, like Charles Leslie a decade earlier, despair of convincing ideologically committed people that the "science" they draw on is spurious. Nevertheless, they argue that the challenge must be taken up and dealt with and not simply set aside as too blatantly ridiculous. In common with an increasing number of social scientists (including other contributors to this volume), the Jefferys are explicit that their work has an engaged political and applied dimension.

Legitimizing knowledge claims

Vincanne Adams, like the Jefferys, writes about the way in which scientific language is made use of locally. In this case medical legitimacy, and even international recognition, is being sought. What is made explicit in Adams' paper, as in several others, is a global engagement. Bibeau and Pederson show how "outsiders" seek to legitimize their evidence about African sexuality by drawing on flawed scientific and thinly disguised racist theories that seem to be impervious to refutation. The work of the demographers these authors study is blatantly political and ideological. The Jefferys show how science, once again flawed science (due to poor methodology rather than to a blatantly ideological stance), is taken up by conservative, "traditionalist," right-wing elements in Indian society, who attempt to use it to forward their political interests. In Tibet, Vincanne Adams notes that although the very meaning of science is hotly debated, claims are nevertheless made by certain practitioners that Tibetan medicine is scientific in order to "prove" its efficacy. These claims have political and economic significance and are addressed to the state as well as to international bodies interested in the "development" of Tibet. Adams' analysis of truth claims extends Leslie's observations regarding how social, historical, political, and economic forces influence the way in which medical traditions and medical knowledge are represented.

Adams argues that proof that Tibetan medical treatment is efficacious in contemporary Tibet is not limited to claims about empirical truth measured by statistical outcomes. Attributions of efficacy and determinations of proof are subject to particular demands placed on Tibetan doctors who skillfully navigate the divide between post-Maoist materialist ideology and attempts of the Tibetan population to maintain its distinct cultural identity. Given a tense political climate, Tibetan medical professionals have learned to "read" evidence in particular ways. Proof, in this sense, becomes not just a question of epistemology (although this is important), but rather a question of the way epistemology is made to speak for politics, history, and free markets in a changing world.

Adams describes a Tibetan doctor who employs ultrasound in her treatment of female patients to whom she administers herbal medicine. She is initially puzzled over the doctor's declaration that all her patients are cured regardless of the findings of a post-treatment ultrasound test. Adams learns that from the perspective of a humoral approach to healing, the signs of having successfully eliminated a disorder are discerned through diagnostic techniques that indicate specific humoral imbalances. Once a healthy humoral balance is restored, a patient is pronounced cured. Obstructions that continue to appear on the ultrasound test are often deemed to be residual traces of a problem that has not fully abated, or scars from a past disorder.

Such reasoning is commonly encountered in India as well as Tibet. What is insightful about Adams' study is that she questions why the ultrasound test was used in the first place, and why the Tibetan doctor was so particular about describing her treatment of patients as practical rather than driven by abstract humoral theory. Notably, the doctor juxtaposes her modern scientific approach to Tibetan medicine with Tibetan medicine that incorporates ritual and mystical elements. In this sense, her treatment is in line with government ideology at a time when religion is associated with political dissent, and legitimacy is associated with the visible practices of "outside medicine." Her use of ultrasound is conditioned by Tibet's internal political history that requires Tibetan medicine to be "scientific" in its "own" way and to align itself to a singularly complex form of modernity. As in Nichter's case study of the social uses of diagnostic testing in India, the use of ultrasound in Tibet serves metamedical purposes.

Adams' analysis of the micropolitics of Tibetan medicine is also attentive to forces of globalization (see also Jones 2001). Practitioners and producers of Tibetan medicine have a vested interest in appearing scientific not just as a result of internal state politics, but because of new economic liberalization policies that make Tibetan medicine a marketable commodity in an international arena. Given the exigencies of this market, there is an incentive to popularize single drug therapies for named disorders rather than a need, as was formerly required in the practice of Tibetan and Chinese medicine, to continuously tailor medications to individuals' distinctive constitutions (Farquhar 1994b; Lock 1980).

The papers by Adams, Bibeau and Pederson, the Jefferys, and Nichter direct our attention to both the production and appropriation of scientific truth for social and political ends. These papers, in concert with a growing number of publications (e.g., Arnold 1993; Comaroff 1993; Lock 1993; Young 1995), illustrate that scientific and medical knowledge has a life of its own as a legitimating force quite independent of the institutional settings, disciplinary knowledge bases, and laboratories where it is habitually produced and practiced. This raises an important research agenda for medical anthropologists, namely how the public interprets "scientific" and "quasi-scientific" claims of efficacy. Such an approach requires research into the semantics of efficacy as well as considerations of how efficacy is assessed within the scientific community and talked about by practitioners, the press, and those marketing products and promises.

Establishing the efficacy of healing modalities has become a central issue at this time of rapid globalization and of growing medical pluralism and hybridization in the West. The Institute for Complementary Medicine, a recent addition to the US National Institutes of Health, has been assigned the task of figuring out the best scientific methods enabling the assessment of so-called complementary and alternative (CAM) medical practices (National Center for Complementary and Alternative Medicine five-year strategic plan, 2000). This is no mean feat because there is considerable confusion among researchers about methodologies that test efficacy versus ones that shed light on mechanisms of action of a therapeutic modality. Consider for a moment the evaluation of medications. The basic assumption of a double blind study employing a placebo control (the present methodology of choice) is that the effect of a medication consists of two components, a specific physiological and a nonspecific psychological component, whereas the effect of a placebo consists of only one, the nonspecific psychological component. It is not the total effectiveness of a medication that is being evaluated, but the extent to which the physiological component adds significantly to the psychological component.

The reason for using placebo control groups is to identify why treatments are effective, not whether they are effective. Yet many researchers, practitioners, and members of the general public tend to think of placebo studies as a means of setting minimum standards of effectiveness for treatments. More misguided yet, they understand such studies to be testing whether a therapy actually works or if its action is no better than chance. The placebo response of all therapeutic actions (including the attention received from a practitioner, the treatment setting, memories triggered by sensual cues) is overlooked and it is forgotten that what the placebo response indexes is the interdependency of body and mind and the latent capacity of the mindful body to engage in self cure (Kirsch 1999). It is also forgotten that the placebo response may be adverse (Hahn 1997; Weihrauch and Gauler 1999) and that there is a difference between tests that employ a double blind design where a subject does not know whether they have taken placebo or trial medication and a design using deceptive administration of a placebo where a subject thinks he is taking the "real thing," testing the effect of expectation (Kirsch and Weixel 1998).

Efficacy, effectiveness, and placebo response is a complex area of study, and one in which anthropologists need to become more actively involved. Our reason for dwelling on the subject is to point out that attributions of efficacy, however determined, and be they positive or negative, influence treatment expectations and thus effectiveness in their own right. Social facts influence the production of "scientific facts," and the production and appropriation of social facts is often motivated by stakeholders having subtle and not so subtle agenda.

Another observation is worth noting and brings to mind Weber's writing on the tension between routinization and disenchantment versus charisma and the need for higher meaning in a mundane world. The need to appear scientific is a social phenomenon that both legitimates status and challenges the boundaries of science. Consider, for example, the way in which the epistemology of biomedical knowledge is presently under siege. Advocates of other forms of medical knowing and religious belief are currently attempting to prove the efficacy of their practices using "scientific criteria" and yet at the same time question the primacy of scientific criteria to establish truth. One is reminded of a recent article published in *Science* where the usual grounds for establishing scientific efficacy are severely challenged by a research project in the United States involving prayer. Entirely unbeknownst to the patients involved in the project, some religious believers were asked to pray for cancer patients living in a different state. The study used a small sample, but showed a statistically significant improvement in those patients who were prayed for as opposed to the control group for whom no prayers were said (Harris et al. 1999). Does science legitimate religion at times, or is it perhaps that religion legitimates science?

Politics of science and medicine

Yet another vision of science is addressed by Young's essay in which he comments on an earlier paper by Charles Leslie about a well-respected practitioner of Ayurveda. This practitioner is one of those who claims that science, as it makes progress, confirms the "perfect truths of Hindu theory" and that the telos of Hindu philosophy is where science is heading. Charles showed that such an argument could only be remotely sustained by ignoring the way in which Ayurveda itself had undergone a "revival," central to which was the incorporation of some aspects of scientific knowledge. In other words, the timeless, "perfect truths" of Hindu theory are grounded in shifting sands – as are other similar claims, including those associated with science.

Young sets about showing how the relatively recent emergence of evolutionary psychiatry is one such example of claims based on flawed postulates. He discusses the assumptions on which this new psychiatry is based and then proceeds to deconstruct them as so many *Just so* stories – plausible, but essentially "conjectural and often based on problematic mechanisms." Young shows that hidden debates about values, especially about the naturalization and medicalization of morals, is what makes evolutionary psychiatry so provocative and, to some, so attractive.

That values are embedded in science has been shown repeatedly (Daston 1992; Hacking 1985; Latour 1993; Lock 1993; Young 1995) and it was perhaps the work of Fleck (1935) on syphilis that first opened up this line of inquiry in the social sciences. Fleck argued that a scientist's phenomena are products of his technologies, practices, and preconditioned ways of seeing. Even so, scientific tests, standards, systems of measurement, and so on are understood as neutral and objective, and their efficacy is based on this objectivity. However, increasingly the self-vindicating "styles of reasoning" (Young 1995) used by scientists and physicians are being laid bare as the assumptions built into supposedly neutral arguments are exposed (Berg 1997; Cambrosio and Keating 1995; Lock 2001; Lock et al. 2000).

Science and medicine are called into question in another more obvious way by the almost daily exposure in the media of political interest at work and how it so often orchestrates scientific and medical practice. A further difficulty is, of course, that biomedicine has not proved itself effective for a large spectrum of disease and distress. Under these circumstances we are witnessing on the one hand a turn toward "complementary" medicine in the "developed" world, one that forces recognition of an engaged pluralism but in which scientific monitoring is a government requirement. On the other hand, as several of the essays in this book make clear, the dialectic of pluralism in those parts of the globe where "development" took off more recently usually takes a rather different turn, one where the assumed "truth" of science is being used to buttress tradition. This is the case even though science and biomedicine come as part of the package of modernization and globalization, whose intrusion and challenge to social and political order many people and governments at local sites are trying to avert (see Appadurai 1996a on global cultural economies in general).

This apparent difference between those countries where science and biomedicine have a long tradition as opposed to those whose experience is relatively recent is largely one of emphasis, however. In all cases, the activity is one of boundary making and disputes over power, which have direct implications for the health, well-being, and identity formation of peoples everywhere.

The promise of progress: social engineering revisited

The politics of biopower proposed by Foucault, and so evident in many of the essays in this book, is taken up by Lock in her paper on utopias of health and germline engineering. Utopias of health have a very long history, but it is only since the last century that the idea of progress and notably the enhancement of health through technological intervention has come to the fore. Closely associated with programs for health enhancement are social eugenics, and one aspect of governmentality from the end of the nineteenth century until well into the twentieth century was to manipulate populations through "negative eugenics" – through the active control of reproduction of those people designated as "inferior." Lock argues that we are now in an age of *laissez-faire* eugenics. This is made possible by the new genetics in which individuals and partners are increasingly encouraged to participate in genetic testing and screening programs central to a new form of preventive medicine designed to ensure that only "healthy" babies are born. Germline engineering, banned for the present time, makes it possible through a manipulation of germ cells to control not only the offspring of individuals, but of all their ensuing generations. Lock's essay, similar to that of Young, questions how truth claims about science, in this instance germline engineering, are produced. She highlights the intersection of government interests in producing only healthy people with those of scientists who are keen to make use of innovative technologies and with those of that most powerful of new players in the global economy, the private-sector biotechnology enterprise. Petersen (2001) adds to this analysis by considering the role of the media in propagating "biofantasies" and shaping public thinking and debate about genetics and its medical possibilities.

A driving force behind eugenics has always been the idea of betterment of the society of the future, and to this end some individuals must be sacrificed for the greater good of all. Most utopian visions of future life have a eugenic component to them and involve sacrifice on the part of the living, often of their lives, or else the removal of defective and unsuitable elements. Trawick's paper exposes the utopian myth in Sri Lanka that incites young people to sacrifice themselves in war for the benefit of future, happier generations purged of unsavory elements. Smaller, less dramatic sacrifices are imposed on people everywhere through the numerous ways in which social and political orders reproduce value systems, supposedly for the good of society and often in the name of economic health, that perpetuate inequalities and often misery in the daily lives of numerous citizens.

Confronted with massive social change and economic destablization, uncertainty prevails worldwide. This is not the tedious but ordered modernity that Weber visualized but, on the contrary, a massive erosion of any semblance of control accompanied by a protean spread of inequality and exploitation. This is "disorganized capitalism" (Lash and Urry 1987). It is not surprising under these conditions of uncertainty that ethnic lines harden, violence is common, claims for a return to the "traditional" order and the values it espouses are frequently heard, and pluralism flourishes. This is the situation even as the merits of modernity, science, and new technologies of all kinds are lauded, adopted piecemeal, and indigenized. Charles alerted us with prescience several decades ago to this future in which we now live.

Violence and healing

Several medical anthropologists (Linda Green, Nancy Scheper-Hughes, Arthur Kleinman, Carolyn Nordstrom, Veena Das, to name a few) have been compelled by their field experience to consider human suffering at the site of the individual body and within larger social formations as part of the purview of their research.[6] In her paper about war, violence, and healing in Sri Lanka, Trawick, too, confronts racism and hatred, this time between Sinhalese and Tamils, and the way in which these sentiments are inculcated into young people and reproduced from one generation to the next through the retelling of myth. Trawick shows how these myths are transmitted in part through poetry and song, rather than by claims to scientific legitimacy as is the case in the papers by Bibeau and Pederson and by Jeffery and Jeffery. Appeals to the emotions and hence to the "truth" of inner experience to justify exclusion and violent action against peoples designated as less-than-human are, of course, much older, and perhaps ultimately more powerful, than are truth claims that appeal to scientific verity.

Trawick discusses the paradox of the ongoing war between Sinhalese and Tamils that is waged ostensibly for purposes of healing. She shows how ethnicity is essentialized as part of the mythology of warfare in order to provoke hatred on one side and martyrdom on the other. Trawick's claim is not that people use myth to make sense of the chaos and suffering of war, but rather that myth is evoked (sometimes deliberately, sometimes not) by stakeholders to motivate people to join in war in the first place, and to keep them fighting. The sacrificial sentiments contained in Sinhalese and Tamil myths are quite distinct, one centered on ridding a homeland of affliction through sacrifice of a demonized "other" and the other on redeeming a subjugated homeland through self-sacrifice. In both cases, myths motivate people to kill and to be killed in what has become an all-out war, in order that their own nation and society be healed of the affliction that is the war itself. Over time, these two communities have increasingly become "unimaginable" to each other (Hayden 1996).

Trawick's approach to ethnocidal warfare may be juxtaposed to Arjun Appadurai's (1998) analysis of ethnocidal violence. Appadurai, in an essay on ethnocidal violence between social intimates (originally delivered in Colombo Sri Lanka), suggests that ethnic violence is rooted in long-standing, festering feelings of ethnic insecurity and paranoia wherein ethnic identity is established in opposition to an "other" at the site of the body. Left out of Appadurai's discussion is the extent to which governments, ruling classes, and multinational and transnational organizations are responsible for creating the conditions for ethnic warfare. Trawick does not discount Appadurai's position, but suggests that ethnic conflicts are orchestrated by those in positions of power who perpetuate war through the work of culture wherein myth is called upon to justify violence, and death takes on meaning within a larger cosmology. For Appadurai, responsibility for violence lies in the hands of the masses, whose ethnic identity is threatened at times when cosmologies and social structures are in flux, whereas for Trawick the responsibility for violence largely lies in the hands of power brokers who profit from the conflict.

Why is this important for medical anthropology? Trawick calls on anthropologists to recognize that analyses of ethnic conflict that attempt to rationalize and find culturally functional "meaning" diverts attention away from the fact that conflicts, such as that found in Sri Lanka, are perverse and out of control. In a manner analogous to Arthur and Joan Kleinman's work on suffering in clinical settings (1991), Trawick warns anthropologists not to reason away the stark reality of terror, torture, and displacement one encounters in the field. To do so is to delegitimate the experience of those whose lives we witness.

Anthropologists who push interpretations of meaning alone, Trawick argues, inadvertently contribute to a negative feedback loop that prevents those in the global community from recognizing both the barbarism that is occurring and the global political circumstances that motivate it. Does this enable the global community to identify the problem as local and not become involved? Trawick, like Linda Green (1999) who has documented atrocities in Guatemala, calls on anthropologists to "give voice to sight" (Sider 1989: 14) to describe the darker side of the human condition and to engage the global community through descriptions that are not driven by partisan agendas. To "heal" such a thing as modern warfare, it is necessary to identify its true causes, Trawick argues, that are political, and not the natural outgrowth of local cultures or cultural differences.[7]

The maturation of medical anthropology

The essays in this volume represent a spectrum of the current research in medical anthropology that Charles Leslie has inspired during his long career as teacher, researcher, and editor. Anthropological research into health, illness, medicine, identity, and the body provide remarkable insights into the social and political domains of the past, present, and even of the future. Above all, such research reveals the ways in which ideologies associated with science and modernization, particularly an obsession with control through categorization, rarely "fit" with the realities of everyday life, and actually inflame divisiveness, notably when taken up by causes devoted to nationalism, racism, or social eugenics. These essays also show how although, in theory, pluralism like modernism, brings increased possibilities for individual agency, because it is inevitably associated with politics, in practice, it is often structured from above, albeit frequently disguised as increased choice or fulfilling the rights of individuals. For example, increased choice with respect to medical technologies may well coalesce with individual interest and desire, but if the hegemonies in which such choice is embedded pass unnoticed there might well be untoward repercussions for society at large. These dilemmas are grist to the mill of medical anthropology and for research that portrays the realities of the everyday lives of informants, many of whom actively take on, or are pushed into, the trappings of modernism and then must live with the consequences. These changes are occurring worldwide in environments where local governments are eviscerated by the policies of international institutions such as the World Bank and multinational organizations, and where corruption passes unheeded, taking away any semblance of protection the State might afford its subjects. The essays in this book document increasing inequalities, uncertainties, rigidities, and violence directly associated with globalism, modern economies, and scientific rationalism that informants everywhere are subject to today. The contributors to this book have been inspired by Charles Leslie's urging that we embrace issues with an "informed heart" as well as some measure of reflexivity. In his own words:

> My argument is that scientific work requires passion. Particularly in the social sciences we must examine what we are passionate about, and how our passions influence our work.
>
> (Leslie 1990: 912)

Notes

1   Foucault's concept of biopower, as is well-known, has two poles – that of anatomopolitics directed at individual bodies and, at the other pole, the manipulation and control of populations which began to be systematized from the end of the nineteenth century through techniques of the survey (1979, 1980a, 1980b). Biopower affects both the ways populations are monitored and the ways individuals engage in self-surveillance and bodily discipline. Knowledge about risk makes social institutions as well as individuals accountable.

2   Ulrich Beck (1992, 1996) and Anthony Giddens' (1991) theories of reflexive modernization draw a distinction between early and late modernity. Early modernity is characterized by the invention of risk which transformed a radically indeterminate cosmos into a manageable one, through the myth of calculability (Reddy 1996). The later period is characterized by a growing sense of uncertainty and ambivalence, distrust of rapidly changing and contradictory expert knowledge, and the globalization of doubt. In late modernity, risk is not easily calculable and the politics of responsibility become more, not less complex. Scientific skepticism turns inward, risk factors are contested, and progress is questioned in the wake of experiments in modernity gone awry. Beck's writings on "risk society" present us with a population which increasingly questions authority and conducts searches for alternative explanations. They are left with a condition of chronic doubt and insecurity which has both an up and down side. The up side is that they are: a) compelled to engage in reflexive biographies in which they exercise agency by choosing courses of action based on the facts they choose to accept at any given time and, b) question the authority and the relevance of oppressive structures and institutions. On the down side they are left with a growing sense of uncertainty and threat. Giddens recognizes a complementary state of internal self-doubt and suggests that this state may make expert opinion look attractive, perhaps in the form of trusted filter newsletters stamped with the names of Harvard or Johns Hopkins (e.g. in the health field). For a good introduction to social theories of risk, see Lupton (1999), and for a critique of reflexive modernity see Caplan (2000), Maffesoli (1995), Mellor (1997), and Touraine (1995). For medical anthropologists it is the diversity in the experience and response to risk which is important. This requires a consideration of power relations and hegemonic process as they influence the selection of risk factors, the production of knowledge about risk, and the means by which biopower is contested as well as exercised.

3   This is a subject that begs greater investigation given the importance of such issues as acquired bacterial resistance to antibiotics (see for example Okeke, et al. 1999).

4   Stephen J. Gould (1987) has alerted us as to how biological determinism is often masked by the language of interactionism and reference to the bidirectionality of biology – culture influence. Context is paid lip service, but a determinist rather than a potentialist view of genetics is advanced.

5   Images of hypersexuality in Africa deflect attention from other factors contributing to HIV transmission, such as iatrogenic medical practices (Minkin 1990).

6   Three recent volumes on violence and social suffering (Kleinman et al. 1997; Das et al. 2000, 2001) provide a good introduction to this area of study.

7   Trawick's study differs from other studies of violence in Sri Lanka which have documented how the experience of suffering, uncertainty and loss associated with warfare have been assimilated through religion and ritual (Lawerence 2000; Perera 2001).

References

Adams, V. (2001). Particularizing Modernity: Tibetan Medical Theorizing of Women's Health in Lhasa, Tibet. In *Healing Powers and Modernity*, edited by Linda Connor and Geoffrey Samuels, pp. 222–246. Westport: Bergin and Garvey.

Adleson, N. (2001). Reimagining Aboriginality: An indigenous people's response to social suffering. In *Remaking a World: Violence, Social Suffering, and Recovery*, edited by Veena Das, Arthur Kleinman, Margaret Lock, Mamphela Ramphele and Pamela Reynolds, pp. 76–101.University of California Press.

Appadurai, A. (1996a). Disjuncture and Difference in the Global Cultural Economy. In *Modernity at Large: Cultural Dimensions of Globalization*, edited by Arjun Appadurai, pp. 27–47. University of Minnesota Press.

—— (1996b). Number in the Colonial Imagination. In *Modernity at Large: Cultural Dimensions of Globalization*, edited by, pp. 114–138. University of Minnesota Press.

—— (1998). Dead Certainty: Ethnic Violence in the Era of Globalization. *Public Culture* 10(2): 225–247.

Arce, A. and Long, N. (2000). Reconfiguring modernity and development from an anthropological perspective. In *Anthropology, Development and Modernities: Exploring discourses, counter-tendencies and violence*, edited by A. Arce and N. Long. New York: Routledge.

Arnold, D. (1993). *Colonizing the Body: State Medicine and Epidemic Disease in Nineteenth Century India*. Berkeley: University of California Press.

Bates, D. (Editor) (1995). *Knowledge and the Scholarly Medical Traditions*. Cambridge: Cambridge University Press.

Beck, U. (1992). *Risk Society. Towards a New Modernity*. London: Sage.

Beck, U. (1996) World risk society as cosmopolitan society? Ecological question in a framework of manufactured uncertainties. *Theory, Culture and Society*, 13 (4): 1–32.

Berg, M. (1997). *Rationalizing Medical Work: Decision-support Techniques and Medical Practices*. Cambridge, Mass: The MIT Press.

Boonmongkon, P., Pylypa, J. and Nichter, M. (1999). Emerging Fears of Cervical Cancer in Northeast Thailand *Anthropology in Medicine* 6(3): 359–380.

Boonmongkon, P., Nichter, M. and Pylypa, J. (2001). Women's "*Mot Luuk*" Problems In Northeast Thailand: Why Women's Own Health Concerns Matter As Much As Disease Rates. *Social Science and Medicine* 53: 223–236.

Briggs, C. (1994). The Sting of the Ray: Bodies, Agency, and Grammar in Warao Curing. *Journal of American Folklore* 107(423): 139–166.

Bujra, J. (2000). Risk and Trust: Unsafe Sex, Gender and AIDS in Tanzania. In *Risk Revisited* edited by Pat Caplan, pp. 59–84. London: Pluto Press.

Bukhman, G. (2001). Reform and Resistance in Post-Soviet Tuberculosis Control. Ph.D dissertation, Department of Anthropology, University of Arizona, Tucson. Ann Arbor: University Microfilms.

Cambrosio, A. and Keating, P. (1995) *Exquisite Specificity: The Monoclonal Antibody Revolution*. Oxford: Oxford University Press.

Caplan, P. (editor) (2000). *Risk Revisited*. London: Pluto Press.

Cassey, E. (1993). *Getting Back into Place: Toward an Understanding of Place – World*. Bloomington: Indiana University Press.

Chatterjee, P. (1993). *The Nation and its Fragments: Colonial and Postcolonial Histories*. Princeton: Princeton University Press.

Comaroff, J. (1993). The Diseased Heart of Africa: Medicine, Colonialism, and the Black Body. In *Knowledge, Power & Practice: The Anthropology of Medicine and Everyday Life*, edited by Shirley Lindenbaum and Margaret Lock, pp. 305–329. Berkeley: University of California Press.

Comaroff, J. and Comaroff, J. (1993). Introduction. In *Modernity and its Malcontenets : Ritual and Power in Postcolonial Africa*, edited by Jean Comaroff and John Comaroff, pp. xi–xxxvii. University of Chicago Press.

Csordas, T.J. (1996). Imaginal Performance and Memory in Ritual Healing. In *The Performance of Healing*, edited by C. Laderman and M. Roseman, pp. 91–113. New York: Routledge.

Das, V., Kleinman, A., Ramphele, M. and Reynolds, P. (2000). *Violence and Subjectivity*. University of California Press.

Das, V., Kleinman, A., Lock, M., Ramphele M. and Reynolds, P. (2001). *Remaking a World: Violence, Social Suffering, and Recovery*. University of California Press.

Daston, L. (1992). Objectivity and the Escape from Perspective. *Social Studies of Science* 22: 597–618.

Desjarlais, R. (1992). *Body and Emotion*. Philadelphia: University of Pennsylvania Press.

—— (1995). Presence. In *The Performance of Healing*, edited by Carol Laderman and Marina Roseman, pp. 145–164. New York: Routledge.

Dunn, F. (1976). Traditional Asian Medicine and Cosmopolitan Medicine as Adaptive Systems. In *Asian Medical Systems: A Comparative Study*, edited by Charles Leslie, pp. 133–158. Berkeley: University of California Press.

Farmer, P. and Kim, J. (2000). Resurgent TB in Russia: Do we know enough to act? *European Journal of Public Health* 10(2): 150–153.

Farquhar, J. (1994a). Eating Chinese Medicine. *Cultural Anthropology* 9(4): 471–497.

—— (1994b). *Knowing Practice: The Clinical Encounter of Chinese Medicine*. Oxford: Westview Press.

—— (1995). Re-writing traditional medicine in post-Maoist China. In *Knowledge and the Scholarly Medical Traditions*, edited by Don Bates, pp. 251–276. Cambridge: Cambridge University Press.

Farrington, J. and Lewis, D., with Satish, S. and Michat-Teves, A. (1995). *Non-Governmental Organisations and the State in Asia: Rethinking Roles in Sustainable Agricultural Development*. London and New York: Routledge.

Fisher, W.F. (1997). Doing Good? The Politics and Antipolitics of NGO Practices. *Annual Review of Anthropology* 26: 439–464.

Fleck, L. (1935). *Genesis and Development of a Scientific Fact*. Chicago and London: University of Chicago Press.

Foucault, M. (1979). *Discipline and Punish: The Birth of the Prison*. New York: Vintage.

—— (1980a). *Power and Knowledge: Selected Interviews and other Writings*. Brighton, England: Harvester.

—— (1980b). *The History of Sexuality:* Vol. 1. New York: Vintage.

Geschiere, P. (1998). Globalization and the Power of Intermediate Meaning: Witchcraft and Spirit Cults in Africa and East Asia. *Development and Change* 29: 811–837.

Giddens, A. (1991). *Modernity and Self-Identity: Self and Society in the Late Modern Age*. Cambridge: Polity Press.

Ginsberg, F. and Rapp, R. (1995). *Conceiving the New World Order: The Global Politics of Reproduction*. Berkeley: University of California Press.

Gould, S.J. (1987). *An Urchin in the Storm*. New York: Norton.

Green, L. (1999) *Fear as a way of life*. New York: Colombia University Press.

Gupta, A. (1998). *Postcolonial Developments: Agriculture in the Making of Modern India*. Durham, NC: Duke University Press.

Gutierrex, E. and Kendall, C. (2000). The Globalization of Health and Disease: the Health Transition and Global Change. In *Handbook of Social Studies in Health and Medicine*, edited by Gary Albrecht, Ray Fitzpatrick, and Susan Scrimshaw, pp. 84–99. London: Sage.

Hacking, I. (1986). Making Up People. In *Reconstructing Individualism*, edited by Thomas Heller, Morton Sosna, and David E. Wellbery, Stanford: Stanford University Press.

—— (1990). *The Taming of Chance*. Cambridge: Cambridge University Press.

Hahn, R. (1999) Expectations of Sickness: Concept and Evidence of the Nocebo Phenomenon. In *How Expectancies Shape Experience*, edited by Irving Kirsch, pp. 333–356. Washington, DC: American Psychological Association.

Harris, W., Gowda, M., Kolb, J., Strychacz, C., Vacek, J., Jones, P., Forker, A., O'Keefe, J. and McCallister, B. (1999). A Randomized, Controlled Trial of the Effects of Remote, Intercessory Prayer on Outcomes in Patients Admitted to the Coronary Care Unit. *Archives of Internal Medicine* 159: 2273–2278.

Hayden, R. (1996). Imagined Communities and Real Victims: Self-Determination and Ethnic Cleansing in Yugoslavia. *American Ethnologist* 23(4): 783–801.

Horton, R. (1967). African Traditional Thought and Western Science. *Africa* 38: 50–71, 155–187.

Janes, C. (1999). The Health Transition, global modernity and the crises of traditional medicine: the Tibetan Case. *Social Science and Medicine* 48: 1803–1820.

—— (2001). Tibetan Medicine at the Crossroads: Radical Modernity annd The Social Organization of Traditional Medicine in Tibet Autonomous Region, China. *Healing Powers and Modernity*, edited by Linda Connor and Geoffrey Samuels, pp. 197–221. Westport: Bergin and Garvey.

Janzen, J. M. (1978). *The Quest for Therapy in Lower Zaire*. Berkeley: University of California Press.

Jeffery, R. and Jeffery, P. (2000). Religion and Fertility in India, *Economic and Political Weekly* September 2: 3253–3259.

Kavanagh, A. and Broom, D. (1998). Embodied Risk: My Body, Myself? *Social Science and Medicine* 46(3): 437–444.

Kaufert, P.A. (2000). Screening the body: the pap smear and the mammogram. In *Living and Working with the New Medical Technologies*, edited by Margaret Lock, Alan Young and Alberto Cambrosio, pp. 165–183. Cambridge University Press.

Kirsch, I. (1999). *How Expectancies Shape Experience*. Washington DC: American Psychological Association.

Kirsch, I. and Weixel, L.J. (1988). Double-Blind Versus Deceptive Administration of a Placebo. *Biomedical Therapy* 16(3): 242–245.

Kleinman, A.M. (1980). *Patients and Healers in the Context of Culture*. Berkeley: University of California Press.

Kleinman, A. and Kleinman, J. (1991). Suffering and Its Professional Transformation: Toward an Ethnography of Interpersonal Experience. *Culture, Medicine, and Psychiatry* 15(3): 275–301.

Kleinman, A., Das, V. and Lock, M. (1997). *Social Suffering*. Berkeley; University of California Press.

Lash, S. and Urry, J. (1987). *The End of Organized Capitalism*. Madison: University of Wisconsin Press.

Latour, B. (1993). *We Have Never Been Modern*. Cambridge, Mass: Harvard University Press.

Lawrence, P. (2000). Violence and suffering, Amman: The work of oracles in Sri Lanka's eastern war zone. In *Violence and Subjectivity*, edited by Veena Das, Arthur Kleinman, Mamphela Ramphele and Pamela Reynolds, pp. 171–204. Berkeley; University of California Press.

Leslie, C. (1980). Medical pluralism in world perspective. In *Medical Pluralism*, edited by Charles Leslie. Special issue of *Social Science and Medicine* 14B(4): 190–96.

—— (1989a). Indigenous Pharmaceuticals, the Capitalist World System, and Civilization. *Kroeber Anthropological Society Papers* 69–79, pp. 23–31.

—— (1989b). India's Community Health Workers Scheme: A Sociological Analysis. *Ancient Science of Life* IX(2): 40–53.

—— (1990). Scientific Racism: Reflections on peer review, science and ideology. *Social Science and Medicine* 31(8): 891–912.

—— (1995). The Blind Anthropologist and the Elephant of Traditional Asian Medicine. In *Proceedings, Part 9, The 4th International Congress on Traditional Asian Medicine,* published by the Department of the History of Medicine, Juntendo University, Tokyo.

Leslie, C. and Young, A. (1992). *Paths to Asian Medical Knowledge*. Berkeley: University of California Press.

Lock, M. (1980). *East Asian Medicine in Urban Japan: Varieties of Medical Experience*. Berkeley: University of California Press.

—— (1984). Licorice in Leviathan: The Medicalization of Care for the Japanese Elderly. *Culture, Medicine, and Psychiatry* 8(1984): 121–139.

—— (1990). Rationalization of Japanese Herbal Medication: The Hegemony of Orchestrated Pluralism. *Human Organization* 49(1): 41–47.

—— (1993). *Encounters with Aging: Mythologies of Menopause in Japan and North America*. Berkeley: University of California Press.

—— (1998). *Twice Dead: Organ Transplants and the Reinvention of Death*. Berkeley: University of California Press.

Lock, M., Young, A. and Cambrosio, A. (2000). *Living and Working with the New Medical Technologies: Intersections of Inquiry*. Cambridge: Cambridge University Press.

Lock, M. and Gordon, D.R. (1988). *Biomedicine Examined*. Dordrecht: Kluwer Academic Publishers.

Lock, M. and Kaufert, P. (1998). *Pragmatic Women and Body Politics*. Cambridge: Cambridge University Press.

Lovejoy, O.C. (1990). Comments on Scientific Racism: Reflections on Peer Review, Science and Medicine Ideology. *Social Science and Medicine* 31: 909–910.

Lupton, D. (1999) *Risk*. London: Routledge.

Lyttleton, C. (2000). *Engendered Relations: Negotiating Sex and AIDS in Thailand*. Amsterdam: Harwood Academic Press.

Maffesoli, M. (1995) *The time of tribes: the decline of individualism in mass society.* London: Sage.

Mellor, P. and Schiiling, C. (1997) *Re-forming the body: Religion, community and modernity.* London: Sage.

Mencher, J. (1999). NGOs: Are they a force for change? *Economic and Political Weekly,* July: 24–30.

Miles, A. (1998a). Radio and the commodification of natural medicine in Ecuador. *Social Science and Medicine* 47(12): 2127–2137.

(1998b). Science, nature and tradition: The mass-marketing of natural medicine in urban Ecuador. *Medical Anthropology Quarterly* 12(2): 206–225.

Minkin, S.F. (1990). Medical research on AIDS in Africa. *Social Science and Medicine* 33(7): 786–790.

Mudimbe, V.Y. (1988). *The Invention of Africa. Gnosis, Philosophy and the Order of Knowledge.* Blomington and Indianapolis: Indiana University Press.

Nandy, A. (1994). *The Illegitimacy of Nationalism.* Bombay: Oxford University Press.

Nayar K.R. (2000). Public Medicare: Unhealthy trends. *Economic and Political Weekly* July 29-August 4.

Nguyen, V.K. (2001). Epidemiology, Interzones and Biosocial Change: Retrovirus and Biologies of Globalization in West Africa. Doctoral Thesis, Department of Anthropology, McGill University.

Nichter, M. (1978). Patterns of curative resort and their significance for health planning in South Asia. *Medical Anthropologist,* 1978 2: 2, 29–58.

—— (1992a). Commentary. In *Anthropological Approaches to the Study of Ethno-medicine,* edited by Mark Nichter, pp. 223–259. Philadelphia: Gordon & Breach Publishers.

—— (1992b). Ticks, Kings, Spirits, and the Promise of Vaccines. In *Paths to Asian Medical Knowledge,* edited by Charles Leslie and Allan Young, pp. 224–256. Berkeley: University of California Press.

—— (1994). Illness Semantics and International Health: The Weak Lungs/TB Complex in the Philippines. *Social Science and Medicine* 38: 5, 649–663.

—— (1996a). Self-medication and STD prevention. *Sexually Transmitted Diseases* Sept/Oct: 353–356.

—— (1996b). Pharmaceuticals, the commodification of health, and the health care-medicine use transition. In *Anthropology and International Health: Asian Case Studies,* edited by Mark Nichter and Mimi Nichter, pp. 265–328. Amsterdam: Gordon and Breach.

—— (1998). The Mission Within the Madness: Self-Initiated Medicalization as Expression of Agency. In *Pragmatic Women and Body Politics,* edited by Margaret Lock and Patricia Kaufert, pp. 327–353. Cambridge University Press.

—— (1999). Introduction to the American Anthropological Association Forum on Health and Ethnicity sponsored by the Public Policy Committee. Washington D.C.

—— (2001a). Risk, Vulnerability, and Harm Reduction: Preventing STIs in Southeast Asia by Antibiotic prophylaxis, A Misguided Practice. In *Cultural Perspectives on Reproductive Health,* edited by C. Makhlouf Obermeyer, pp. 101–127. Oxford University Press.

—— (2001b). India and the Political Ecology of Health: Indigestion as sign and symptom of defective modernization. In *Healing Powers and Modernity*, edited by Linda Connor and Geoffrey Samuels, pp. 85–108. Westport: Bergin and Garvey.

Nichter, M. and Kendall, C. (1991). Beyond Child Survival: Anthropology and International Health in the 1990's. *Medical Anthropology Quarterly* 5: 3, 195–203.

Nichter, M. and van Sickle, D. (2002). The Challenges of India's Health and Health Care Transition. In *India Briefing*, edited by Philip Oldenburg and Alysia Ayres, in press. New York: M.E. Sharpe.

Nichter, M. and Vuckovic, N. (1993). Agenda For an Anthropology of Pharmaceutical Practice. *Social Science and Medicine* 39(11): 1509–1525.

Okeke, I.N., Lamikanra, A. and Edelman, R. (1999). Socioeconomic and behavioral factors leading to acquired bacterial resistance to antibiotics in developing countries. *Emerging Infectious Diseases* 5(1), http://www.cdc.gov/ncidod/eid/vol5no1/okeke.htm

Oths, K. (1994). Health Care Decisions of Households in Economic Crises: An Example from the Peruvian Highlands. *Human Organization* 53(3): 245–254.

Perelman, M. (2000). Tuberculosis in Russia. *International Journal of Tuberculosis and Lung Disease* 4(12) S208-S214: pp. 1098–1103.

Petersen, A. (2001). Biofantasies: genetics and medicine in the print news media. *Social Science and Medicine* 52: 1255–1268.

Peterson, A. and Lupton, D. (1996). *The New Public Health: Health and Self in the Age of Risk* London: Sage.

Pigg, S.L. (1992). Inventing Social Categories Through Place: Social Representations and Development in Nepal. *Comparative Studies in Society and History* 34: 491–513.

—— (1997). Found in Most Traditional Societies: Traditional Medical Practitioners between Culture and Development. In *International Development and the Social Sciences: Essays on the History and Politics of Knowledge*, edited by F. Cooper and R. Packard, pp. 259–290. Berkeley: University of California Press.

Prakash, G. (1999). *Another Reason: Science and the Imagination of Modern India*. Princeton, New Jersey: Princeton University Press.

Qadeer, I. (2000). Health care systems in transition III. India, Part I. The Indian Experience. *Journal of Public Health Medicine* 22(1): 25–32.

Reddy, S. (1996). Claims to expert knowledge and the subversion of democracy: the triumph of risk over uncertainty. In *Economy and Society*, 25(2): 222–54.

Roseman, M. (1988). The Pragmatics of Aesthetics: The Performance of Healing Among Senoi Temiar. *Social Science and Medicine* 27(8): 811–818.

—— (1991). *Healing Sounds from the Malaysian Rainforest: Temiar Music and Medicine*. Berkeley: University of California Press.

—— (1996). Pure Products go Crazy: Rainforest Healing in Nation-State. In *The Performance of Healing*, edited by Carol Laderman and Marina Roseman, pp. 233–269. New York: Routledge.

—— (2001). Engaging the Spirits of Modernity : The Temiars. In *Healing Powers and Modernity*, edited by Linda Connor and Geoffrey Samuels, pp. 109–129. Westport: Bergin & Garvey.

Rushton, P.J. (1999). *Race, Evolution, and Behavior: A Life History Perspective*. Port Huron, MI: Charles Darwin Research Institute.

Rushton, J.P. and Bogaert, A.F. (1989). Population Differences in Susceptibility to AIDS: An Evolutionary Analysis. *Social Science and Medicine* 28(12): 1211–1220.

Sider, G. (1989). A Delicate People and their Dogs: The Cultural Economy of Subsistence Production – A Critique of Chayanov and Meillassoux. *Journal of Historical Sociology* 2(1): 14–40.

Sivin, N. (1995). State, cosmos and body in the last three centuries, B.C.. *Harvard Journal of Asiatic Studies* 55(1): 5–37.

Stoler, A. and Cooper, F. (1997). Between Metropolis and Colony: Rethinking a Research Agenda. In *Tensions of Empire: Colonial Cultures in a Bourgeois World*, edited by R. Cooper and A. Stoler. Berkeley: University of California Press.

Trawick, M. (1987). The Ayurvedic Physician as Scientist. *Social Science and Medicine* 24: 12, 1031–1052.

Touraine, A. (1995). *Critique of Modernity*. Oxford: Blackwell.

Unschuld, P. (1985). *Unification of the Empire, Confucianism, and the Medicine of Systematic Correspondence*. Berkeley: University of California Press.

Van der Geest, S. and Whyte, S.R. (1989). The charm of medicines: Metaphors and metonyms. *Medical Anthropology Quarterly* 3(4): 345–367.

Vasavi, A.R. (1994). Hybrid Times, Hybrid People: Culture and Agriculture in South India. *Man* 29: 283–300.

Vuckovic, N. and Nichter, M. (1994). Agenda for an Anthropology of Pharmaceutical Practice. *Social Science and Medicine* 39(11): 1509–1525.

Weihrauch, T. and Gauler, T. (2000). Placebo-Efficacy and Adverse Effects in Controlled Clinical Trials. *Arzneim-Forsch Drug Research* 49: 5, 385–393.

Wood, K., Jewkes, R. and Abrahams, N. (1997). Cleaning the womb: constructions of cervical screening and womb cancer among rural Black women in South Africa. *Social Science and Medicine* 45(2): 283–294.

Wright, P.W.G. and Treacher, A. (1982). *The Problem of Medical Knowledge: Examining the Social Construction of Medicine*. Edinburgh: University of Edinburgh Press.

You, H. (1994), Defining Rhythm: Aspects of an Anthropology of Rhythm. *Culture, Medicine, and Psychiatry* 18: 3, 361–383.

Young, A. (1982). The Anthropology of Illness and Sickness. *Annual Review of Anthropology* 11: 257–280.

—— (1995). *The Harmony of Illusions: Inventing Post-Traumatic Stress Disorder*. Princeton: Princeton University Press.

Chapter 2

Governing bodies in New Order Indonesia

Steve Ferzacca

> Medical systems are social and cultural. In contrast to health systems,
> their boundaries are not those of biological populations, species and
> ecological networks, but of political organization and cultural exchange.
>
> (Charles Leslie 1978: xii)

Charles Leslie's now classic *Asian Medical Systems* (1976) came to
mind during the early days of my fieldwork in Yogyakarta, Indonesia
(1991–1993). Leslie's research on Asian medical systems drew attention
to the ways in which modernizing movements resulted in a search for
supposedly lost authentic traditions, revealed in the spirit and practice
of medical revivalisms. At the same time, he observed the place of
"medical revivalism," particularly in China and India, as "an aspect
of cultural nationalism in these societies" (Leslie 1976: 319, 1977). Like
Leslie, I noted both trends in Indonesia as I set out to study how diverse
local medical practices were characterized by both the population and
the state.

In this essay I explore medical pluralism as a form of state rule. In this
regard, the pluralism of medical practice and perception I encountered in
Yogya (short for Yogyakarta) that I once described as constituting a hybrid
medical system (Ferzacca 1996) is examined here as a form of *governmentality* that represents a modern "art of government" (Foucault 1991
[1978]) concerned with "the art of *managing* the economy" of a demographically defined population "for the common welfare of all" (Gupta
1998: 320; emphasis added).[1] I argue here that medical pluralism for
Suharto's New Order regime in Indonesia was a crucial element for a
political organization based upon an ideology and pragmatics of development (*pembangunan*). The introduction of colonial medicine, and so
science, in the late nineteenth and early twentieth centuries when
Indonesia was the Netherlands East Indies is the point at which the peoples
of Indonesia become defined as a population that can be managed as a

"collective mass of phenomena" (Foucault 1991 [1978]: 102), particularly in demographic terms, and in terms of health and disease as demographic variables, and so as targets of intervention. With the Suharto regime (1966–1998), scientific medicine becomes an important technique of development and nation building. This history of this form of governmentality in the Indonesian archipelago illustrates ways in which this art of government is "at once internal and external to the state" (ibid. p. 103) – Leslie's linkage of political organization and cultural exchange. Evidence of this linkage, echoing loudly from the development politics of Suharto's New Order government was the localized universal grammar of modernity inherent within state projects of development. Medical pluralism, I argue, became one of the few spaces in Indonesia for everyday forms of "political struggle and contestation" (ibid.).[2] In this way, the provisioning of a range of health care and the character of this range, indicative of creative, agentive transgressions of practitioners (and so their clients), work to reproduce the discursive and practical categories that were essential for state rule and governance during the Suharto regime.

Stated concerns

It is by now commonplace for anthropologists and historians to reveal within grand designs and mega-movements like global modernity the uneven appearances of these designs and movements in different sites. Some attention has been given to the migration of Western science to the rest of the world as a course through which global modernity flows.[3] For parts of the "developing world" Western science often piggy-backed its way into political affairs and peoples lives on the back of scientific medicine. Based on applied bioscience, scientific medicine with its technique and efficacies was at the same time a remedy of the consequences of colonialism and underdevelopment, and a sign of the modern. For many a colonial history, scientific medicine begins proto-forms of governmentality cloaked in the guise of "humane imperialism" (see Arnold 1988, 2000; Comaroff and Comaroff 1992). Scientific medicine becomes a significant feature of postcolonial forms of governmentality because of its technological, qualifying, and practical relations with many of the demographic measures that define the economy and health of a population. These measures, for example, rates of fertility, infant mortality, life expectancy, disease prevalence, among others, not only make up a population's profile, but are also the targets as well as the efficacious indices of scientific medicine, and so the targets and efficacious indices of the presence or lack thereof of development. Because of the urgent realities of health conditions in a majority of the new nations emerging after World War Two, it is not surprising that medicine and health became central to the strategies for nation building of postcolonial governments. Here the heroics of scientific medicine often find a place in nationalist histories. What remains un-*stated* (so to speak) is the way medical provisions operate as forms of state rule. Indonesia provides a case in point.[4]

Boomgaard (1993: 86), working from Dutch sources, claims that the "popularity of shots" in Java that began with the anti-yaws campaigns after 1900, left a "lasting impression" of the efficacy of scientific medicine on the medical *mentalité* and practices in colonial Indonesia. Even though in the early years of the twentieth century the majority of Indonesians were not treated by doctors trained in scientific medicine, it was quickly becoming a "phenomenon *su generis*" in the daily lives of colonized Indonesians and particularly the Javanese (ibid., p. 87).

The increasing presence of scientific medicine had the effect of demarcating, both cognitively and practically, in a thoroughly modern way, the plurality of medical practice and perception. In the case of the influenza pandemic of 1918, debates regarding the efficacy of "traditional" versus scientific, "colonial" medicine appear in colonial reports and the popular vernacular press (Brown 1987: 243–246). A colonial era publication written in Bahasa Indonesia and distributed just after the 1918 flu pandemic illustrates these debates. The plot of the story is based on the Ramayana epic in which the hero Rama wins the hand of Dewi Sinta in a contest of skill. In this story, the hero must successfully treat the flu in order to win the hand of the "sweet" Si Seriati.

FATHER OF SERIATI: Whoever can dispel this danger (the flu) can marry my daughter si Seriati. Isn't si Seriati sweet, abang Gendoet?

ABANG GENDOET: Oh, very good. She seems sweet, beautiful and well behaved, disciplined, likes to work, and has love and affection for all people.

FATHER OF SERIATI: Seriati certainly would very much like to be married to a husband who is clever about treating sickness. So much the better if that person has a handsome and strong body, is beautiful and likes to work.

However, our prospective hero, Abang Gendoet, treats the flu, referred to at this point in the story as a common disease (*sakit kromo*), or the fever-cough disease, with traditional medical science (*ilmu tabib*). He uses an amulet of last resort. Enter, Si Pandjang, who comes along in the nick of time and speaks to the gathering crowd.

SI PANDJANG: Are you sick with this common disease? Why are you just brooding, like a bunch of wet chickens? Oh, ya. When you are sick with a fever and a cough, that is influenza (*penyakit influenza*). Don't you get too much fresh air. Don't be struck by air. Eat porridge, and if you wish to drink water drink hot tea. If after one week's time your body feels strong, you may go out of your house, but you can not open your shirt.

Si Pandjang goes onto explain that *penyakit* influenza is a disease spread by microbes found in the saliva of people sick with the flu. Microbes enter through the nose and into their blood stream. Because the flu is spread through the air people should reduce their risks for catching the flu by watering down the earthen floors of the homes so that flu germs that cling to airborne dust are kept to a minimum. He also explains that once flu germs enter the body they go to war with white blood cells. His advice is to treat the flu by covering the body with blankets, applying a cool compress on the head for fever, eating soft food like porridge, eggs, milk, finely chopped vegetables (but without chili peppers, coconut, or sour condiments), soup, broth, and drinking hot tea to speed up recovery; but he also recommends taking a chemical pharmaceutical, *tablet Bandoeng*. Not surprisingly, Si Pandjang walks off with the prize (*Awas! Penjakit Influenza* 1920).

While the Dutch colonial regime celebrated the efficacy of its medicine in vernacular terms, it too saw the need for an array of medicines and medical practices to meet the health needs of its far-flung colony that encapsulated an amazing diversity of curious indigenous materia medica.[5] Since declaring Independence (1945) from Dutch rule, and especially since 1960, the Indonesian state has shown interest in the array of medicines and medical practices available among the diverse peoples of this archipelago. At the time of my fieldwork the efforts of Suharto's New Order regime to "develop" health care in Indonesia were continuing in basically the same form with similar goals. For Suharto's New Order regime, *pembangunan*, the Indonesian word for development, operated as the ideological apparatus and practical legitimacy used to champion the presence of the Indonesian government in the daily lives of its citizens – a presence that can only be characterized as immediate in every sense of the word. "Developmentalism" (Heryanto 1990), the discursive regime for Indonesian state rule during the Suharto years, served as the universal langue for a local parole of Indonesian modernity. Suharto adopted the development paradigm complete with the denominations of the modern and its phantasmagoric companion, tradition, that became, like for many other newly emerging nation-states, vital signs of the health of the social body and heuristic measures of the advancement of the nation-state toward the global status of a developed modern country.

During the time I was working in Yogya, a great deal of national and local attention was given to both the promotion and regulation of *pengobatan tradisional* as a key element in the delivery of primary health care. The Indonesian government considers *pengobatan tradisional* an essential resource in the cause of development. The logistical issues inherent in the New Order's engineering of an Indonesian flavored *modernisasi* (modernization), an element or outcome of the development process, have set limits on the ability of the government to provide scientific medicine to a diverse and dispersed national citizenship. Since the transnational discourse on development that the Indonesian government employs as a gold standard uses the health of the nation as a measure of progress, health concerns and health care delivery are central for nationalist projects of development. Yet, for a developing country like Indonesia, technologically advanced scientific medicine can not always be made available to the Indonesian population overall. Nor, given the diversity of ethnic groups and their nearness to or distance from the centers of modernity, is scientific medicine always an appropriate technologic intervention. Given these contingencies, classic Indonesian development rhetoric expressed in the 1992 Republic of Indonesia legislation "about health" (*Tentang Kesehatan*) clearly outlines the role of *pengobatan tradisional* as a development, and therefore, nationalist issue:

> Health development is basic to all aspects of life, and concerns a healthy physical and mental as well as social economy. As the expansion of health development occurred there were changes in orientation resulting in a better set of values as well as thinking particularly about the efforts towards solutions of problems in the health field that are influenced by political, economic, social, and cultural factors important for stability and safety that accompanies development science and technology. These changes in orientation will influence the process of coordinating health development. In addition to these ideas the planning of health development needs to pay attention to the totality of a large Indonesian population made up of a variety of ethnic groups and customs that occupy thousands of islands that are dispersed with various levels of education and society.
>
> (Undang-Undang Republik Indonesia No. 23 1992: 2)

In order to plan "health development" in a rational manner, the variety of medical practices and perceptions found in this archipelago needed to be considered and standardized for utilitarian purposes. The Department of Health outlined the defining characteristics of traditional medicine and the role these medicines and medical practices should have in the National Healthcare System.[6] Governmental legislation, along with the 1960 National Medicine Policy, was to establish a "strong legal foundation" for the provisioning and use of traditional medicines and practices in order to ensure a wider set of health care provisions, spread evenly to all, that at the same time protected and developed medical pluralism as a national cultural inheritance.[7] This legislation planned for the development of traditional medicines and practices using the rational manner of scientific medicine (*secara medis*) forged from a nexus of expertise, research, and testing.

In addition to these internal legislative developments relevant to medical pluralism has been the promotion of medical pluralism in the market place for which cultural exchanges of all kinds are engaged in a lively, competitive empire of signs, so to speak. For the marketing of traditional medicine, scientific medicine as a foil for comparison is both embraced and condemned. Jaya Suprana, Secretary General of the Federation of Jamu and Traditional Medicine Manufacturers, a major manufacturer of factory-produced traditional medicine (Jamu Jago), and often-quoted *jamulog* (jamu expert), engages in some story-telling of his own to illustrate these points:

> "*Si Amir is sick. His mother immediately carries him to the doctor. After the doctor has examined Amir he writes him a prescription for medicine. Amir takes the prescription to the pharmacy for his medicine. Three days pass and Amir is still not cured. Then, Amir is cared for in the hospital.*" The plot of this story is similar to the customary ones taught in school, as a part of health education for generations of Indonesian youth. Rarely is there a school teacher in Indonesia that will tell a story like, "Amir is healthy and safe because each day he routinely drinks jamu."[8]
>
> (Suprana 1993: 4)

Nevertheless, in order to compete as a medical commodity in these increasingly modernist times in a local and hopefully global marketplace, jamu and traditional medicine as legitimate therapeutic alternatives to chemical pharmaceuticals need to be highlighted for their complicity with state projects of regulation, development, and rationalization.

> We don't need to debate this any further about the absolute innovative will and effort required in order to survive if not prosper in the middle of this critical stage of globalization! There is already a precise calculated effort by the Republic of Indonesia Department of Health to build a jamu industry in order to develop the forms of traditional Indonesian medicine into one new standardized form recognized by pharmaceutical experts all over the world, for example, fitofarmaka [phytopharmaceuticals]. These innovative steps fit with international agreements of competition that are ideal for the ability to compete in the international business marketplace. Bravo, Department of Health, Republic of Indonesia!
>
> (ibid.)

In addition to this celebration of the role of the state for the marketing of traditional medicine is the important message that medical pluralism must be packaged in nonconfusing ways for the global market. Here, cultural exchange is central for the shape of medical pluralism. Locally, nonconfusing cultural content for medical pluralism is an interest of the state as well.

Post-traditional medicine

The 1992 laws "about health" define *pengobatan tradisional* as "medical practices or health care with approaches, pharmaceuticals, and medical treatments that refer to experience and expertise that have been passed down (*turun-temurun*), and when applied fit with the norms to be in effect in society."[9] *Pengobat tradisional* include "substances or medical substances from plant, animal, and mineral sources, available manufactured naturally occurring essences, or a mixture of all of these as they have been passed down to be used for treatment based on experience."[10] Once again, Jaya Suprana provides some insight into this absence:

> Jamu is often proudly considered as one of the artifacts of Indonesian national culture from the field of health care like no other in this world. Jamu's acclaim draws from the same breath as batik or gamelan as artifacts of a culture noble, exquisite, and exalted [*adiluhung*], resulting in prestige and a role that needs to be raised up not only for social life in Indonesia, but outside the country as well.
>
> (ibid.)

Suprana situates *jamu*, health tonic drinks made from mostly spices, and traditional medicine with the *adiluhung*, or what Florida (1987) describes as "veritable icon(s) of Javanese High Culture."[11] Medicines as artifacts of exquisite traditions in this sense are easily located (and re-located) as signifiers among others in a cultural politics that Florida suggests is informed by "the myth of the *adiluhung*" (ibid., p. 2). Pemberton (1994) also describes the manner in which Suharto's New Order regime's heightened attention to and willful manipulation of representations of the past and the traditional became essential for a "New Order *adiluhung* rhetoric." This rhetoric had linkages to a "late Colonial voice" (Florida 1987: 3). The postcolonial voice continues to be one in which things Javanese are reproduced as the identity of the nation-state. Situating traditional medicine with the other "veritable icons" of Javanese culture in order to establish their authenticity and cultural heritage imbues medicine as both a medium and instrument of Indonesian political organization. The medicines themselves occupy spatially dispersed ethnically diverse bodies that reside in this archipelago in ways that the "Javanization of medical personnel" during the Dutch colonial period and later with Indonesian independence spatially dispersed Javanese throughout the archipelago in the name of the Dutch Colonial Public Health Service and the Indonesian National Health System (Brown 1987). The marked features of traditional medicine are determining factors for defining the presence of medical pluralism within a local medical *system* that governs bodies for purposes of state rule as modern health care. In both cases state occupation across space through bodies is taking place.

The following vignettes show how perceptions and practices, knowledge and technique, discourse and power are "redistributed" among social relations and how a particular political order is defined and sustained in terms of development in a post-traditional world.[12] With a consideration of some of the practitioners I encountered, a "relations of governmentality" (Newberry and Ferzacca 1999) inherent in the plurality of medical practice provides insight into the spaces for everyday forms of "political struggle and contestation" that at the same time constitute relations of state rule. Several examples help to show this form of governmentality at work.

Practicing medical pluralism

It is interesting that practitioners of *pengobatan tradisional* are left out of the formulations of nationalist health policy. They are, perhaps, implied by the marked categories of inheritance and experience as key reference points for determining whether some medical practice or pharmaceutical used by a healer is traditional. It is more difficult to predict how practitioners will behave as artifacts, particularly since many practitioners of *pengobatan tradisional* are often too traditional compared to the veritable icons in a cultural politics important for a "New Order *adiluhung* rhetoric" of rule. In these cases, as we will see in the following, development efforts in Indonesia directed toward practitioners, as in most other "Third World" countries, have sought to improve and update their practices to be scientifically rational ones, rather than to celebrate existing practices as icons of a refined, civilized past. In other cases, unrecognizable traditional medicine either is made to be recognizable, or censored. In this way, *pengobatan tradisional* is post-traditional and is a symptom of an emergent post-traditional society (Giddens 1994) within which medical pluralism represents a reflexive project of modernization (Beck 1994) that embeds traditions – creatively transgressive, accommodatingly innovative, or stubbornly conservative – within centers of power.[13]

One example I encountered during my fieldwork was a meeting I attended with a healer I worked with extensively that was held at the primary health care center that serviced our subdistrict. The meeting was given the title, *Rapat Pengobatan Tradisional* (Traditional Medicine Meeting). Bu Pijet, a masseuse, escorted me to this and other monthly meetings of local practitioners who use *pengobatan tradisional*. Those who came were predominantly traditional midwives (*dukun bayi*), and all women. Besides midwives, there were also several women who made *jamu*. The primary health care center's doctor, also a woman, attended the meeting. She was there to listen, but also to guide and educate, or improve the methods and techniques of this front line of health care delivery and practice.

During our introductions I was asked the common question of whether or not Janice and I had children. I replied as always, "not yet," but we were trying with some difficulty. This spurred a good deal of discussion. One of the midwives mentioned that a woman had come to her who wanted a child, even though she already had eight. The others attending shook their heads and whispered to each other. The doctor turned her attention toward the midwife regarding this case – the midwife then realized that perhaps she had stirred up something inadvertently. The doctor asked for the name of the woman, the name of the husband, the address and location of the house, all the while writing down everything.

The doctor lifted her head from her writing tablet and said that there should be no fear of competition among each of the women at the meeting. A spirit of mutual aid and sharing should be present as colleagues in the art of healing. Each woman was asked to share her experience (*pengalaman*) in front of the group. No one seemed to pay much attention to these monologues. As Bu Pijet spoke, however, the group became attentive, and the doctor wrote down several of her recipes for herbal, plant-based medicines that she uses in her practice. Bu Pijet reminded the group several times that she did not "inherit" her knowledge, but obtained it through study and experiential learning. From here the doctor took over the discussion as it shifted from exchanging experiences, styles of healing, *jamu* and medical recipes, to a discussion of primary health care knowledge that these front line healers needed to improve their knowledge and practice. The doctor covered the common areas of improvement – sanitation, clean knives for cutting the umbilical cord, information about breast feeding, immunizations, and other government directives, and the meeting ended.

This brief vignette shows how development practice and post-traditional traditions facilitate the redistribution of power as state rule that is essential, as Foucault notes (1991 [1978]: 104), for a "governmental state, essentially defined no longer in terms of its territoriality, of its surface area, but in terms of the mass of its population with its volume and density."[14] It is a classic example of ways in which so-called traditional medical practices enter into development schema. The vital statistics of the population are brought to bear into the lives of individuals. Secondly, in order to understand medical pluralism as a form of governmentality, Moore (1996: 12) suggests we consider how governmentality operates as "mechanisms (techniques of knowledge, power and subjectification) through which social authorities seek to administer the lives of individuals and collectivities, and the ways in which individuals and collectivities respond." The state's presence in this act of welfare is obvious – the meeting was state sponsored, it took place in a government primary health care center, and an agent of the state, the doctor (doctors are government civil servants), was present. However, the presence of the state was also indexed by Bu Pijet's apology that although her practice is based on experience, one of the important elements the state uses to define *pengobatan tradisional*, her knowledge and technique were not inherited (*keturunan*), the other important element. It was precisely her apology that led my attention closer toward an understanding of medical pluralism as governance and state rule.

In my work with various practitioners of *pengobatan tradisional*, I encountered formulaic life histories, which seemed to legitimate their practice of medicine (Ferzacca 2001). These histories referenced, but went beyond inheritable knowledge. For example, the owner of a *warung jamu* (*jamu* shop) famous for its traditional medical tonics for treating children told me that both his business and his recipes were inherited from his grandparents and their ancestors. He then emphasized that while his expertise had origins in this inheritance, his practice was also influenced by divine inspiration (*ilham*). He possessed an intuitive potency, or as he referred to it, *instink yang kuat* (a strong instinct). I asked him about the notion of *instink*, and he explained:

> In the past people had morally good and strong instincts because there were many who practiced [asceticism and Javanese knowledge] (*banyak nglakoni, banyak prihatin*). What is meant by pengobatan tradisional is a medicine that is put into practice based upon the ways (*cara*) that have been passed along (*naluri*) or inherited (*keturunan*) from our ancestors (*nenek-moyang*), and doesn't use chemicals, but only natural ingredients (*bahan alam*) from all kinds of plants (*tumbuh-tumbuhan*).

The owner incorporates the major themes that run through the everyday discourse on traditional medicine in Yogyakarta and illustrates the essential relationship between inheritance and experience. The question is, then, does the state definition of traditional medicine inform on-the-ground folk theories of traditional medicine as a contrasting portrait to scientific medicine? Or, is it the reverse? Or both?

Two final vignettes may help us find some answers. The term *terkun* represents a combination of the Indo-English word, *dokter*, with the Javo-Indonesian term *dukun* that is used for the Javanese shaman. *Terkun* is a hybrid title and healing practice that has fallen out of favor in recent times. In the history of medical pluralism in Java, the case of Gunawan Simon, a Chinese-Indonesian who practiced as a terkun in the West

Javanese city of Bandung, is cited as the watershed case that led to the downfall of the *terkun* as a legitimate figure.[15] The similarities with the flu story are reflected in reverse.

The story goes that when Gunawan's younger brother became sick with dysentery his mother took his younger brother to the doctor for treatment, only to find the doctor was playing badminton. The doctor became angry with Gunawan's mother for interrupting his recreation, but reluctantly prescribed some medicine. Gunawan was stunned when he was told of what happened and his "heart revolted." His mother suggested that he should become a doctor, but a just and fair doctor.

Gunawan graduated from the Faculty of Medicine at the University of Padang in 1972 as a general practitioner. However, because of his reaction upon hearing of his mother's experience with a practitioner of scientific medicine and her wishes that he become a just and fair doctor, Gunawan decided to practice an eclectic mix of scientific medicine and traditional medicine that would serve the masses. It was at this moment that he became a *terkun*. Gunawan's services as a *terkun* became well-known, so much so that the former Indonesian vice president, Adam Malik, sick with liver cancer, consulted him. Gunawan treated him with a "blended medicine" that included opium, steroids, antibiotics, and several substances that generally are grouped together as controlled substances (*obat-obatan daftar G*). His "new way" (*cara baru*) for curing cancer was scrutinized by the Administrative Board of Indonesian Doctors for breaking the medical code of ethics. The Board explained that Gunawan Simon was not a cancer expert, nor was he a specialist. The Board recommended the withdrawal of his license to practice medicine and suggested that he continue to practice, perhaps as a *sinshe* (Chinese herbalist), but not as a *dokter*, or in this case as a *terkun*. The Board's edict that he practice as a *sinshe* revealed Gunawan's Chinese heritage, which certainly was no small issue in this affair, even if hidden from view. And although his license to practice scientific medicine was withdrawn, he continues to have duties as a *sinshe* at the Emanuel Hospital in Bandung.

One wonders if Gunawan had referred to himself in the first place as a *sinshe* whether or not he could have avoided this scrutiny. The Board questioned his expertise as a trained cancer specialist. But this was not the true point of contention. Practitioners, entrepreneurs, and consumers of *pengobatan tradisional* are known for their miraculous claims of curing all forms of disease and malady which are accepted without trepidation. For practitioners of traditional medicine, having expertise in a particular field of medicine or healing is not necessary, nor expected.

In the case of Gunawan, the discursive parameters that outline the characteristic features of the traditional *vis-à-vis* the scientific shaped the actions of the Board. Here the state and scientific medicine, as in state sponsored development, are melded together. As an example of the "professionalization of indigenous healers" (Last 1996), Gunawan over-steps professional boundaries and becomes a victim of a politics of professionalization operating as a rationalizing body politic. However, it is not only the fact that a bureaucratic arm of the state discharged penal-ties and punishment that instantiates the presence of the state in medical affairs. It is Gunawan's use of *cara*, which can be translated as a way, manner, method, that did not fit, or *cocok*, with the claims of being a *terkun*.[16] Pemberton (1994: 65) noted that in the context of the Javanese court chronicles he examined the term *cara* "easily blends toward reifi-cation as 'style' and even more so as 'custom'". He sees this reification in context with historically contingent "epistemological shifts" and "a particular form of reflexivity" that further adds to this concept to denote a sense of "culture" (ibid., p. 66). Remember the owner of Jampi Asli made *cara* a point of significance when he said, "What is meant by *pengo-batan tradisional* is a medicine that is put into practice based upon the ways (*cara*) that have been passed along or inherited from our ancestors." Gunawan misapprehended the consequences of his appropriation of *cara*. Gunawan's eclectic medicine was determined by the state to be an unvi-able hybrid. It was not the product of social and cultural reproduction, and so his medicine could not reproduce viable offspring of its own. In the end, the Board simply directed Gunawan to continue his healing within *recognizable* and reproductive traditional approaches for a Chinese Indo-nesian – the *sinshe*.

Another vignette specific to Yogya will offer some insight as well. For any researcher interested in *pengobatan tradisional* in this Central Javan-ese city, the name of Bu Dewi is heard with the most frequency – she is legendary. Her ability to attract clients is considered a sign of her extreme potency. Bu Dewi practices one day each week in Yogya (Monday) and in Solo (Wednesday), the other court city just to the north, and two days of each week (Friday, Sunday) in the Indonesian capital city of Jakarta; on Tuesdays, Thursdays, and Sunday afternoons she travels. Saturdays are her days of rest. At the time of our interviews she was thirty-two years old, and had been a practicing healer for twenty-one years. I found that a calling to heal at a young age was a common feature in the life histo-ries of healers I worked with in Yogya.

The location of her practice in Yogya is just to the east of the city in an area where rice fields are giving way to modern suburban homes. She moved to her current location, a suburban *kampung* known as the "Green House," from the neighborhood where I lived, where she had practiced for nine years. Many of our neighbors worked for Bu Dewi as aides. She is a Muslim, and the title included in her full name, *Raden Ajeng* (RA), signifies not only her noble blood lines, but also that she was, at the time, an unmarried aristocrat. While Bu Dewi carries the *ningrat* suffix that marks again her genealogical relationship to the *kraton*, and in her case the Yogya *kraton*, she says she refuses to live in the *kraton* because she feels that her associations with everyday people would be limited by her residence in the court. She sees and treats hundreds of patients daily, and, according to her, thousands come to her practice in Jakarta on a daily basis.

Her patients gather in a waiting room. After signing in, each patient pays rupiah 500 (0.25 US$) and is given a number. Before they move into the waiting room, the attendants who sign-in patients ask them to explain their need or desire to see Bu Dewi. Their answers are written on a small card for Bu Dewi to read when she meets the patient for treatment. I was told by the attendant that Bu Dewi rarely speaks to patients. Patients are also asked at this time of sign-in if they have been examined through laboratory measures, and if so, they are asked for the results of these examinations. The waiting room walls are covered with photographs of Bu Dewi and framed government documents that "officially" sanction her to practice *pengobatan tradisional*. A television is tuned into the early afternoon soap operas that many enjoy.

First and foremost, the menu of her services that hangs in the waiting room reads that she uses *pengobatan tradisional* and particularly is an expert in *kebathinan*, or Javanese mysticism. Under the entry "medicine practiced in the way of kebathinan" there are listed various medical techniques that she incorporates in her practice, including: ayurvedic/unani medicine, Chinese herbalism, shamanism, acupuncture, and religious spiritualism. Her stock and trade, however, is that of nearly every other healer of *pengobatan tradisional* in Yogya that I met, herbalism and massage. The menu reads that her diagnoses are derived from examining the pulse (*urat nadi*) and considering the results of doctor and laboratory examinations. It claims that she can treat a wide variety of internal and external illnesses and diseases. Finally, the menu heralds that she has inherited her ability to heal.

Kebathinan, usually referred to as Javanese mysticism, is lauded as the most authentic and indigenous example of *kejawen* (Javanese) knowledge and technique – it is one of the veritable icons of Javanese culture. *Kebathinan* is described in the literature as a Javanese "science of life," "range of mystical beliefs," and the disciplining of a person's *batin*, inner realm, as it exists within the rises and declines of human life (*sangkan paraning dumadi*).[17] *Kebathinan* is associated with the revivalist mystical cults that emerged in the 1970s (see Stange 1992). Its public presence on Bu Dewi's menu of services represents relationships between various state mandated governing orders in the process of rationalization for purposes of development, in this case the modern secularization by modern nation-states of religious orders.[18]

But moreover, Bu Dewi, and her "medicine practiced in the way of *kebathinan*," combines in her practice all that is sublime and appropriately refined that is expected of a Javanese aristocrat nurtured in the realm of the *adiluhung*.[19] Her composure and controlled sense of self as she meets with her clients is the same technique of self promoted and required by New Order rhetoric and rule as a normative discipline of the self expected of the ideal Indonesian citizen. On a national level, mass mediated descriptions, always censored by Suharto's government, often described outbreaks of protest or social criticism as examples of *amuk* that located political resistence and social critique in terms of loss of composure and control of the self. But, such composure in also valued by Javanese as expressions and evidence of power. Bu Dewi exemplifies normative Javanese concepts of self-mastery and control that have become makers of an ideal Indonesian cultural citizenship.[20]

In this way, Bu Dewi, and the medical practices and perceptions she embodies and provisions, are, in Pemberton's (1994: 10–11) terms, *recognizable* as a "manifestation of what it is assumed to be" – Javanese culture (*kebudayaan Jawa*) that is authentic (*asli*), inherited (*keturunan*), and iconically sublime (*adiluhung*). Pemberton calls this the "culture effect" (ibid.), reflective of an obsession on the part of New Order authorities and the citizens of Indonesia, particularly the Javanese with traditional Javanese culture. However, this aesthetic and practical disposition of the self that Bu Dewi performs and reproduces in the context of her medical practice is also laden with the potential for power and agency. Her traditional medicine is post-traditional as a reflexive project on the Javanese "idea of power" within the nation-state project of modernity.

Governing bodies

Scholars of medical pluralism have observed an increased plurality of health care, practices, and perceptions with the emergence of complex state societies. Frohock (1992) suggests a necessary relationship between increasing medical plurality and the ideals of neutrality and tolerance of the liberal state that ideally allows the occupation of public space by multiple realities and related levels of competence. Baer (1995: 493), in a review article, remarks that, "in contrast to indigenous societies, which tend to have a more or less coherent medical system, state societies are characterized by an array of medical systems – in other words, medical pluralism" (see also Baer et al. 1997).[21] The dependent variable here is the presence of patterns of social hierarchy that the content and forms of medical pluralism reflect (Baer et al. 1997: 10). Crandon-Malamud (1991), in work on medical pluralism in Bolivia, notes the role of medicine in identity formations and social change. Last (1996), using the concept of a "national medical culture," describes an array of competing medical systems for which there is usually, but not always, some dominative system essential for defining the terms of competition. Importantly, he also specifies the lesser and greater degrees of state regulation for national medical cultures. Finally, as stated at the outset, Leslie's approach sees a processual plurality of health care for countries like Indonesia in the throes of modernizing and entangled in modernist projects that have come to embrace identifications of the "traditional dimensions of modernization" (Leslie 1974: 70).

In all cases medical pluralism is observed as a *function* of a complex society. Medical pluralism, especially outside Europe and the United States, is also examined as a predictable outcome of a universally contingent classificatory system of *modernity*. The universality of such a system is either identified as a cognitive one for which categories of the "modern" and the "traditional" operate as organizing principles, or as modern social forms and practices related to identity formations. For example ethnicity, or nationalism and regionalism of all kinds shape the boundaries of medical practice and perception.[22] While these boundaries of medical systems are important to identify from an ethnographic point of view (Kleinman 1980), it is also important to consider, again from an ethnographic point of view, that such boundaries are themselves instrumentalities of and for political organization.

I would like to return to Moore's (1996: 12) suggestion that I cited earlier that if we are to consider how governmentality operates as a particular art of governance, we should direct our attention to the "mechanisms (techniques of knowledge, power and subjectification) through which social authorities seek to administer the lives of individuals and collectivities, and the ways in which individuals and collectivities respond." Attention to the social and cultural boundaries that delineate "sectors" of a medical system provides important descriptive terms. Locating these descriptive terms in sites of the production, reproduction, and redistribution found within the bounds of formal state institutions, as we saw with the meeting of traditional midwives at the primary health care clinic, and within the realm of everyday practice and life, reveals ways medical pluralism as *political organization* governs bodies. The "cosmo-politics" (Cheah and Robbins 1998) of this local knowledge reflect transnational histories of global modernity embraced by political regimes. Suharto's New Order rationalized pluralistic medical practice and perception within a universal grammar of scientific method and reason, and appropriated the peoples of Indonesia within the model of a population.

Moreover, medical pluralism locates the state in the intimate cleavages and crannies of people's lives through their own agency, as people make the state and enact state rule. The state is lived in this sense, not as false consciousness, but as reflexive projects within definitive fields of regulation.[23] Giddens (1994: 75) suggests that with post-traditional society, "we have no choice but to choose how to be and how to act." Choices, then, become obligatory within a "medium of power and of stratification" (ibid., p. 76). Post-traditional medicine in Yogya compels choice within stratified networks of social practices that are culturally informed by a logic of development and welfare. Medical pluralism, from this point of view, is not only some juncture of a modern hybridity-at-large dependent upon deterritorialized cultural circuits trafficking places like Indonesia. Disguised as state-sanctioned social welfare, medical pluralism is also part and parcel of rhetorical practices and discursive formations often originating from and supported by the State, in this case, the New Order state. In this way medical pluralism operates as an instrument of state rule brought about by the "rationalization" of health practices and perceptions as a local medical *system* with, as Foucault (1991 [1978]: 102) noted, "its primary target the population and as its essential mechanism the apparatuses of security" (see also Atkinson 1989; Taussig 1987; Thomas and Humphrey 1994).

Recent ethnographic work on medical systems, often with great delight, celebrate scores of "eclectic practitioners of traditional and modern therapies" (Leslie 1976: 6) who are involved in the creative process of either reinventing traditions or vernacularizing scientific medical practice. These eclecticisms, often heralded as flurries of bricolage or pastiche, rely heavily on agency and resistance models. Although many critical medical anthropologies note medical pluralism as a "therapeutic alliance" that should be viewed as a "new colonialism", particularly in the so-called developing world (Singer 1977), it seems to me that a conceptualization of the social structural arrangements in any instance of medical pluralism should consider the "duality of structure" that explains human action as simultaneously a "moment" of production and reproduction.[24] What we see with medical pluralism in Yogya is the refashioning of modernity in local and cosmopolitan terms through medical practice and perception both as state rule, or political organization as Leslie described it, and agentive response toward and for an other modernity.

Medical pluralism can be viewed as emergent product of universal processes of this most recent modernity. It can also be seen as the consequence of an equally emergent public sphere associated with complex state societies. Medical pluralism certainly is manifest of hierarchical social relations and differentiated access to an array of available health care, and the product of market forces among competing forms of medical practice. I argue here that medical pluralism must also be viewed, as Leslie suggested, as a crucial element for political organization. From this perspective, all of these vantage points on medical pluralism illustrate how the plurality of medical practice and perception operates in the governance and management of a population, and so in the lives of people.

Acknowledgments

This research was supported by a Fulbright IIE Award (1991–1992) and a Fulbright Institute of International Educators Extension Award (1993). I would like to thank the people of Lembaga Ilmu Pengetahuan Indonesia (LIPI), and Dr Tonny Sadjimin at the Clinical Epidemiology and Biostatistics Unit (CEBU), Dr Sardjito General Hospital in Yogyakarta, Java. I am particularly grateful to the American-Indonesian Exchange Foundation (AMINEF). My most heartfelt thanks go to Mark Nichter for being the kind of mentor and friend who has made a difference in my scholarly and personal life. I also appreciate the comments and suggestions of the reviewers who made this a better essay that I hope speaks as a celebratory tone to the works and life of a major influence in my own studies of "Asian Medical Systems," Charles Leslie. Finally, thanks to my companion in all of this, Janice Newberry, who continually reminds me to pay attention to the political and the places where power resides. Special thanks to many friends and co-workers in Yogyakarta, especially Pak Gembong, Bu Dewi, Bu Aseh, Mas Nurwijaksono, Mbak Ning Raswani, Mbak Mei Sugiarti, Joan Suyenaga, Hirdjan, Bu Yono and family, to name a few, who informed me about things that appear in this essay. Of course all misrecognitions are entirely due to my own failures and incompetencies.

Notes

1 Escobar (1995) and Ferguson (1990) also provide in-depth considerations of the governmentalization of life in the Third World and Africa respectively. Moore (1996) offers a succinct summary of Foucault's ideas on governmentality, with a discussion of anthropological engagements with governmentality that "actually take account of the complexities and techniques of knowledge production within and between societies, groups and regions" (p. 14).

2 Foucault (1991 [1978]: 103) suggests that the "only real space for political struggle and contestation" becomes mapped out by "problems of governmentality and the techniques of government" due to the fact that these, in the governmentalization of the state, become the only "political issues" that matter. This, he remarks, is a "singularly paradoxical phenomenon" and problem of governmentality (ibid.).

3 See Leslie (1974, 1976), but with particular attention to the migrations of science with biomedical practice and perception also see Arnold (2000), Crandon-Malamud (1991), Farmer (1992), Hess (1995), Mendelsohn and Elkana (1981), Romanucci-Ross (1977), or Gieryn (1999), Nader (1996), Prakash (1999), or Shinn, Spaapen, and Krishna (1997) for science in general across cultures. For science in the Dutch East Indies see Pyenson (1989).

4 An interesting comparative example is Reynaldo Ileto's (1995) study of the war against cholera in the Philippines (1902–1904) that even for nationalist writers of colonial history remains an example of American colonial benevolence. What remains unexamined are the "original moorings in colonial war and pacification campaign" (Philippine – American War of 1899–1902) of these public health efforts in favor of a "universal history of medical progress" that

disregards the historical relationships between medicine, disease, and war during the American colonial period in the Philippines (ibid. p. 52).

5 See Schoute (1937) for a description of the array of medical practice and perception during the Dutch colonial period, and the reliance on this array to meet the health needs of both the colonizer and the colonized.

6 See Ordinance Number 23 1992 (*Undang-Undang Republik Indonesia Nomor 23 Tahun* 1992).

7 See Ordinance Number 9 1960 (*Undang-Undang Republik Indonesia Nomor 9 Tahun* 1960).

8 Emphasis in the original.

9 *Undang-Undang Republik Indonesia Nomor 23 Tahun* 1992: 3.

10 Ibid.

11 Florida (1987: 3–4) translates *adiluhung* as meaning "the beautiful sublime," and shows its relationship to the "alleged 'high' arts, 'traditional' rituals, linguistic etiquette, and the like" of a refined Javanese culture from a golden-age past that is "imagined" in the present through iconic forms and practices. Florida remarks, "One is tempted to call this dominant modern image of Javanese culture, based as it is on the *adiluhung* and extremely refined or *halus* vision of life, the '*halusination*' of Javanese culture" (ibid., p. 3).

12 I am referring to Moore's (1994) analysis of power and ideology within "patterns of production, consumption, distribution and investment" for which she suggests that it is "the mechanisms of redistribution rather than production and reproduction which are crucial for understanding relationships" (p. 101).

13 Giddens writes: "The post-traditional society is quite different [from traditional societies]. It is inherently globalizing, but also reflects the intensifying of globalization. In the post-traditional order cultural pluralism, whether this involves persisting or created traditions, can no longer take the form of separated centres of embedded power" (1994: 104–105).

14 This essay of Foucault's on "Governmentality" (1991 [1978]) is a rare rumination on his part of the global context of the modern European state. See Gupta (1998) for a similar observation.

15 Much of this story is drawn from *Apa & Siapa: Sejumlah Orang Indonesia 1985–1986*, and "Jampi-Jampi Dokter 'Plus'", in *Tempo* 18 Juli 1992: 82–83.

16 The notion of fit, or *cocok*, carries great significance in Java (see Geertz 1960). Notions of the Javanese self as it relates to Javanese ideas about personhood are based on ideas of the appropriate fit between the two (Suparlan 1978). Taking on a name, title, status, role, occupation, and so forth that does not fit with one's already predetermined capacity to fill any of these can lead to sickness, misfortune, and catastrophe. This is especially true for those who want to take on the name, title, status, role, occupation of healer. A common explanation for the failure of someone to become a healer is that there were problems with fit.

17 For *kebathinan* as "science of life" see Weiss (1977: 13); Mulder (1984: 39) on kebathinan as "range of mystical beliefs;" and Keeler (1987: 21) on its concern with "inwardness of human life." Another important source is Hadiwijono (1967).

18 The Suharto government officially recognizes five religions acceptable to its Pancasila ideology – Islam, Catholicism, Christianity, Hinduism, and Buddhism. Several "wild sects" have been domesticated over the years with the support of Suharto (see Geertz 1960: 349–352). Kebathinan, as an organized outgrowth of what Koentjaraningrat (1985: 398–405) refers to as *Agama Jawi*, or indigenous Javanese religion, began in the late nineteenth century, gained strength

and membership in the dawn of Indonesian nationalism in the early twentieth century, lost favor during the years of the failed coup in the mid-1960s because of associations with the Indonesian Communist Party (PKI), and was once again revitalized in the 1970s "aliran debates" as a religion based on *kepercayaan*, or beliefs, largely because of New Order lobbying efforts (see Stange 1992). A spirit medium in our neighborhood was also a leader of a small *kebathinan* group who met from time to time. At one of the meetings I attended she assured me that President Suharto himself was aware of the group and practiced *kebathinan* himself. In fact, many Javanese cited with pride, satisfaction, and a sense of vindication Suharto's relationships with Javanese mysticism and shamanism. Indonesia's current president (2000) is a Muslim *Kiai*, or religious specialist and teacher, whose associations with Javanese mysticism are not known, but predictably absent.

19 This *"halusination"* of *pengobatan tradisional* earmarks a postcolonial voice in Java that continues to echo a late-colonial one Florida (1987) suggests has been the voice of the New Order government in Indonesia. Pemberton (1994), Tsuchiya (1990) and others have noted that the inspirations that became known as "Javanology" that were crucial in the figuration "Java" were co-authored by Dutch and Javanese alike. Tsuchiya (1990: 92) discusses the contributions of the court literati known as *pujangga*, who played an important role in the development of Dutch Javanology. The *pujangga* not only wrote the court chronicles that documented turbulent, glorious, or not so glorious dynastic histories, but scripted esoteric knowledge, court literatures, local histories, and traditional Javanese learning – things *adiluhung*.

20 Others have noted "Malay–Javanese primordialism" as significant in the construction of an Indonesian national identity. For example, see Anderson (1990), Florida (1987), and Pemberton (1994), Bowen (1986), Hitchcock and King (1997), and Tsing (1993), just to mention a few.

21 The classic anthropological works on medical pluralism include, but are not limited to: Dunn (1976), Feierman (1979), Janzen (1978), and the various essays in Leslie's (1976) edited volume. Ohnuki-Tierney (1984) and Lock (1980) offer studies of medical pluralism in highly industrialized Japan, and so have relevance to this essay in that both are ethnographies of medical pluralism in the context of "urban medical systems" (Ohnuki-Tierney 1984: 6).

22 Appadurai's modernity-at-large is built on a "theory of global cultural interactions predicated on disjunctive flows" (1996: 46). In the process, he suggests that "modernity is decisively at large, irregularly self-conscious, and unevenly experienced" (ibid., p. 3). He seems most interested in how the engine of modernity, modernization, becomes "domesticated by the micro-narratives of film, television, music, and other expressive forms, which allow modernity to be rewritten more as vernacular globalization and less as a concession to large-scale national and international policies" (ibid., p. 10). Leslie is also concerned with modernization as a "long-term and self-conscious historical movement" (1974: 70). It is with this self-consciousness that "modernity has developed its own traditions," characteristic of an "experimental attitude" summoned by the continual backward looking and reinvention of "more authentic traditions" (Ibid.). From this perspective the making of tradition is a redundant process of "selective retention" even though such retentions may not fully resemble the objects of mimesis. It is not that Appadurai and Leslie are necessarily at odds here, in fact Leslie's thoughts pre-date contemporary anthropological thinking on the subject of invented traditions and the role of Western medicine in the inventing of medical traditions. They do differ somewhat in their representations of "culture" – Appadurai (1996: 46) choosing

the disjunctive and "fractal metaphor," and Leslie, not surprisingly given the time of these writings, employing the "system" metaphor that considers the function this aspect of modernization plays in change and equilibrium.

23 See Newberry (1997) and Newberry and Ferzacca (1999) on the lived Indonesian state.

24 This is an essential piece to Gidden's (1984) notion of "structuration" that he proposes as a corrective for the errors of both phenomenology that registers society as a "plastic creation of human subjects" and the mistakes of functionalism and structuralism that offer "a deficient account of human agency and a deterministic conception of structure" (pp. 26, 217).

References

Anderson, B.R.O'G. (1990). *Language and Power: Exploring Political Cultures in Indonesia*. Ithaca: Cornell University Press.

Apa & Siapa: *Sejumlah Orang Indonesia 1985–1986*. (1986). Disusun oleh mjajlah berita mingguan TEMPO, Jakarta: Pustaka Grafitipers: 849–850.

Appadurai, A. (1996). *Modernity at Large: Cultural Dimensions of Globalization*. Minneapolis: University of Minnesota Press.

Arnold, D. (1988). Introduction: Disease, Medicine and Empire. In *Imperial Medicine and Indigenous Societies*, edited by David Arnold, pp. 1–26. Oxford: Oxford University Press.

—— (2000). *Science, Technology, and Medicine in Colonial India*. Cambridge; New York: Cambridge University Press.

Atkinson, J.M. (1989). *The Art and Politics of Wana Shamanship*. Berkeley: University of California Press.

Awas! Penjakit Influenza (1920). Balai Poestaka. Serie No. 480. Weltevreden: Drukkerij Vokslectuur.

Baer, H.A. (1995). Medical Pluralism in the United States: A Review. *Medical Anthropology Quarterly* 9(4): 493–502.

Baer, H.A., Singer, M. and Susser, I. (1997). *Medical Anthropology and the World System: A Critical Perspective*. Westport, CT: Bergin & Garvey.

Beck, U. (1994). The Reinvention of Politics: Towards a Theory of Reflexive Modernization. In *Reflexive Modernization: Politics, Tradition and Aesthetics in the Modern Social Order*, edited by U. Beck, A. Giddens, and S. Lash, pp. 1–55. Stanford: Stanford University Press.

Boomgaard, P. (1993). The Development of Colonial Health Care in Java: An Exploratory Introduction. *Bijdragen Tot De Taal, Land-En Volkenkunde* 149: 77–93.

Bowen, J. (1986). On the Political Construction of Tradition: *Gotong Royong* in Indonesia. *Journal of Asian Studies* 45(3): 545–561.

Brown, C. (1987). The Influenza Pandemic of 1918 in Indonesia. In *Death and Disease in Southeast Asia: Explorations in Social, Medical, and Demographic History*, edited by Norman G. Owen, pp. 235–256. New York: Oxford University Press.

Cheah, P. and Robbins, B. (editors) (1998). *Cosmopolitics: Thinking and Feeling Beyond the Nation*. Minneapolis: University of Minnesota Press.

Comaroff, J. and Comaroff, J. (1992). *Ethnography and the Historical Imagination*. Boulder: Westview Press.

Crandon-Malamud, L. (1991). *From the Fat of Our Souls: Social Change, Political Process, and Medical Pluralism in Bolivia*. Berkeley: University of California Press.

Dunn, F.L. (1976). Traditional Asian Medicine and Cosmopolitan Medicine as Adaptive Systems. In *Asian Medical Systems*, edited by Charles Leslie, pp. 133–158. Berkeley: University of California Press.

Escobar, A. (1995). *Encountering Development: The Making and Unmaking of the Third World*. Princeton: Princeton University Press.

Farmer, P. (1992). The Birth of the Klinik: A Cultural History of Haitian Professional Psychiarty. In *Ethnopsychiatry: The Cultural Construction of Professional and Folk Psychiatries*, edited by Atwood Gaines, pp. 251–272. Albany, NY: SUNY Press.

Feierman, S. (1979). Change in African Therapeutic Systems. *Social Science and Medicine* B13: 277–284.

Ferguson, J. (1990). *The Anti-Politics Machine: "Development," Depoliticization, and Bureaucratic Power in Lesotho*. Cambridge: Cambridge University Press.

Ferzacca, S. (1996). In This Pocket of the Universe: Healing the Modern in a Central Javanese City. Doctoral dissertation, University of Wisconsin, Madison.

—— (2001). *Healing the Modern in a Central Javanese City*. Carolina Academic Press.

Florida, N.K. (1987). Reading the Unread in Traditional Javanese Literature. *Indonesia* 44: 1–15.

Foucault, M. (1991 [1978]) Governmentality. In *The Foucault Effect: Studies in Governmentality*, edited by Graham Burchell, Colin Gordon and Peter Miller, pp. 87–104. Chicago: University of Chicago Press.

Frohock, F.M. (1992). *Healing Powers: Alternative Medicine, Spiritual Communities, and the State*. Chicago: University of Chicago Press.

Geertz, C. (1960). *The Religion of Java*. Chicago: University of Chicago Press.

Giddens, A. (1984). *The Constitution of Society: Outline of the Theory of Structuration*. Berkeley: University of California Press.

—— (1994). Living in a Post-Traditional Society. In *Reflexive Modernization: Politics, Tradition and Aesthetics in the Modern Social Order*, edited by Ulrich Beck, Anthony Giddens and Scott Lash, pp. 56–109. Stanford: Stanford University Press.

Gieryn, T.F. (1999). *Cultural Boundaries of Science: Credibility on the Line*. Chicago: University of Chicago Press.

Gupta, A. (1998). *Post-Colonial Developments: Agriculture in the Making of Modern India*. Durham; London: Duke University Press.

Hadiwijono, H. (1967). *Man in the Present Javanese Mysticism*. Baarn, Netherlands: Bosch & Keuning N.V.

Heryanto, A. (1990). The Making of Language: Developmentalism in Indonesia. *Prisma* 50 (September): 40–53.

Hess, D.J. (1995). *Science and Technology in a Multicultural World: The Cultural Politics of Facts and Artifacts*. New York: Columbia University Press.

Hitchcock, M. and King, V.T. (1997). Introduction: Malay-Indonesian Identities. In *Images of Malay-Indonesia Identity*, edited by M. Hitchcock and V.T. King, pp. 1–17. Kuala Lumpur: Oxford University Press.

Ileto, R.C. (1995). Cholera and the Origins of the American Sanitary Order in the Philippines. In *Discrepant Histories: Trans-Local Essays on Filipino Cultures*, edited by Vicente L. Rafael, pp. 51–81. Philadelphia: Temple University Press.

Jampi-Jampi Dokter 'Plus' (1992). *TEMPO* 18 Juli: 82–83.

Janzen, J.M. (1978). *The Quest for Therapy in Lower Zaire*. Berkeley: University of California Press.

Keeler, W. (1987). *Javanese Shadow Plays, Javanese Selves*. Princeton, NJ: Princeton University Press.

Kleinman, A. (1980). *Patients and Healers in the Context of Culture: An Exploration of the Borderland between Anthropology, Medicine, and Psychiatry*. Berkeley: University of California Press.

Koentjaraningrat (1985). *Javanese Culture*. Oxford; New York: Oxford University Press.

Last, M. (1996). The Professionalization of Indigenous Healers. In *Medical Anthropology: Contemporary Theory and Method*, edited by C. F. Sargent and T. M. Johnson, pp. 374–395. Praeger.

Leslie, C. (1974). The Modernization of Asian Medical Systems. In *Rethinking Modernization: Anthropological Perspectives*, edited by John J. Poggie, Jr. and Robert N. Lynch, pp. 69–108. Westport, CT: Greenwood Press.

—— (1977). Pluralism and Integration in the Indian and Chinese Medical Systems. In *Culture, Disease, and Healing: Studies in Medical Anthropology*, edited by David Landy, pp. 511–517. New York: Macmillan Publishing Co.

—— (1978). Forward to John Janzen's *The Quest for Therapy: Medical Pluralism in Lower Zaire*. Berekely: University of California Press.

Leslie, C. (editor) (1976). *Asian Medical Systems: A Comparative Study*. Berkeley: University of California Press.

Lock, M. (1980). *East Asian Medicine in Urban Japan*. Berkeley: University of California Press.

Mendelsohn, E. and Elkana, Y. (Editors) (1981). *Sciences and Cultures: Anthropological and Historical Studies of the Sciences*. Dordrecht, Holland: D. Reidel Publishing Co.

Moore, H.L. (1994). *A Passion for Difference: Essays in Anthropology and Gender*. Bloomington and Indianapolis: Indiana University Press.

—— (1996). The Changing Nature of Anthropological Knowledge: An Introduction. In *The Future of Anthropological Knowledge*, edited by H.L. Moore, pp. 1–15. London; New York: Routledge.

Mulder, N. (1984). *Kebatinan dan Hidup Sehari-Hari Orang Jawa: Kelangsungan dan Perubahan Kuturil*. Jakarta: PT Gramedia.

Nader, L. (editor) (1996). *Naked Science: Anthropological Inquiry into Boundaries, Power,and Knowledge*. New York: Routledge.

Newberry, J. (1997). Making Do in the Imagined Community: State Formation and Domesticity in Working Class Java. Doctoral dissertation, University of Arizona, Tucson.

Newberry, J. and Ferzacca, S. (1999). It Takes a Village to Make A State: Reproduction in New Order Indonesia. Paper presented at the 98th Annual Meeting of the American Anthropological Association, 20 November, Chicago.

Ohnuki-Tierney, E. (1984). *Illness and Culture in Contemporary Japan: An Anthropological View*. Cambridge: Cambridge University Press.

Pemberton, J. (1994). *On the Subject of "Java"*. Ithaca: Cornell University Press.

Prakash, G. (1999). *Another Reason: Science and the Imagination of Modern India*. Princeton, NJ: Princeton University Press.

Pyenson, L. (1989). *Empire of Reason: Exact Sciences in Indonesia, 1840–1940*. Leiden; New York: E.J. Brill.

Romanucci-Ross, L. (1977). The Hierarchy of Resort in Curative Practices: The Admiralty Islands. In *Culture, Disease, and Healing*, edited by David Landy, pp. 481–487. New York: Macmillan.

Schoute, D. (1937). *Occidental Therapeutics in the Netherlands East Indies during Three Centuries of Netherlands Settlment (1600–1900)*. Publications of the Netherlands Indies Public Health Service.

Shinn, T., Spaapen, J. and Krishna, V. (editors) (1997). *Science and Technology in a Developing World*. Dordrecht: Kluwer Academic.

Singer, P. (editor) (1977). *Traditional Healing: New Science or New Colonialism*. London: Conch Magazine Limited.

Stange, P. (1992). Religious Change in Contemporary Southeast Asia. In *The Cambridge History of Southeast Asia, Volume Two: The Nineteenth and Twentieth Centuries*, edited by Nicholas Tarling, pp. 529–584. Cambridge: Cambridge University Press.

Suprana, J. (1993). Jamu Terancam Punah? *Kompas* 28(192) 10 Januari 1993: 4.

Taussig, M. (1987). *Shamanism, Colonialism, and the Wild Man: A Study in Terror and Healing*. Chicago: University of Chicago Press.

Thomas, N. and Humphrey, C. (editors) (1994). *Shamanism, History, and the State*. Ann Arbor: The University of Michigan Press.

Tsing, A.L. (1993). *In the Realm of the Diamond Queen: Marginality in an Out-of-the-Way Place*. Princeton, NJ: Princeton University Press.

Tsuchiya, K. (1990). Javanology and the Age of Ranggawarsita: An Introduction to Nineteenth-Century Javanese Culture. In *Reading Southeast Asia*, edited by Takashi Shiraishi, pp. 75–108. Ithaca: Southeast Asia Program, Cornell University.

Undang-Undang Republik Indonesia Nomor 9 (UU RI 9) (1960). Kebijaksanaan Obat Nasional.

Undang-Undang Republik Indonesia Nomor 23 (UU RI 23) (1992). Tentang Kesehatan.

Weiss, J. (1977). Folk Psychology of the Javanese of Ponorogo. Doctoral dissertation, Yale University, New Haven, CT.

Chapter 3

Too bold, too hot

Crossing "culture" in AIDS prevention in Nepal

Stacy Leigh Pigg

Charles Leslie's insistence that medical systems in Asia must be understood as dynamic products of history led to an analysis of the professionalization of Ayurveda in India that showed how claims about knowledge were situated within struggles over colonialism, nationalism, and
modernization in India. This vision first spawned important work on
medical pluralism and the dynamic of "conflict and accommodation
between [Asian medical] traditions and the world system of cosmopolitan
medicine" (Leslie and Young 1992: 7; see also Leslie 1976). Now, as the
era of overt colonial domination, underpinned by self-confident ideologies of progress and civilizing missions, shades into an era of international
development that is grounded in planning rationality in the name of social
welfare, it is harder to separate what were previously conceptualized as
endogenous and exogenous forces. Yet Leslie's insight that medical practices themselves are not the only thing at stake in discussions of illness
remains key for research on medical cosmopolitanism.

In the bland bureaucratic language of international AIDS intervention
efforts, all local values and meanings are "cultural" and all services,
methods, models, and interventions should be "appropriate." But the
notion of culturally appropriate AIDS intervention is an ambiguous
promise. It simultaneously offers the particularistic hope of practical
actions, each perfectly suited to its context, and a contradictory commitment to transcendent solutions, in need of only minor re-packaging for
export. Every important question about knowledge, power, and cultural
meaning in relation to bodies and their health goes begging when a phrase
like "culturally appropriate" stands as our only way of stating the issues
presented by the facts of difference and inequality.

AIDS intervention work in South Asia struggles with the gap between
two kinds of "appropriateness:" what *can* be done and what *should* be
done. And assessments of "can" and "should" are bound up with views
of the "culture" in question, assessments of its boundaries, its integrity,
its authenticity, its very location "in" some places, some practices, and

some knowledges but not in others. Claims about cultural values and suitability have been political claims from the beginning in discussions of AIDS, whether in New York or New Delhi, because claims about culture can be used as easily to censor as to express a perspective. In South Asia, for instance, it has sometimes been claimed that AIDS need not be a concern of government because traditional social values will protect the population. Measures such as condom promotion and sex education are sometimes opposed by officials and the public on the grounds that they are socially unacceptable. Reports on sexual practices relevant to the risk of HIV transmission have been condemned as obscene and denigrating to local populations. Assertions about social organization and values anchor these arguments, and these assertions effectively define the debate at home while also commanding at least polite respect in international arenas. From the point of view of international AIDS activists, in contrast, such assertions look not only dangerously conservative but also absurdly naïve in the light of both the epidemiology of AIDS as well as experience with strategies of prevention. AIDS activists bemoan such attitudes as short-sighted prejudices that should be countered on both pragmatic and ideological grounds, not respected as differences that are merely "cultural." Where does this contestation over characterizations of "culture" leave the goal of a "culturally appropriate" AIDS intervention? A controversy in Kathmandu, Nepal surrounding one rather atypical AIDS prevention initiative suggests the complicated ways international public health priorities intersect with local social experiences and debates to produce claims about local norms and values.[1]

Talking about sex

A live radio call-in show captured the attention of Kathmandu's middle-class in the spring and summer of 1997. It was this show's startling content that set people talking: never before had matters of sex been dealt with so explicitly in a public forum. Between March, when the DJ's invitation for listeners' questions on sex, AIDS, and family planning was answered with an unexpectedly frank and intense enthusiasm, and late July, when the Minister of Communications himself was threatening to ban the show, the Hotline had arguably become the single most popular show on radio. It had also become a problem for its sponsor (a company that markets contraceptives), for the AIDS intervention program to which it was linked as a partner agency, and for the FM radio station whose broadcasting license was threatened because the show's sexual content was said to violate standards of decency. The debate raged: was the show entertainment or health education?

The Hotline brought to the fore an already contentious issue: whether to talk about AIDS requires talking about sex, and whether talking about sex is possible, appropriate, or even necessary in Nepal. "Sex" – in particular, certain forms of public attention to sex perceived as new to Nepal – was singled out in mid-1990s Nepal as the most problematic social challenge posed by the specter of an AIDS epidemic.[2] In the AIDS-and-reproductive-health circles of Nepal's development bureaucracy, "Nepali society" and the "difficulties" its secrecy, embarrassment, and morality were said to pose for their health work were constantly reiterated against the contrasting image of the "openness" toward "sex" in the West – an openness that figured ambiguously in this discourse as both the proper starting point for AIDS education and the cause of the AIDS epidemic itself.

The Hotline was an urban, middle-class phenomenon, closely linked to the very economic and cultural processes that were creating a bourgeois class occupying a distinctive cultural space.[3] The ways in which people in this class saw the Hotline as being "about sex" and how they evaluated its treatment of "sex" as a topic indicate something about the shifting matrices in which sexuality is being constructed for the middle class. And it is from the middle-class that the planners, bureaucrats, and NGO workers who interact with foreign donors and manage public understandings of AIDS come.

What was at stake in claims about the (in)appropriateness of sex talk on the Hotline? To answer this question, I offer an interpretation that does not take as its starting point essentializing characterizations of "cultures" and the organization of sexuality within them. Sexuality in Nepal is produced in social matrices and through organized sets of meaning that are varied and changing.[4] The sexuality to which discussions on and of the Hotline constantly referred is actually a moving target, itself partly but problematically captured for some Nepalis in a new type of public attention to "sex". The question to ask about the Hotline's discussion of sexual matters is not how far it deviates from some baseline of accepted values and behaviors, but how the grounds for a public discussion in terms of something called "sex" come to be established.[5]

"Are you making us into America?" the Hotline was accused at one point. The commotion around the Hotline was presented by critics as a sign of upheaval in a traditional moral society confronted with alien values thrust upon it by too-rapid exposure to global modernization. This portrait of the social context pits a deceptively homogenous set of Nepali values against foreign (mainly Western) influences. Critics of the Hotline thus used the same logic of absolute difference that has guided international health efforts since colonial times. International AIDS prevention efforts habitually draw on this way of thinking when they use stereotypes of shared norms and values to determine what is culturally appropriate. This rather flat and static way of characterizing "culture" is common in mainstream international development, but it is, interestingly, at odds with the recognition among AIDS activists worldwide that discussions of AIDS are almost always controversial because they force a recognition of the transgressive, marginalized, and unsanctioned elements within the social order. AIDS interventions in the south are increasingly channeled through the international development apparatus, and one consequence of this is a de-politicization of the stakes in defining community values. To begin to address this issue, I trace here how particular representations of the social context in which AIDS interventions take place become, themselves, a part of the social context. This is important to note because these characterization of "Nepali society" have a real impact when accepted at face value by powerful institutions such as foreign aid donors.

The challenge "are you making us into America?" also reflects very real questions about how social relations and values are changing across different segments of Nepali society as a result of the proliferating tendrils of globalization and modernization. These questions are not best addressed by assuming that modernity lies solidly outside the social space identified as Nepal. To begin with that sort of assumption is to close off from the start any sustained consideration of the effects of many people's uneven and partial engagements with a diverse set of abstract and concrete phenomena: discourses of medicine, sexology, or self-fulfillment; daily life as it incorporates schools, shopping, TV and video viewing, and international pop music; and changing family arrangements and the expectations of love, marriage, and generational authority that go with them. In this paper I suggest that middle-class experiences with Nepali modernity explain both the enthusiastic reception of the Hotline's explicit discussion of sexual matters as well as the seemingly contrary sense of moral panic its broadcast also fed.

In the debate over the Hotline, we can see the sometimes contradictory effects of a medicalization of sexuality in the name of development and a sexualization of consumption in the name of modernization. To take these cross-cutting pathways into account is to complicate our understanding of the social terrain on which AIDS interventions actually intervene. It leads us, moreover, to think about the ways AIDS prevention activities themselves enter into the production of local meanings. The terms on which the Hotline was debated, and the tensions these debates signaled, can show us something about the multiple, partially discontinuous processes that are forming people as sexual subjects and structuring their location in a politics of citizenship and exclusion.

Bold and hot

> Hi, I'm Bimal. Why don't you join me every Sunday at 9 pm for the CRS Hotline on Kantipur FM. I'll be playing HOT music and talking about HOT issues. Are you tired? Frustrated? Unsatisfied? Inquisitive?

> *Scared, jealous, lovesick? Confused? Or is there any issue that is really*
> *BOLD and daring that you have no one to share your feelings with?*
> *Then talk to me, Bimal, your listening ear, on CRS Hotline every Sunday*
> *at 9 pm – on Kantipur FM.*
>
> (Radio ad, in English, for the Hotline, July 30, 1997)

The Hotline was broadcast on an FM radio band whose signal range was limited to the Kathmandu Valley area. Its style of music and presentation addressed a mostly young, urban, relatively affluent audience. Whereas Radio Nepal was restricted in the amount of foreign music and English language content it broadcast, the new FM radio stations were able to build a broadcasting image around the hip sounds of international pop music, slangy mixtures of English and Nepali, tie-ins to other activities like dance parties, fashion shows, and advertising for goods and services (such as schools and tutoring services) catering to a middle-class niche market. Indeed, "FM" – newly established little more than a year before the Hotline went on the air – stood as a symbol of a kind of cultural and social identity. The Hotline was distinctively "FM" in this sense, and opposition to it in part reflected discomfort with the new bourgeois youth culture to which it spoke most powerfully (see Liechty 1995).[6]

In earnest and urbane tones, the DJ Bimal would invite listeners to write in with their questions. During the hour-long show, Bimal read the questions from letters by listeners, and helped the guest expert field live phone calls too, all the while reminding listeners of the sponsor "CRS, suppliers of quality contraceptives." Some questions from listeners recounted very personal worries or sexual difficulties, while others were presented as matters of abstract curiosity. Most, though not all, of the questions came from teenage boys or men. The guest expert doctor would explain, reassure, and clarify, dealing sometimes with very specific technical issues of physiology and illness, sometimes with issues of sexual function, sometimes with the social context and meaning of sexual behaviors. Factual accuracy in an answer was often at odds with the psychological subtext of many questions, which often ostensibly asked one thing but suggested another concern. Likewise, the answer that would come from western sexology and sex education traditions was often at odds with the moral organization and social realities of sexual lives in Nepal.

All this was punctuated by breaks to listen to pop music hits *("... pretty woman, walking down the street, pretty woman ..."*); plugs for CRS *("18 years of unselfish dedicated service to the nation")*; jingles in English advertising CRS-distributed condom brands *("the touch of her hands, the look in her eyes, is magic tonight ... Panther condoms for pleasure and safety)* that would be followed immediately by ads promoting depo-provera; and catchy AIDS prevention slogans *("with AIDS there is no second chance")*.

This mixture of entertainment, AIDS prevention messages, confessional, expert advice, family planning promotion, titillation, information, and guidance counseling set a tone entirely unlike any previous radio show with a public health or family planning mandate. To the dismay of many officials, listeners did not ask the sorts of questions that many planners felt would lead to "knowledge" about AIDS – questions like the quiz contest favorite "What do the letters in the acronym AIDS stand for?" Instead, listeners were interested in topics such as masturbation, female orgasm, and oral sex, and they presented worries about their homosexual, premarital, marital, and extramarital sexual relationships. This kind of sex talk in the name of health was uncharted territory.

"So we thought, why not do a show like that in Nepal?"

The eclectic sound of the show reflected its hybrid bureaucratic origins as a development-commercial-government-private sector collaboration. Kantipur FM was one of the new commercial radio stations that recently had been given permission by state-sponsored Radio Nepal to broadcast out of its studios. The airtime for the one-hour Hotline was paid for by CRS, Nepal Contraceptive Retail Services Pvt, Ltd., a company charged with marketing contraceptives, and the show was to serve as an advertisement for its products. CRS, in turn, is heavily subsidized by USAID (who set up the company in 1979). It receives "tied aid" in the form of US-made condoms. USAID also ran AIDSCAP, a global AIDS prevention program organized around strategies of condom promotion and STD awareness and treatment. The administration of the AIDSCAP program was contracted out to the private non-profit firm Family Health International. CRS happened to also be one of the "implementing agencies" AIDSCAP-Nepal used for its condom promotion component. Private enterprise, foreign aid, profit, and state-sponsored development were thoroughly mingled at every level in the organizations that together put the Hotline on the air.

It was during a trip to East Africa that the managing director of CRS and an American official of USAID-Nepal observed in Kampala a live radio show in which listeners could call in with their questions about sex. "So we thought, why not do a show like that in Nepal?," the managing director said (interview July 18, 1997). "If we had been in Nepal, we wouldn't have even contemplated the idea of something like this," the USAID official said (personal communication, July 17, 1997). A couple of consultation meetings were held between the key figures at AIDSCAP-Nepal, USAID-Nepal, and Kantipur FM to hammer out a format for the show, and within a few weeks, it was on the air. Had the CRS Hotline idea been subjected to the normally lengthy development planning process, it probably never would have gotten on the air in the form it initially took. In the inevitable rounds of consultation and review, it would surely have been set up along the lines of accepted forms of didactic development communication, its message thoroughly rationalized and strongly controlled from the center. The debate about the "acceptability" of the show in the "Nepali context" would have taken place behind closed doors, where no voices that would contradict planners' judgments could be heard.

As it was, the show plunged into unexplored terrain, live, on air, and what happened during that first broadcast took everyone, including those putting on the show, by surprise. They were inundated with calls, some with questions so frank and personal they stunned the DJ and doctor and left them, by their own account, in a cold sweat at the thought of addressing matters such as anal intercourse and oral sex on the airwaves. The first show was such a stunning surprise because no one, including the show's programers and sponsors, anticipated that the listening public could behave in a way so different from the way this public, imagined as a generalized "our Nepali society" and as "targets" of AIDS prevention messages, was characterized in the normal round of program planning consultations.

By July of 1997, after the show had been on the air for four months and the crisis around it had come to a head, the CRS officials who sponsored the show were absolving themselves of responsibility by saying, "we never expected the show to go in that direction! It is too much for Nepali society" (interview, July 18, 1997). CRS's involvements in the social marketing of contraceptives and in the AIDS-oriented promotion of condoms were supposed to converge in their sponsorship of the Hotline, but more often these two efforts diverged as CRS executives worried about their "company image" if they became associated with AIDS in people's minds. The DJ was complaining that he had been instructed, impossibly, not to use the word "sex" on the show, and letters from listeners piled up because there was never enough time to address them all on the air. Some AIDSCAP-Nepal officials worried that the controversy over the show might jeopardize the acceptance of more mainstream mass media AIDS awareness campaigns.

All these expressions were set in a larger context of ambivalence toward AIDS prevention as an area of investment for foreign aid resources. Why give so much attention to AIDS?, many skeptics wondered. There had been an abrupt upsurge in donor interest in AIDS prevention in Nepal in the early 1990s. In 1992 and 1993, several million dollars of assistance came in for programs specifically targeting AIDS, even though at that time there were only around 100 individuals in the country known to be HIV positive.[7] Epidemiological predictions that South Asia would soon experience a dramatic epidemic explosion seemed compelling to donors but abstract to Nepali officials. To the extent that anyone in development circles was thinking about AIDS in the late 1980s and early 1990s, the widespread impression was that AIDS was a foreign problem which affected deviants.[8] Early fears about AIDS entering Nepal focused on foreign tourists and later shifted to "Bombay returnees" (Nepali women who had worked in brothels in India).[9] If the state was to play a role in AIDS prevention, it seemed to many commentators at that time, it would be by introducing quarantine measures and strict HIV antibody testing at the border with India. Guarding the public's health was equated with guarding the border.

By 1997, when the Hotline went on the air, there had been several years worth of AIDS awareness conferences in plush Kathmandu hotels for journalists, officials, politicians, and NGO leaders. Mass media campaigns promoting condoms and explaining HIV transmission and prevention had done their work. The funding, technical training, and program support provided by donors did much to make AIDS a more publicly visible and familiar issue. Frequent newspaper articles appeared, endlessly recirculating the same statistics, such as estimates from WHO on the number of HIV infections and guesses of the number of Nepali women working in brothels in Bombay. Yet, with the exception of a few highly sensationalized cases, actual Nepali people sick with HIV/AIDS remained largely invisible even to those professionals most involved in AIDS intervention activities.[10] What constituted meaningful AIDS prevention remained under debate. The larger question – why should we be concerning ourselves with AIDS at all? – hung silently in the air. NGOs funded by donors to develop AIDS prevention programs became proponents for AIDS intervention, while the rest of the health development community merely tolerated the inevitability of the attention given to this new donor priority. If USAID was backing AIDS prevention, through their AIDSCAP program, then the question of whether to devote energy to AIDS prevention was already settled, at least formally. The magnitude of the HIV problem in Nepal was a statistic to be recited, not a matter to be debated. The Hotline did not have to defend itself on these grounds. What was debatable was the form of attention to sexuality. The debate about the sexual content of the Hotline was embedded within the larger politics of international donor funding agendas and national priorities.

The controversy

"Not just for 'lovebirds' but also for the development of the country"

Was it pornography or education? It was around this question that much of the discussion about the Hotline swirled. "It is too bold," critics said. "This is simply indigestible to Nepali society!" opponents claimed. These condemnations notwithstanding, listeners, mostly young people, not only tuned in but also flooded the radio station with letters and calls. The number of phone calls taken live on air had to be cut back because too many people were calling in with personal questions about the very sexual activities many officials claimed "no one in this society talks about" or "do not exist in Nepal." What, wondered many critics, does this kind of discussion of sex have to do with AIDS? People are mistakenly taking this show as entertainment, in the words of one Radio Nepal programmer, and "they don't realize that it is for education." [e] The problem, he said, was that "people think it is a sex program, not an AIDS program." "It is whetting their curiosity" [e].*

Fans countered with arguments about the Hotline's role in producing an enlightened citizenry, as in this fan letter:

> ... Kantipur FM is doing a good job giving awareness to us about sex education which is a necessity in developing country like Nepal where people feel shame talking about sex ... [CRS Hotline] has proved that FM is not just for "lovebirds" but also for development of country [e].

To claim that something is necessary for national development is a rhetorical tactic with extraordinary force in Nepal, where, for more than forty years, development has been the rallying cry for national unity, patriotism, and citizenship. To many observers, however, it was not entirely obvious how answering questions from young men about masturbation and nocturnal emissions (the most common questions posed to the Hotline) was to be construed as a step toward national development. The airtime devoted to what many critics saw as inappropriately personal and individual concerns clashed, they felt, with the features of the show that marked it as public education in the name of development. Commercials promoting family planning were one such sign; the constant invocation of the need for education, information, and awareness was another.

By allowing listeners to present all sorts of questions about sex to the show, the Hotline was viewed by some as abdicating its authority to enforce certain standards of public language and personal disclosure. A development aesthetic exists in Nepal, an aesthetic that guides, among other things, what a "development message" should look and sound like: it runs to slogans like: "safe sexual behavior is the basis for a healthy life" (*surakchit yon byabahaar nai swasthya jibanko aadhaar ho*); "do not have sexual intercourse with many people" (*dherai janaasanga yon sambandha raakhnu hundaina*); "treat sexually transmitted diseases promptly!" (*turanta yon rogko upachaar garaun*). The Hotline programmers eschewed the typical top-down exhortations that send standardized health messages out to a passive public in favor of an interactive style of broadcasting. But the show went a step further. By doing too good a job in its social marketing of safe sex (and in the process, marketing Kantipur FM's racey image), it blurred the line between development and commercialism. It criss-crossed two ways that middle-class Nepalis experience their modernization: as national citizens/leaders and as middle-class consumers. The family became the focus of this ambivalence about the kind of civic self one was to be.

"The right kind of sex education should be given"

When not advertising the Hotline as "hot" and "bold," Kantipur FM's programmers portrayed the show as "teaching people about their bodies." The show easily fit into a set of other debates about the necessity of "sex education." Parents, teachers, and youth with whom I spoke expressed the view that sex education should be given in the "right" [e] way, while often leaving ambiguous what the "right" way would look like and what its purpose would be.

By answering questions about techniques for attaining sexual satisfaction, often very specific personal questions from listeners, the Hotline included techniques for pleasurable fulfillment in its definition of sex education. Calling this "explicit, even perverse at times," one critic asked "does each and every person need to be informed about everything that can be called sex education?" [e]. But for a male teacher I interviewed, sex education is good because "it is because those things are unknown that people get AIDS and all these other kinds of diseases" [n]. The readiness with which many people in 1997 offered "disease prevention" as the rationale for sex education reflects the rapidity with which aspects of AIDS prevention discourse became pervasive. The category of Sexually Transmitted Disease was introduced only with the intensified AIDS awareness programs of the mid-1990s. Though the idea that sexual activities might make one ill is not new in Nepal, a discourse linking disease prevention, sex education, and right living arguably is.

Sex education seemed like a good thing to many people when they assumed that "awareness of AIDS and STDs" would be its focus, not because they saw themselves or their children as actually at risk, but because, implicitly, disease could mark the boundaries of proper sexual conduct.[11] Expectations that AIDS awareness was and should be a form of moral education pervaded AIDS education efforts but also came into conflict with the prevailing international public health wisdom that moral approaches to AIDS and STD prevention do not work. Thus posters and pamphlets suggesting that AIDS could be prevented by "only hav[ing] sex between husband and wife" (*pati patni bich maatra yon sambandha simit raakhera*) or "avoid[ing] sex with prostitutes" (*beshyaabrittimaa lageko ... byektiharu yon sambandha raakhnu hundaina*) – messages that made intuitive sense to many, even those in charge of AIDS programs – vied with the more strictly orthodox "use condoms," a message many felt actually endorsed and promoted not AIDS prevention, but sexual promiscuity. The Hotline condensed these contradictions. Its origins lay in the public health philosophy that people should be given the information they need and want because, in the words of one Nepali official with advanced training in public health, "who knows who is going to do what?" [e]. Yet as official outcry against the show coalesced around its purported "unacceptability in Nepali society," the broadcasters became more careful to talk about abstinence, responsibility, and the importance of marriage. The show at times veered rather erratically between slogans like "don't condemn sex, condom it!" [e] and responses to listener questions concerning their premarital sexual relationships that were prefaced with judicious assertions about the benefits of delaying sexual intercourse until after marriage. The moral need to reinforce traditional values organizing sexual expression seemed to many all the more necessary in the face of a younger generation increasingly exposed to modernizing influences.

"It can't be listened to in a family setting"

Sex education was thought of as a tool to keep young people from acquiring "bad habits," or *bigreko baani*. Said another teacher, "it is our responsibility to stop [young people] from taking <u>sex</u> in the <u>wrong</u> way" [n]. The Hotline violated some of these expectations for the "right kind of sex education." "I am a bachelor boy of 25 years and I am one of the victims of homosexuality," wrote one listener. "I have a boy partner of the same age with whom I have had a sexual relationship for about 4 years. We have never had anal sex like other homosexuals do . . . Do we have risk of HIV or STDs? Can we have oral sex?" [e]. Your sexual orientation is normal, replied the doctor, before giving information on certain sexual practices and risk of HIV infection. The Hotline dealt with a small but steady stream of questions from young men about their sexual relations with other men, as well as premarital sexual relations with girlfriends. Homosexuality, premarital sex, and matters such as incest (about which the Hotline received at least one letter from a teenage girl) were never recognized, let alone discussed, in other AIDS education programs. The newly formed AIDS intervention bureaucracy recognized only two types of sexual encounters: between husband and wife, and between man and prostitute. The open secret of the existence of homosexual, premarital, and incestuous sexual relations was ignored in discussions about AIDS prevention, but continually reaffirmed by conversations between listeners and the expert on the Hotline.

Of exchanges like these, critics said "there has to be a limit." "No matter how advanced we might be," in the words of one official critic, "there are certain things that are simply unacceptable." "No matter how developed" or "modern," in the words of many others, "we are still embarrassed by this kind of discussion." "We are just not that free yet" [n], it was often said. The continued existence of the proper "limits" is indicated by the "awkwardness" people say they would feel if listening to the Hotline in front of the rest of their family. Similar reservations are also expressed about many US-made TV shows, such as Santa Barbara and Baywatch, newly available via satellite, as well as many western films, widely available on video since the mid-1980s (see Liechty 1998). This image of the family, together and unembarrassed by the programs on TV or radio, is a symbol that Nepal still maintains the "limits" that "the West" has discarded.

These references to "the limits" that the Hotline "pushed too far" asked people to interpret the Hotline as a particular kind of moral threat to the social order. Everyone is expected to know where "the limit" is through a visceral response to certain words and topics that would bring to mind that which should remain hidden. And there was, in fact, universal agreement that one would indeed feel laaj, or "awkwardness," listening to discussions of sex on the Hotline in front of family members.[12] There is a psychosocial logic here that is inescapable in this social context. Holding back and keeping silent are ordinary ways of enacting the respect one owes to certain others. Restraint itself thus marks status asymmetries, asymmetries that are understood as the moral foundation of the social order. Limits on speech are thus often presented as signs of more pervasive limits on behavior. Importantly, the association between speech set loose and the loss of proper behavioral restraints also surfaced frequently in commentaries about the social transformations since the restoration of multiparty democracy in 1991. It was not uncommon for people to make an association between the expanded sphere of political expression (freedom of speech) and perceived increases in corruption, social unrest, and a lack of law and order. When people can say anything, it is thought, they can also do anything. The Hotline was thus portrayed as a specter of chaos.

When critics of the show argued that it "couldn't be listened to in a family setting," they were asserting the ubiquity of a certain kind of "family setting" that the very popularity of the show belied. There was an image not only of the family grouped around the radio or TV, but also of patriarchal control over what women and children would see or hear. This family was implicitly understood not to need a show discussing sexuality, and especially not one focusing on problems or worries, pleasure or desires. Against this image there exists an emerging middle-class family reality in which children might have their own rooms, their own radios, and enough freedom and privacy to encounter programming that they could not, indeed, listen to in a family setting. The privacy of one's own room was what enabled people to listen to the Hotline and perhaps to some degree what made many young people feel they needed this kind of discussion of sexual matters. The new forms of spatial privacy that mark middle-class privilege also isolate young people of this class. Unlike their poor or rural contemporaries, they do not learn about sexuality in the intimacies of a crowded one-room house. The "family setting" invoked by critics of the Hotline was one where middle-class privilege could render sexuality invisible, but without any lessening of the traditional forms of familial regulation of the sexual lives of its members.

The Hotline's popularity arguably stemmed from its use of the airwaves to create an ambiguously open space for a discussion of sex that could be entered anonymously. This virtual space offered not just an evasion of the familial management of sexuality, but a new kind of sexual sociality that went beyond the silent fantasy space created by, for instance, Hindi films. Like most public spaces, it was understood to be the domain of men (see Liechty 1995). Not only did teenage boys and men come forth more readily with all kinds of questions, but the discussion of AIDS and STD prevention as led by the guest experts and the DJ assumed an active agent with control over whether or not to expose himself to the risk of infection. This did not prevent teenage girls and women from finding their own reasons why the show was valuable. A married woman, for instance, said that she thought information given about oral sex and HIV transmission was good "because some <u>husbands</u> like <u>oral sex</u> and women are afraid." Some high school girls I spoke to approved of instructions on condom use because "so many boys in our country don't have this knowledge and that's how people end up with AIDS." Others said that listening to the show was worthwhile for them because it helped them understand how boys thought. Thus the Hotline became, to some degree at least, an indirect vehicle for communication about sex between men and women.

Moreover, in the name of disease prevention, it introduced a language of health and hygiene around sex. Framed as knowing about one's body, presented as education, and mediated through the expertise of a doctor, the Hotline offered a language in which sex could be discussed, potentially, at arm's length.

"You can just go out on the street and buy any kind of magazine"

When asked whether the Hotline was "too bold" for Nepal, young fans shrugged and replied blandly that nowadays you can easily buy a magazine with pictures of naked women or rent any kind of video. The incipient medicalization of sex through the AIDS intervention projects of development is emerging simultaneously with the sexualization of consumption. The last decade has witnessed an unprecedented intensification not only of media and commodity consumption, but also the increased visibility of "sexy" ads, music, and fashions. When people talked about the Hotline, they did so in relation to other new features of the urban landscape such as beauty pageants, miniskirts, dating, satellite TV, and *Femina*, the Indian women's magazine.

It is in this intertextual field that the Hotline was actually understood by listeners. But the planners and agency representatives who were discussing the Hotline's fate ignored this larger representational context of which the show was clearly a part. The authorities spoke of the Hotline as if it were the only way that its audience would be coached in how to understand their sexual selves – aside, of course, from the traditional "family." In doing so, they designated a whole set of activities, images, pleasures, and ideals in the lives of the middle-class as not "Nepali." The rhetorical effect was to police a boundary of pure national identity so as to create a clear divide between a Nepali inside and a westernizing outside. The persuasive force of this rhetoric came at the cost of seeming out of touch with the everyday life of the Hotline's target audience.

Consumer identities are embodied for middle-class youth through a complex interpenetration of consumption practices, media images, and gendered self-fashioning in everyday life, according to Mark Liechty's research in Kathmandu (Liechty 1994). Young men imagine their pursuit of body-building and martial arts in relation to action-adventure films, and young women use beauty parlors and fashion to cultivate feminine images that equally self-consciously emulate those depicted in films and advertising. Although individuals move in and out of these "selves" in the course of daily life, these gendered consumer identities (as Liechty calls them) have become the form for a new kind of self-hood. Importantly, when middle-class men and women fashion themselves through their consumption practices, they do not see themselves as "Western." Instead, they are carving out a middle-class identity, distinguished from what they depicted as both the vulgarity of the poor and the promiscuity of the high elite by an ethos of moral restraint. Liechty (1995) found that restraint in sexual practices was frequently the focus of definitions of middle-class identity, even as middle-class consumer practices were sexualized. What then does it mean when this middle class speaks for the nation as a whole?

"no one in Nepal says these things"

> . . . community practices surrounding sexuality represent more than local traditions, for communities are also termini of worldwide economic, social, and political and cultural patterns.
>
> (Ross and Rapp 1997: 157)

The Hotline was controversial precisely to the extent that it condensed a contradiction in middle-class understandings of self. This was a contradiction between the middle-class self-definition in terms of a morality of sexual restraint and the shifting frameworks within which sexuality was actually understood and experienced. This sense of a shift was perhaps best expressed by one professional who – in response to accusations of hypocrisy leveled against critics said to condemn the Hotline in public but praise it in private – commented,

> this is a new area for everyone and we really don't know how to judge it. We are not hypocrites for that reason. The fact is we are dealing with a new set of situations and we have mixed feelings about it and we aren't sure how to go forward. I advocate the show as a professional, but in the privacy of my home I judge and question these things on a different wave length [e]. (meeting on 13 July 1997).

These kinds of uncertainties are expressed – more and more publicly, it seems – in relation to an object called "sex" that now seems to people to be everywhere and more problematically visible. Donor-funded AIDS intervention work has made "sex" a development problem. In its attempts to alert people to the sexual transmission of HIV, it has also intensified a certain medicalization of sexuality by promulgating a discourse of sexual health and hygiene. At the same time, the middle-class consumer world has become increasingly "sexy." Families become a private space into which this "sex" may be allowed (as the pursuit of "personal" pleasure) or disallowed (as a threat to collective values). The realms of family, medicine, national welfare, and popular consumption intersect, albeit unevenly, in middle-class lives, to pose dilemmas that the middle class then extrapolates to all Nepalis.

To raise critical questions about the way the middle-class attempts to speak for all requires more than stating the obvious: that the Nepali urban middle-class is not Nepali society. To simply acknowledge the diversity of class and ethnic positions within Nepal only replicates the notion of cultural bubbles with distinctive sensibilities. Recognize difference, we certainly must. But the crucial political issue lies in how those points of view established as "different" come to be connected.

The views about sexuality the middle-class expresses inevitably become the standard of respectability against which other Nepalis' lives and values will be measured. Significant but often subtle exclusions are enforced when the AIDS intervention work is assessed through the middle-class lens. Repeated assertions that "no one in Nepal" says these things, does these things, has the implicit effect of laying the blame for the spread of AIDS on those, such as prostitutes, who can be depicted as outside the "real" Nepali sexual norms. The effect is more subtle when, for instance, middle-class AIDS intervention workers comment that the carpet factory workers their programs target are "franker than us" and "much more open than we are." Propriety is defended; AIDS is figured as a problem of people who are already outside "the limits."

Local assertions about what is "acceptable in Nepali society" get filtered through international health development's own discourse of difference, in which Nepal figures as "other" to western expertise. When middle-class Nepali AIDS workers report to foreign donors and their representatives why discussions of sexual matters in AIDS education are so "difficult," they honestly convey a sociological truth. It *is* difficult. But their reports are almost always taken at face value by foreign donors. Rather than opening up an examination of the complex dynamics of these "difficulties," their observations are converted into a vacuous global-babble about "cultural sensitivities." These are not simply overgeneralizations. They are overgeneralizations that do a particular kind of work. They stake out a subject position: to be "Nepali" is not to be "open" about sex; to be "open" about sex is to be the kind of person who spreads AIDS. National identity and middle-class sensibilities become conflated in a move that simultaneously marks two exclusions: those who do not belong and those who could/do have HIV.[13] What is most sobering, I believe, is the way the international language of "cultural appropriateness" moves in lock-step with ideological assertions within Nepal about where the "limits" of acceptability lie.

The complex transnationality of projects of international health pose political and interpretive challenges that we have only begun to consider. Recent international agreements, such as the 1994 International Conference on Population and Development, call on activists and researchers to understand and help change the dynamics of social and cultural practices that undermine reproductive and sexual health. By placing sexuality within a framework of health promotion and development, these initiatives make sexual matters into objects of international and national interest in new ways. Always shaped by modes of social and moral regulation within communities and nations, sexuality is now also politicized at the juncture of international health doctrines, donor funding, and state responsibility. In this situation the state juggles potentially contradictory roles: guardian of public health, worthy recipient of foreign aid, and champion of national honor and order. States that take up the banner of sexual and reproductive health (sometimes by merely fitting existing population control policies into this new language), may do so only within limits that ensure that the normative is neither undermined nor questioned. The discussions of sexuality and sexual practices brought to the fore by the new international interest in "sexual and reproductive health," of which AIDS intervention is a part, are potentially disruptive. Not only might they, as radical activists hope, lay bare an edifice of inequality and its consequences for individual health, but these discussions may be absorbed into public consciousness and dispersed through the mass media in unpredictable and potentially threatening ways. Hence the desire on the part of many authorities to frame discussion of sexual health as a matter of the preservation of social units such as the family or the national social order itself.

Modern sex education and sexual health campaigns have, for more than a century, been vulnerable to charges that they are obscene and threatening to the moral basis of the social order (see Brandt 1987; Porter and Hall 1995; Weeks 1989). This reaction is neither new nor particular to so-called traditional societies. Nor is it unusual to discover (as I have shown here) that the normative moral order is in reality less unitary, seamless, and bedrock firm than its defenders claim. My analysis of the controversy around the Hotline in Kathmandu registers another case of the by now easily recognized moral-medical debate on sexuality, and it shows how this debate was unfolding within the particular circumstances of late twentieth-century Nepal. Yet I have sought here to do more than provide a description of the Nepali version of the same old story of conservative resistance to certain approaches to sex education. For one thing, the Nepali case cannot be understood apart from the power relations inherent in international development and donor agendas on the one hand, and the lasting colonial symbolics of images of Western modernity, on the other. Struggles over the regulation of sexuality evident in the reactions to the Hotline are inseparable from dependency on donor aid, influence of international mass-media, and formation of a middle-class increasingly defined through its consumption practices. AIDS intervention efforts are inextricable from institutional relations of development and are imbricated in anxieties around social identity, status, and power. To imagine that the difficulties in implementing a sexual health program will be resolved when the right balance of "cultural sensitivity" is achieved is to misapprehend the social dynamics at play.

The Hotline exposed several points of tension in middle-class views of sexuality. Much of the debate revolved around the criteria for distinguishing between pornography and legitimate health education, a distinction felt to be necessary but whose very basis was contested in the debate itself. At issue was the relation between the public good, gauged in terms of national development, and personal desires and pleasures. The Hotline imploded the ideological edifice separating the middle-class's experiences of increasingly sexualized consumer self-fashioning from its embodiment of the sober aim of national advancement. Viewed in this context, the obscenity that some saw in the show lay not simply in the words said and the topics raised, but in the unseemly mixing of "health messages" with youth pop culture and personal sexual concerns, a mixing that confounded the accepted representations of the citizen. The show also made public a density of talk about and interest in sexual matters.

It not only transposed "private" thoughts and circumscribed discussions into a form of public interaction, but it created a virtual space in which discourse could appear to be very much like intercourse and could therefore appear to threaten the very social demarcations that regulate sexuality. If people are talking in this way, the reasoning went, what might they be doing? In this sense, the show itself could be seen as promiscuous because of the interminglings it facilitated. The show trespassed numerous boundaries – those defining the development aesthetic, those ordering relations between old and young, those defining proper conduct, those circumscribing the moral meanings of modern consumption. And yet, although these transgressions were clearly startling, they were not universally unwelcome nor completely unacceptable, despite some gatekeepers' claims to the contrary. That these moves were highly charged does not mean that they were culturally inappropriate. The debate around the Hotline thus directs our attention to cross-cutting claims about norms and values and to the uses to which these claims are put. Claims about culture are claims about social boundaries.

Concerns about "cultural sensitivities" mark the need for a diplomatic maneuver in interactions between foreign donors and recipient agencies, between program planners and government gatekeepers, or between educators and their targeted groups. There are many differentials of power and perspective to bridge, and these cannot be reduced to a simplistic opposition between the possible imperialism of "western donors" and the authenticity of a shared national "culture." It might be more useful, therefore, for practitioners to think in terms of politically appropriate AIDS intervention, for the formulation of "appropriate" (and achievable) AIDS intervention is a thoroughly political process. As I have suggested here, instead of asking about the "cultural" acceptability of sexual discussions, we might more usefully inquire into the social and historical processes that shape the modes of sexual debate and the stakes of sexual regulation. These processes are open-ended, and they can and do shift the basis for consensus and contestation. The ideas and interventions originating in the transnational community of international health are part of these processes and part of the context. Indeed, this case shows that the "cultural attitudes" the public health planners may find may be shaped in significant ways by their own actions.

Notes

* Code-switching between English and Nepali prevailed in the interviews and commentary I record here. Statements made predominantly in English are indicated as [e]; those made predominantly in Nepali as [n]. English words and phrases within Nepali utterances are underlined. In some cases, where it seemed to me that the Nepali and English versions of the phrase or concept were interchangeable and equally frequent, I have not indicated language.

1 I came to follow the fate of this radio show during my 1997 ethnographic research in Kathmandu focusing on the production of public knowledge about AIDS. The show and the controversy around it was a common topic in my conversations with Nepali NGO workers and others during this research. In July 1997, I was contracted by Family Health International, managers of the AIDSCAP-Nepal program that had provided seed funding for the show, to interview stakeholders and listeners and prepare a brief assessment of the show. I use data from these interviews with the permission of Family Health International and the interviewees, to whom anonymity was guaranteed. Because many of the individuals I interviewed in conjunction with this project have a continued professional, personal, and political stake in the contested field of AIDS and public health, I have sacrificed some ethnographic precision in order to protect individual identities. I am grateful to Abana Onta for organizing and conducting focus groups with school teachers and high school youth as part of the assessment of the Hotline.

   The research on which this paper is based was made possible by a grant for the Joint Committee on South Asia of the Social Science Research Council and the American Council of Learned Societies with funds provided by the National Endowment for the Humanities and the Ford Foundation. The Social Sciences and Humanities Research Council small grants program administered by Simon Fraser University supported the background research on public representations of AIDS. I alone am responsible for the interpretation presented here.

2 Contentions around sexual behaviors and sexual relationships, as well as the representation of these behaviors and relationships in various discourses of AIDS have been central to the politicization of HIV/AIDS. This can be seen in the early epidemiological hypotheses about "gay-related immunodeficiency" in North America (Oppenheimer 1992) and early gay activists' debates about whether to condemn the sexualization of urban gay male cultures or to embrace it as a route of "safe sex" (Crimp 1988; Shilts 1987); in speculations about African promiscuity; and in the concerted targeting of prostitutes as the "source" of HIV infection in many countries. It should be noted, however, that AIDS poses many other social challenges, namely around issues of inequality, marginalization, gendered power relations, and human rights (see Farmer 1992; Farmer et al. 1996; Mann and Tarantola 1996; Lurie et al. 1995). For instance, an alternative interpretation of the social challenge of AIDS to Nepal – one rarely discussed in Nepali newspapers or the plans of AIDS-related INGOs and NGOs – would center on the massive labor migration of Nepalis to other countries (see Seddon 1999).

3 The debate about the Hotline was a middle-class debate, and I do not mean to imply that it was everyone's debate. Nor is the point of my analysis to underscore the cleavage between the concerns of Kathmandu's bourgeoisie and the rest of the country's population. How these concerns resonate in other social contexts, or how concerns about sexuality and social change might be articulated from other social locations is a question for empirical investigation. I have argued previously that the "difference" between the elite and villagers is often overdrawn in discussions of Nepali society, in ways that tend to underemphasize villagers' involvement in cosmopolitan engagements with modernity while continually bracketing off any serious consideration of the formation of local modernities as an integral part of contemporary Nepali society (Pigg 1992, 1996). While my discussion here is restricted to the

ethnographic space of my research, I want to leave open the question of the relation of what I describe here to other social positions in Nepal. Differences are to be expected, but a sheer and unbridgeable difference should not be presumed.

4 The question of how understandings and experiences of sexuality are actually constructed at the intersections of gender, kinship, economic production, and state intervention in diverse Nepali contexts is well beyond the scope of this paper.

5 I explore other facets of this question more extensively elsewhere (Pigg 2001). To what does the term "sex" refer in these Nepali discourses? Why must the domain of "sex" be labelled in English, and what does this imply for the discussion of sexual matters in Nepali? What relation does this discursively constructed domain of "sex" have to varied Nepali experiences of sexuality? I refer here to "sex" (in quotes) to suggest that we must explore a distinction between a particular way of representing a domain of life (as "sex") and experiences of sexuality and sexual relations.

6 English words and phrases are mixed with Nepali on the Hotline, as it is on many FM shows, because this ease with English marks both a style and a privilege that distinguishes the middle class. On the Hotline, English words are doubly important because they allow people to say things they feel they cannot say easily in Nepali, because Nepali terms either seem too rude or are not even known. Pigg (2001) contains an extensive discussion of this code-switching and the language ideology around the use of English.

7 By 1992, the total number of HIV infections reported was 114 and by July 1997 it had only risen to 675 (National Centre for AIDS and STD Control statistics; see also Suvedi et al. 1994; Seddon 1999). These official numbers are more significant in terms of how they function as artifacts in representations of AIDS than as indices of actual rates of infection. Problems of access to medical care, testing and reporting make it obvious that the number of reported cases is lower, probably much lower, than the actual number of persons with HIV. In 1999, UNAIDS estimated the total number of adults and children living with HIV to be 26,000, for an adult rate of 0.24% (UNAIDS and WHO 1999).

Just as elusive as the epidemiological facts is a reliable estimate of donor funding for AIDS prevention in this period. The World Health Organization provided modest funding to establish a small National AIDS Programme and to support a sentinel surveillance program in the late 1980s through the Global Program on AIDS. Between 1990 and 1993, the World Bank, UNDP, the EEU, USAID, and AmFAR (the American Foundation for AIDS Research) and several other multilateral and bilateral donors either commissioned preliminary studies (in the case of the World Bank) or funded active AIDS prevention programs in Nepal.

8 The first recorded AIDS-related death, widely publicized, was that of a foreign tourist. In 1985 I saved a clipping from a newspaper that called on the government to ban Indian second-hand clothes sellers as a means of protecting Nepalis from AIDS.

9 The focus on prostitutes, in particular, as the "source" of AIDS has overshadowed any appreciation of the role the massive labor migration of both men and women might play in structuring the epidemic.

10 In contrast to parts of Africa or Haiti (Farmer 1992), where the impact of illnesses and deaths was being felt more or less simultaneously with the first

epidemiological, clinical, and scientific research that built our understanding of AIDS, in Nepal expert knowledge and the accompanying imagery around AIDS has far outstripped a share public sense that AIDS is affecting people in Nepal. At the time of my research in 1997, I was told that public hospitals and nearly all doctors were refusing to treat people with HIV. At the same time, some leaders of AIDS-related NGOs were being contacted personally for help by individuals diagnosed as HIV positive, often their first encounter, after several years of AIDS intervention work, with persons known to have tested positive for HIV. Despite an outcry against several NGOs involved in supporting a group of young women who had been "repatriated" from brothels in Bombay, many of whom were then discovered to be HIV positive, AIDS was regarded mostly as a hypothetical epidemic, and actual people living with HIV/AIDS as a rarity. The newness of the epidemic upsurge in South Asia, coupled with difficulties of recognition, biomedical diagnosis, testing, and reporting, made AIDS difficult to discern in the Nepali population.

11 Writing on the USA, Patton (1996: 7) speaks of a "national pedagogy" whereby "the AIDS epidemic became a vehicle through which to renegotiate the meaning of being a good American." The compassionate citizen was constructed as not at risk for contracting HIV. Frankenberg (1992) also points out how AIDS serves to mark boundaries of affinity and difference among people.

12 *Laaj* is typically translated into English as "shame" or "embarassment," but the people whose views I discuss here used *laaj* more or less interchangeably with the English words "awkward" or "odd." I have followed their own code-switching choice here.

13 This symbolic connection between social marginality, or "otherness," and a marked status as "AIDS carrier" is far from unique to Nepal. Indeed, it is extremely pervasive. Nonetheless, it is important to understand the particular ways this logic takes shape in specific sociopolitical circumstances around the world and to appreciate how the structure of AIDS intervention expertise may inadvertently contribute to this logic.

References

Brandt, A.M. (1987). *No Magic Bullet: A Social History of Venereal Disease in the United States Since 1880*. Expanded Edition. New York: Oxford University Press.

Crimp, D. (1988). How to Have Promiscuity in an Epidemic. In *AIDS: Cultural Analysis, Cultural Activism*, edited by Douglas Crimp, pp. 237–271. Boston: MIT Press.

Farmer, P. (1992). *AIDS and Accusation: Haiti and the Geography of Blame*. Berkeley: University of California Press.

Farmer, P., Connors, M. and Simmons, J. (editors) (1996). *Women, Poverty, and AIDS: Sex, Drugs and Structural Violence*. Monroe, Maine: Common Courage Press.

Frankenberg, R. (1992). The Other Who is Also the Same: The Relevance of Epidemics in Space and Time for Prevention of HIV Infection. *International Journal of Health Services* 22(1): 73–88.

Leslie, C., and Young, A. (editors) (1992). *Paths to Asian Medical Knowledge*. Berkeley: University of California Press.

Leslie, C. (1976). *Asian Medical Systems*. Berkeley: University of California Press.

—— (1992). Interpretations of Illness: Syncretism in Modern Ayurveda. In *Paths to Asian Medical Knowledge*, edited by Charles Leslie and Allan Young, pp.177–208. Berkeley: University of California Press.

Liechty, M. (1994). Building Body, Making Face, Doing Love: Consumer Practice and Consumer Identity in Kathmandu, Nepal. Unpublished manuscript.

—— (1995). Media, Markets, and Modernization: Youth Identities and the Experience of Modernity in Kathmandu, Nepal. In *Youth Cultures: A Cross-cultural Perspective*, edited by Vered Amit-Talal and Helena Wulff, pp. 166–201. London: Routledge.

—— (1996). Paying for Modernity: Women and the Discourse of Freedom in Kathmandu. *Studies in Nepali History and Society* 1(1): 201–230.

—— (1998). The Social Practice of Video-viewing in Kathmandu. *Studies in Nepali History and Society* 3(1): 87–126.

Lurie, P., Hintzen, P. and Lowe, R.A. (1995). Socioeconomic Obstacles to HIV Treatment and Prevention in Developing Countries: The Role of the International Monetary Fund and the World Bank. *AIDS* 9(6): 539–546.

Mann, J. and Tarantola, D. (editors) (1996). *AIDS in the World II: Global Dimensions, Social Roots, and Responses* New York: Oxford University Press.

Oppenheimer, G. (1992). Causes, Cases, and Cohorts: The Role of Epidemiology in the Historical Construction of AIDS. In *AIDS: The Making of a Chronic Disease*, edited by Elizabeth Fee and Daniel M. Fox, pp. 49–83. Berkeley: University of California Press.

Patton, C. (1996). *Fatal Advice: How Safe-Sex Education Went Wrong*. Durham: Duke University Press.

Pigg, S.L. (1992). Inventing Social Categories through Place: Social Representations and Development in Nepal. *Comparative Studies in Society and History* 34 (3): 491–513.

—— (1996). The Credible and the Credulous: The Questions of "Villagers' Beliefs" in Nepal. *Cultural Anthropology* 11(2): 160–201.

—— (2001). Languages of Sex and AIDS in Nepal: Notes on the Social Production of Commensurability. *Cultural Anthropology* 16(4): 481–541.

Porter, R. and Hall, L. (1995). *The Facts of Life: The Creation of Sexual Knowledge in Britain, 1650–1950*. New Haven: Yale University Press.

Ross, E. and Rapp, R. (1997). Sex and Society: A Research Note from Social History and Anthropology. In *The Gender/Sexuality Reader*, edited by Roger N. Lancaster and Micaela di Leonardo, pp. 153–168. New York: Routledge.

Seddon, D. (1999). HIV-AIDS in Nepal: The Coming Crisis. *Bulletin of Concerned Asian Scholars* 30(1): 35–45.

Shilts, R. (1987). *And the Band Played On: Politics, People, and the AIDS Epidemic*. New York: St. Martin's Press.

Suvedi, B.K., Baker, J. and Thapa, S. (1994). HIV/AIDS in Nepal: An Update. *Journal of Nepal Medical Association* 32: 204–213.

UNAIDS and WHO (1999). Nepal: Epidemiological Fact Sheet on HIV/AIDS and Sexually Transmitted Diseases.

Weeks, J. (1989). *Sex, Politics and Society: The Regulation of Sexuality since 1800*, second edition. London: Longman.

Chapter 4

The social relations of therapy management

Mark Nichter

> More is at stake in the interpretation of illness than a set of medical practices.
>
> (Leslie 1992)

Charles Leslie was the founding editor of the University of California book series entitled "Comparative Studies of Health Systems and Medical Care". The first book in that series was John Janzen's (1978) ethnography *The Quest for Therapy: Medical Pluralism in Lower Zaire,* in which he introduced the concept of the therapy management group. In the foreword to this book, Leslie (1978) encouraged anthropologists to study medical systems as social systems, not just systems of knowledge and treatment practices.[1] The study of medical systems demanded ethnographic inquiry into how meaning was negotiated among the afflicted, concerned others, and practitioners as an illness progressed through time. It also required careful consideration of the broader social and political context in which medicine was practiced and illness experienced. It is in the spirit of such an inquiry that I return to an examination of the social relations of therapy management, a concept in need of refinement. While other essays in this volume attend to the relationship between state politics and therapeutic practice (e.g., Adams and Ferzacca) , This essay focuses on the micropolitics of therapy management and is organized around two case histories that lead us to consider the social relations of sickness in the context of poverty and social transformation.[2]

Therapy management has generally been described as a process that involves diagnosis and the negotiation of illness identities, the selection and evaluation of therapeutic options, and the lending of support to the afflicted (Janzen 1978, 1987). Most studies of therapy management have focused on health care seeking, yet therapy management encompasses much more. Therapy management is multidimensional. It embraces what Straus (1985) has referred to as the many "works of illness" and what

Obeyesekere (1985, 1990) has described as the "work of culture."[3] The afflicted, and members of a therapy management group who coalesce around them, engage in a variety of illness-related "works" that emerge through time. These engagements include the marshalling of material resources, the management of emotions, the performative aspects of "being sick" and relating to the afflicted, participation in the co-construction of illness narratives, and provision of a space where healing or the management of sickness takes place. The work of culture involves a reappraisal and reframing of troubles and negative emotions in terms of publicly accepted sets of meaning and symbols. In the context of poverty and emotionally charged predicaments, the work of culture helps members of a therapy management group cope with actions entailing some measure of selective attention and selective neglect (Howard 1994; Nations and Rebhun 1988; Scheper-Hughes 1985, 1992).

Therapy management invites analyses of transactions that are at once influenced by cultural values, social roles and institutions, power relations, and economic circumstances that influence the ways in which illness is responded to in context over time. The study of therapy management requires close attention to disagreement as well as to the building of consensus, the privileging and manipulation of truth as well as the acceptance of ambiguity, and changes in knowledge about diagnosis and treatment which effect thinking about possible courses of action. To study therapy management one must consider nested contexts. It is important to investigate the social dynamics of households, extended kin groups and larger social networks as they influence one another and are influenced by political economy and globalization. With respect to the household, long held assumptions about the household have been challenged of late by anthropologists as well as by researchers in family studies, household economics, and women's studies.[4] The perception that household members are largely altruistic, that they pool their income and function as a homogenous unit having common goals, has been brought into question (e.g. Bruce 1989, 1988; Folbre 1986a, 1986b; Sen 1990). Studies of therapy management provide insights into priority setting within households, the manner in which gender and generation relations influence resource allocation, circumstances that foster competition and cooperation, and processes of negotiation and accommodation as well as resistance and assertion. They also contribute to the anthropology of self and a growing critique of the simplistic way in which cultures and peoples have been described in terms of sociocentric (collectivist) versus individualist motivations and goals.

In the two cases presented here, therapy management entailed difficult choices and different forms of coping in the form of passive acceptance as well as the taking of action. We are led to consider issues related to entitlement and the manner in which individual and group responses to sickness consolidate as well as challenge social relationships. Insights into both the politics of responsibility and the anthropology of self emerge out of "ethnographies of the particular" (Abu-Lughod 1991) that challenge generalizations about "culture." They bring to our attention conflicts and contradictions as well as doubts and ambivalence. Ethnographies attentive to circumstance as well as happenstance generate more than interesting stories, they provide valuable lessons about how life is lived, how actors reflect upon their experiences, and how the framing of these experiences changes over time.

The two case studies draw upon fieldwork conducted in the Philippines and India. The first, compiled from edited field notes, is based on participant observation in an impoverished Filipino household. Exposed to an infectious and socially stigmatizing disease by a sick relative, household members are faced with physical risk while obliged by cultural values to extend routine hospitality. The second case is constructed out of interviews with an Indian patient and impressions of the patient shared with me by his practitioner, a long-time friend. These notes are supplemented by the observations of my research assistant, who developed a close relationship with the patient.[5] The case considers the health care seeking behavior of an Indian who has returned from working in the Gulf and who is not visibly ill but is engaged in a search for diagnosis. His requests for diagnostic tests mobilize a therapy management group that provides him a space to sort out his social relationships. Diagnostic tests prove to have meaning beyond the physical body. Both cases invite us to examine household dynamics and the issue of entitlement as an important dimension of therapy management.

Case one

The first case is presented as a series of three field note entries made during a three-month period of time. Each field entry was an attempt to summarize pages of notes detailing my observations of a household in which a family member was suffering from tuberculosis. These notes summarized discussions, documented interactions, and contained personal reflections. My initial presence in this household was opportunistic. It coincided with a study I was conducting on local perceptions of acute respiratory infection and tuberculosis. My relationship with Nora, the central figure, developed over time and influenced the way she and her family interacted with me. At first I was related to as Nora's "Peace Corps type" employer and later as a friend as well as a representative of a "West" equated with individuality, autonomy, and opportunity. I was conscious of comments Nora addressed to my double, "Mark as representative of the West" as well as comments Nora addressed to her own double, the dream identity she saw for herself in the mirror my representation provided.

At times our relationship was quite close when measured in terms of attentiveness and emotional appraisal. At other times it involved abstractions that unsettled me. When conducting fieldwork near Nora's house, I slept in her house and contributed food for the day's meals. I resisted being viewed as a safety net for household needs, and in this sense experienced first hand spoken and unspoken pressures to provide resources in a context where there was always need and minor crisis.

Field note entry: Mindoro, Philippines, 18 September 1991

It is late in the afternoon and I am visiting the family of Nora, one of my three research assistants who lives in a hamlet three or four miles from a small town in central Mindoro. Nora has been helping me conduct research on respiratory disease and is a young, single mother of an 18-month old child. Inside her well-swept bamboo structured house, the living space (15 × 20 feet) is subdivided into three sleeping partitions and a hearth. Eleven people routinely occupy the house: Nora's mother, two married sisters, one brother-in-law, and six children. The household survives just above bare subsistence. Sixty to seventy peso ($2.10-$2.80) flow into the house on an average day to cover routine expenses. Half of this amount is spent on rice, with a majority of the remaining spent on a small quantity of fish, cooking oil, sugar, and kerosene all purchased daily at a price 10 per cent above the bulk rate. A small monthly remittance (peso 250) from a married sister living in Manila is sent to Nora's mother whose responsibility it is to use it for special needs and emergencies. In the Philippines, married daughters often send money to their mothers as a means of maintaining affiliation with their natal family and as a "debt of gratitude." The remittance places considerable pressure on Nora's mother, because daily life is marked by requests for this cash reserve from both her own family members and neighbors who know that she has money now and then. The tension this small amount of money causes leads Nora's mother to wonder if she would not be better off without it.

Most of the household's daily income is generated by the one working male in the home, Nora's brother-in-law. He drives a motorcycle taxi in the town and contributes about 70 per cent of his daily earnings to the household. The remainder of his earnings go for personal expenses, which include a pack of cigarettes (peso 6), two beers (peso 15), and petty gambling (peso 10). While his wife and mother-in-law are not happy about his personal habits, they do not question his entitlement to them. The percentage of earnings he contributes to the household is not atypical of other males. They voice the opinion that a man who works hard is entitled to his habits but they nevertheless complain that by quitting work too early to sit with his friends he does not work hard enough to bring in more money to the house.

I have brought some food as a contribution to dinner and Nora is busy boiling rice, preparing banana flower with coconut milk, and frying fish. I lie down and close my eyes, but am snapped back into consciousness by the sound of labored breathing and a strained cough. The coughing from the other side of the bamboo partition comes from one of Nora's mother's elder sisters. Nora's aunt is in her late fifties and lives in a hamlet twenty or so miles away. Her own household is very poor and her husband, a rice agriculturalist, can barely manage to feed the family, which is presently being looked after by a daughter who has returned home after a failed marriage. Nora's aunt often visits Nora's house and is close with all members. This visit is particularly long. She has been at Nora's house for a few weeks and nobody seems to know how long she intends on staying. While at the house, she has been helping with the washing, apologizing about her inability to work hard as a result of *mahina ang baga*, "weak lungs." She spends most of the day playing with the children and gossiping.

Dinner is prepared, Nora's brother-in-law comes home, and the food is consumed by household members in a rather *ad hoc* manner. Food is stored under a bamboo cover and whoever is eating serves themselves. Nora's aunt's food is kept aside, however, and I observe boiling water being poured on a fork and spoon that are reserved for her use. She eats alone.

After dinner Nora's aunt wishes to speak to me as she has learned that I know something about health. Informing her that I am not a doctor, I agree to talk to her about her health problem. She wants to be examined. I touch her neck to see if she has fever and look in her eyes to check for anemia. I ask her questions about her breathing, cough, chest and back pain, appetite, and sweating at night. She answers these questions and additionally tells me her blood pressure, indicating that she has seen a doctor. Based on what she tells me, I suspect that Nora's aunt might have an active case of TB. I ask her what she thinks is her problem. Describing her own illness, she makes reference to weak lungs, a term used by the doctor she has consulted at the government rural health unit in town.

I ask her about the medications she has taken and her answers lead me to believe even more strongly that she has TB. It appears she has been on the WHO standard short course for TB. She has taken Odinah, a brand of isoniazid, which she refers to as *vitamin sa baga* (vitamins for the lungs), rifampicin that she knows is an antibiotic, and a third drug the name of which she does not remember. When I ask Nora's aunt about how long she has been taking these medicines, she informs me that she discontinued taking them shortly before visiting Nora's house. Of the recommended six-month course of TB medicine advised by the doctor, rifampicin was taken for only two weeks and Odinah for a month. I inquire why the course of TB medicine recommended to her by the doctor was not followed. Nora's aunt claims that while the *vitamins sa baga* made her feel better, the Rifampicin made her feel cold and nervous. She describes it as *hindi kasundo*, not compatible for her body.[6]

I question Nora's aunt about her perceptions of contagion related to weak lungs and TB, as well as about the availability and cost of medicines she has taken. I find that she is aware that TB is contagious, but does not think weak lungs is contagious. To my questions about medicine availability, it immediately becomes apparent that it is not just Nora's aunt who is noncompliant. The Ministry of Health, which follows WHO guidelines in its recommendations for short course TB chemotherapy, has been unable to provide an adequate supply of drugs to the rural health unit. After her sputum tested positive, Nora's aunt received a two-week supply of rifampicin and a month supply of Odinah free from the doctor. Upon returning to the clinic two weeks later, she was given an injection (most likely streptomycin), because the other TB medicines were unavailable at the time. She was then advised to purchase rifampicin privately. A daily dose of this medicine costs peso 18 at the pharmacy in town, an expense her household cannot afford.

Nora's aunt tells me that the bottle of Odinah she received made her feel better. Impressed by its effectiveness, she shared it with one of her sister's children who suffered from chronic wheeze (*hapo*) in addition to recurrent cough. For her, hapo also constitutes weak lungs for which "vitamins for the lungs" are useful in strengthening the lungs. She has not purchased Odinah privately and asks me if I think it would be advisable I encourage her to return to see the doctor or to travel to the district hospital in Calapan to have a fresh sputum test taken. Perhaps there they will have a better supply of medicines.

Field note entry: 21 September 1991

I listen to Nora's aunt cough and gasp well into the night. Although the small house is partitioned, there is little ventilation and her aunt sleeps in a space near three other people. Inside the mosquito net, allocated to me as a token of my guest status, I experience a feeling of personal vulnerability. I open a window normally closed by the family at night and mentally distance myself from feeling at risk by reassuring myself that I am physically fit and well nourished. I think of Nora and her baby. Nora and I have discussed TB on several occasions following interviews with community members about a range of respiratory illnesses. Bright and full of questions, she has learned much about TB contagion and management. How is she responding to the situation?

I talk to Nora and her mother in the morning about aunty Faith's health. They are worried and have prayed for her. I directly ask them about their concerns related to contagion. Nora's mother is of the opinion that weak lungs is contagious, an idea she maintained even previous to Nora's working with me. For this reason she has separated Nora's aunt's eating utensils and pours boiling water on them after use. There is an unspoken agreement that Nora's aunt will eat alone. Nora and her mother both believe that weak lungs can be spread by contact with the food or saliva of an ill person as well as other forms of close contact like exhaled breath. They both note, however, that it is impossible, given Filipino customs and values, to physically distance themselves from their kin at a time of illness.

This situation and an interview I conducted with Nora at a local hospital led me to reflect about household response to risk. In the hospital, family members serve as attendants of the ill. I spoke to the wife of a man acutely ill with TB. She slept near his bed and during the day two of her children visited the hospital, brought food, and remained on the ward for some hours. There was no doubt that the man was contagious, and yet they remained with him. A nurse had even scolded the woman for allowing her children to visit the ward, but after one scolding she appeared indifferent. I asked the woman if she was worried about getting TB herself and she commented, "He is my husband and the father of these children. Until a week ago we lived together in a small one-room bamboo house. Is this any different? We live together, to be apart would be sad for everyone. With sadness comes ill health and madness. I trust in Jesus." Nora pointed to the attendants of many patients and said this is how it is in the Philippines. She then asked me whether things were so different in the US. I informed her that family members in the US also felt the need to remain with patients in the hospital, but that they had to wear special masks and gowns and that children were not allowed on an infectious disease ward. I then asked the woman being interviewed whether she or her children were taking medicine to prevent getting TB. She answered that she could not afford vitamins. No one had spoken to her about or offered her a prophylactic regimen. I wondered whether they would do so? I never found out. When I returned five days later, the man had gone to a hospital in Manila, a day's journey away.

Field note entry: 1 November 1991

Nora's young daughter was diagnosed as having "weak lungs" four weeks ago. Following three weeks of coughing, fever and excessive sweating, which Nora treated by over-the-counter medicine (including an antibiotic suspension prescribed by a doctor on a previous occasion), Nora took the child to an *arbolaryo* (herbalist) to see whether the child might have *pilay hangin*. Pilay is a local illness associated with dislocations within the body caused by a child falling or being held too tightly. It is only detectable by this type of folk curer. Pilay is commonly associated with cough and fever among children, so Nora's mother advised her to check out this possibility before spending money on a doctor's consultation. The arbolaryo diagnosed the case as Pilay after massaging the child's chest and back. After three days of herbal treatment and massage, Nora's daughter continued to feel hot and eat poorly. Nora decided the child needed to see a doctor, but had no money to pay for the trip to town or for a consultation. Nora's mother lent her some money ($2.50), but Nora did not feel the money was enough and began asking neighbors for a loan as her sisters had no cash and her brother-in-law's taxi was out of commission. When I arrive at the house, I am immediately asked for a loan.

I am greatly relieved that Nora is taking her daughter to the doctor. I have been visiting her house every few days and am contemplating whether or not I should intervene. Before beginning this research project, I had decided I would intervene in cases of acute dehydration, rapid breathing, and indrawn chest indicative of pneumonia and cases of whooping cough. TB poses a real ethical dilemma to me. Diagnosis requires laboratory confirmation and, in the case of children, it is difficult to diagnose. I had encouraged Nora's aunt to seek medical advice, but she had not followed up on my advice, and now the child might be infected! While the child does not manifest life-threatening symptoms, it is obvious to everyone that her health is rapidly deteriorating. I am afraid of sleeping in the house myself; Nora senses my discomfort, and I feel for her predicament.

I accompany Nora to town, but not to the clinic. Nora does not want to be seen with me for fear that the doctor's charges will increase substantially if he sees me. After the consultation, Nora reports to me that her child was diagnosed as having weak lungs. No tests were performed, but the doctor had felt the child's glands, which were swollen. The doctor had asked whether any family members were ill. Nora had told the doctor about her aunt's weak lungs without mentioning that she had been taking TB medication. Without inquiring further about her aunt (or suggesting that she come in to see him), the doctor started the child on a course of rifampicin syrup and isoniazid.

Field note entry: 10 November 1991

For the past month I have been observing how Nora's family has been responding to the child's illness. So far, no connection has explicitly been made by household members between the child's illness and Nora's aunt's illness. If anything, such a connection seems to be played down by more general talk of how common the condition is in the community due to poverty. Last week I asked Nora's mother and two of her older sisters whether weak lungs was hereditary or whether a child could catch weak lungs from another child or an adult. They spoke about Nora's ex-husband's family having a history of weak lungs (and TB), indexing the commonly held notion that weak lungs and TB are hereditary. No mention was made of Nora's aunt, who was not in the house at the time.

Medication for Nora's child is expensive and she is solely responsible for finding the funds to acquire it. Money has not been budgeted for this expense by the household, nor has Nora's mother been forthcoming in identifying this expense as a burden to be covered by the special purpose remittance money she receives. Nora is expected to tap whatever sources she has access to when the need arises to purchase medicines. Nora's brother-in-law, who contributes additional cash resources to the household in times of medical emergencies, has not been expected (or asked) to forfeit his pocket money when Nora needs medicine for her child. This is an act expected only when an illness is very acute and life threatening. Weak lungs in a child is not judged to be very serious by Nora's family members. Ambiguity surrounds the relationship between weak lungs and TB among children. While it is recognized that weak lungs can lead to TB, tuberculosis is not thought to be a children's disease. TB is a disease perceived to develop later if the symptoms of weak lungs are not treated.

How is Nora handling the situation? Most of her attention is directed toward securing medication and special health-promoting foods for her baby. Perceiving government medicine to be of a lower standard, she prefers to purchase medicines from the market rather than even approach the government midwife to see whether medicine might be available this month. Moreover, she is under the impression that short supplies of medicine are reserved for TB patients, not children with weak lungs and no positive sputum or X-ray to show. Her bottle-by-bottle quest for medicine has become central to her moral identity as a mother who will sacrifice anything for her daughter.

Field note entry: 20 November 1991

Although field research has been completed, I have remained in the area, but will have to leave in the next two weeks. I have been providing Nora questionnaire coding work as a means to help her pay for her daughter's medication, but her family is constantly trying to borrow money from her whenever I pay her. They have an uncanny sense of when she has been given money and I am looking into ways of getting her credit at the drug store as a means of making sure her child gets the medicines she needs.

Nora has expressed extreme frustration with her family members who continue to request "emergency loans" from her, disregarding her own need to save money for her child's medicine and "good foods." She has found it difficult to maintain even a small stock of fruits or vitamins in the house for her daughter because whenever she offers these items to her daughter, her sisters' children gather, waiting to be given their share.

This afternoon I find Nora feeding an expensive (peso 12) imported orange to her baby. At first I am struck by what seems to me to be the frivolity of this action by a woman whose family might only have rice and dry fish to eat the following day. Acknowledging my "more practical than thou look" she explained, "I had the money in my hand at the market and I knew if I returned home with it, it would only be requested by others." Like the purchase of shop medicine, the orange represented the best that she could give to her baby as an act of love.

Nora becomes cynical. She questions the true feelings of her family toward her, assessing these feelings in terms of their inattention to her quest to obtain medicines and foods that her child needs. The sickness of her daughter leads Nora to think critically about the social relations that structure her life. Nora's unanswered plea for financial assistance from those whom she counts on to be supportive members of a therapy management group lead her to think about leaving her mother's household.

Nora tells me she wishes she could be an American like me or go to America where she could be free and choose her own life. "If I remain here," she says, "I will never be able to make a better life for myself or my daughter." She is only half joking when she asks me to look for a husband for her in the States. It seems she had been fantasizing about this fairy tale for some time.[7] Her American husband need not be a prince charming, but someone who would support her economically and encourage her to study and work, much as I had. I ask her whether she would not be lonely, if she got her wish and was far from her family. Tears come to her eyes and she says, now you understand what it means to be Filipina.

This case calls attention to the social relations of therapy management. Social risk (risk to social relationships and social identity) is clearly a factor that mediates cultural response to physical risk. Being a "TB patient" as a result of a doctor's diagnosis or the tell-tale symptom of "spitting blood" is associated with stigma in the Philippines. Not wishing to stigmatize their patients, health care providers often tell patients whom they suspect have TB that they have weak lungs and then place them on TB chemotherapy.[8] The term weak lungs is used in popular health culture to refer to a variety of respiratory complaints by various members of the community. While some view weak lungs as equivalent to TB, many others view it as a precursor condition or a stage of lung illness that can lead to TB. Still others associate weak lungs with asthma or believe this condition is manifest in anyone having a history of recurrent or severe acute respiratory illness (Nichter and Nichter 1994, Nichter 1994).

Most people in the Philippines know that TB is contagious, but many do not think weak lungs is contagious. As in the present case, even those members of Nora's community who are aware that both TB and weak lungs are contagious change their behavior very little when a household member suffers from these illnesses. The most common preventive action undertaken is a cleansing of eating utensils with boiling water. Despite a recognition that the illness may be spread through the breath, sick household members are not segregated. I was told time and time again that Filipino values entailing *pakikisama* (offending as little as possible) precluded alienating family members who are ill. To alienate a family member during illness was not only thought to increase suffering and contribute to ill health, but was seen as a failure to acknowledge debts of gratitude (*utang na loob*) to the person for past sacrifices and favors.[9] Pouring boiling water on utensils was the extent to which family members could act without breaching social relations. This example illustrates to what extent a Filipino family will go to maintain "smooth interpersonal relations" (Lynch 1964), even in the face of personal risk.

In Nora's case, both she and her mother were well aware that her aunt was contagious. Indeed a set of unspoken house conventions were set in motion regarding when she ate and with whom she ate. Yet when Nora's child was diagnosed as having weak lungs, no link was articulated between the two illnesses. When I asked household members about the child's illness, alternative explanations were given. Efforts were made by family members to deflect any responsibility that Nora's aunt might feel toward the child's state of ill health. Other "truths" were privileged, other explanations offered, such as the illness being hereditary.

Responsibility for cure, on the other hand, was squarely placed on Nora's shoulders and not shared by household members who spontaneously contributed cash resources only in episodes of acute, life-threatening illness. Nora's mother did not allocate a monthly allowance for needed medications, nor was her brother-in-law expected to forfeit his personal spending money. Moreover, when Nora acquired cash income she was asked to share it with other family members who viewed their needs as more immediate then those of her child.

Nora's family's response to her quest for medicine and need to accumulate capital for its purchase caused Nora to reflect on the quality of her social relations. Like many young Filipinas, Nora appeared to be caught between competing priorities and obligations, group and individual needs, a personal desire to flee her household, and a feeling that she should contribute more to the family. Nora did not reject her family responsibilities as much as question the integrity of group relations manifest as tangible support. The priority of her daughter's health was clear, but it was her priority alone.

Nora had been socialized to sacrifice for the good of her family members and to cultivate *loob* relationships with others as part of a general survival strategy, which Lynch (1964) has described as "seeking security through interdependence rather than independence." Left open to question was what constituted established need on her part such that resources would flow toward instead of away from her. Given her child's illness, her interpretation and that of other family members clashed. Nora's case illustrates the extent to which households are sites of cooperation as well as conflict and competition for scarce resources. Sickness provides a context in which to witness the social relations of each.

Insights into how cultural concepts are used by the poor to cope with hard choices involving resource allocation emerge from this case. Nora's aunt needed to purchase medicines from the open market because of the short supply at the local government clinic. Her personal need conflicted with the basic needs of the members of her own household. Their existence was hand to mouth. Buying medicine for herself would result in her family having little to eat. Nora's aunt was aware of the paradox she faced. While she stated that her condition was not contagious, she recognized that "weak lungs became TB if not treated." She associated her weak lungs with hard work and lack of food. How could she be cured she asked? If she spent money for medicine she would not have enough food to eat. Wouldn't this cause her weak lungs to return?

Nora's household did not volunteer to pay for her aunt's medicine as they did not have the resources. Nora confided in me that if her aunt was to ask her family for money directly, they would be compelled to give her whatever petty cash was on hand if she was acutely ill. After all, they remained indebted to her in a loob relationship. Nora's aunt did not make such a request.

As Leslie has noted, "moral conflicts dispose people to different interpretations of illnesses" (1992: 205). Conflicts may involve the moral identity of the afflicted as well as members of their therapy management group, moral issues related to the etiology of an illness as well as to therapeutic modalities followed and not followed. In this case, Nora's aunt provided a culturally acceptable rationale for not seeking expensive medicine recommended to her by a doctor. She claimed the medicine was not compatible to her body. She indirectly communicated to members of her therapy management group the choice she had made regarding her health care, given economic constraints. She received no argument or alternative advice from others. Indeed, there was a notable lack of discussion about the problem among members of Nora's household. All her extended family could do was support her with what limited resources they had. They could offer her their hospitality and friendship. Poor in physical resources, they honored their loob relationship to her and maintained close social contact. Being attentive to social risk eclipsed their fear of physical risk.

On an applied note, what is clearly needed for a better health outcome in this case is not a program focusing on community based TB education and medication compliance on the part of patients, although culturally sensitive education is important (Nichter 1994). More immediate is a need for compliance on the part of the health care system in both delivering effective TB treatment to patients and following up on exposed family members. It is not ignorance that lies behind the social relations of therapy management that ended up fostering the transmission of TB in Nora's household, but poverty.[10]

Case two

The second case involves a thirty-year-old South Indian man, Ali, his wife Fatima, and his extended family. I interviewed Ali several times over the course of two months and collected secondary data on his family from several sources. I observed Ali interacting with family members while he was an inpatient at a private clinic (nursing home) owned by a long-standing doctor friend of mine. One of my former research assistants was working at the nursing home and I enlisted his assistance in collecting information about Ali's life.

Ali hailed from a village fifteen miles from Mangalore, South Kanara district, Karnataka State, India. A member of the Mapala (Muslim) caste, Ali was a driver before getting the chance to go to the Middle East to make his fortune. Ali was married for a little more than a year before leaving for the Gulf. During this time he spent less than five months with his wife, who had become pregnant two months after their marriage.

Ali had recently returned to South Kanara after completing three years of contract labor in the Gulf and was contemplating returning to the Gulf for another contract job. I met Ali in a Mangalore nursing home while conducting research on a phenomenon I have come to call the Gulf Syndrome. I began observing this phenomenon in the early 1980s in the course of research on the rise of nursing homes along the Malabar coast of Southern India, especially in South Kanara district.[11] Interested in nursing home clientele and the factors influencing a sudden and visible rise in the use of diagnostic tests in the medical practice of town-based doctors, I found that a disproportionate number of nursing home clients requesting lab tests were Muslims returning from the Gulf. In two Mangalore nursing homes monitored during the mid 1980's, Muslims returning home from the Gulf or their close family member filled an estimated one-quarter of beds not allocated to women delivering babies. What was noteworthy about many of these "patients" was their explicit requests for diagnostic tests related to clinically vague, but culturally relevant symptoms serving as markers of lack of general well-being. Typically, their demand as consumers was for tests of the blood, stomach, and heart, as well as new technology they had heard about in the Gulf: endoscopy, sonograms, gastroscopy, EKG, and even CAT scans.

Ali's case was pointed out to me by the owner of a nursing home, a doctor–entrepreneur who had invested heavily in medical technology as a means of attracting patients. While it was his practice to routinely recommend a battery of diagnostic tests for all patients admitted to the nursing home, he criticized other nursing home owners for milking patients for all they were worth by continuing to recommend unnecessary diagnostic tests after a patient's health status was known. Ali had already paid substantial fees to the nursing home for several diagnostic tests. Now the doctor was trying to convince him that enough diagnostic tests had been done. Ali, he said, was a case for an anthropologist. At first I took his comment to mean "a case for a psychiatrist," but I was mistaken.

Upon interviewing Ali, I found that this was his second stay in the nursing home. During his initial five-day stay, he had received several diagnostic tests. He was informed that the results of these tests were within normal range except for his blood pressure, which was moderately high. Three weeks latter he requested retesting. Additionally, he brought his wife Fatima to undertake a series of tests beyond those suggested by a local doctor for anemia. The nursing home doctor, who had no qualms about giving Ali the first set of tests for a healthy fee, was not keen to retest him when "clearly there was no medical reason." Come back in six months, he had suggested, noting that "a person's lab tests do not change so quickly except when one is very ill." Ali remained steadfast in his demands, complaining of lingering abdominal pain and inquiring about a "heart test" (cardiac stress test).

Upon being readmitted to the nursing home for exploratory testing related to his abdominal complaint (ultrasound and gastroscopy), Ali made no additional requests. Although interested in knowing the results of his tests, he did not become obsessive in knowing details. Finding that his wife had low hemoglobin, he made it a point to request the "best" blood tonic available.[12] In her presence he also inquired whether she should have a sonogram as she "had not had one during her first pregnancy."

My initial interview with Ali focused on his general health before his Middle East experience and after his return home. During the interview and subsequent informal talks, I did not get the sense that he was preoccupied with his body, although he had suffered from a minor case of kidney stones and complained of recurrent abdominal discomfort, especially when upset. This impression was shared by the nursing home doctor who had spoken to Ali at some length about the diagnostic tests he undertook. Was this a case of test fetishism? Why were diagnostic tests so important to Ali, I wondered?

Ali confided in my research assistant, who had himself worked in the Gulf. While in the Gulf, Ali had remained in contact with his wife (who was illiterate) through letters to his family with whom she resided. Remittances were sent to Ali's father who was entrusted with looking after the welfare of Fatima and their child. This had continued for about a year until Fatima had returned to her mother's house for an extended visit.[13] A friend of Ali's who returned to the Gulf following home leave, informed him that jealousies between his wife, mother and sisters had escalated in

Ali's absence.[14] Following this, Ali sent remittances to both his father and Fatima's brother, who looked after her welfare and that of their child. Fatima's younger sister was literate and wrote letters on her behalf to Ali.

Upon returning home, Ali was treated with considerable respect but was aware of tension between his mother, two unmarried sisters, and his wife. This directly affected him. He was expected to adjust to being a husband and a father while resuming his role of son and brother. Additionally, he had to contend with relatives and friends who approached him with various business schemes, all contingent upon his return to the Middle East to accumulate additional capital. Ali had spoken to no one about the family difficulties he had experienced while in the Gulf. He had returned home with a new watch, a gold chain, a portable stereo, and foreign shoes: all tokens of the good life.

Ali told my assistant that visiting the nursing home made him feel better. Relatives who visited him there were concerned about his welfare. It was also good for his wife, whose health had been "neglected" as evidenced by the results of tests. In front of Ali, she was shown respect by her affines when they came to visit the nursing home. They inquired about her well-being daily.

What can we make of Ali's demand for diagnostic tests? To some extent it constitutes an exaggerated expression of a more general trend in South Kanara influenced by two sets of factors. On the consumer side, tests have come to represent an expression of truth in the face of growing doubt about doctors' diagnoses. Increasingly, patients who can afford to do so are seeking the advice and treatment of more than one doctor for complaints that are not routine. Given that doctors generally do not touch patients nor ask penetrating questions, but engage in diagnosis by treatment, tests are viewed as visible traces of the truth in a context where visual literacy is rising with the introduction of television and video cassettes.[15] The following observation by one of Ali's friends, a clerk with a fourth-grade education, is illustrative:

> Our Vaidya, traditional practitioners, used to diagnose by feeling the pulse, then came doctors who listened to the disease and the blood (pressure) with the dikry (stethoscope). Now doctors can see what is inside. We have gone to so many doctors for some diseases with no relief and in the end they send us for tests after many medicines have been purchased. Now doctors ask us to go for tests first. If they ask and you do not have the money, you have to try your luck with the medicine. Sometimes the doctor knows and sometimes it is a lucky dip (lottery).
>
> (12 March 1992)

On the supply side, the increased use of diagnostic tests in South Kanara is driven by economic factors. Ordering a test means that a doctor is assured of collecting a fee for services at least twice: once at the time of ordering the test and then again following the test, which the doctor must interpret in order to tailor treatment appropriately. Actually, the doctors often receive three payments. A nursing home with its own lab generates fees from these tests. Doctors ordering tests from outside often have established arrangements with particular labs from whom they receive a cut of the lab charge or periodic gifts.

Another factor driving supply-side diagnostic test popularity is the dynamics of paying back bank loans for diagnostic equipment. Banks in India have become quite liberal in their advancement of loans to doctors for diagnostic equipment. Purchase of this equipment is advantageous because it can be practically written off through depreciation and bank interest can be deducted from income tax.[16] What is necessary, especially during the first few years following equipment purchase, is to conduct enough diagnostic tests to pay the interest on the equipment and at the same time turn a profit. This leads many doctors and nursing home administrators to recommend tests or respond to the demands of clients when such tests are not clinically warranted except as "exploratory procedures."

The time I met Ali, I was considering two factors that possibly contributed to Muslims having a high prevalence of "Gulf Syndrome" – the phenomenon of Gulf-returned workers checking into nursing homes for vague complaints and requesting diagnostic tests. First, it was possible that the reason Muslims frequented nursing homes more than others was simply because they could afford to do so, having newly acquired cash income.[17] While this factor no doubt contributed to nursing home consultation, it did not explain the form of consultation or the specific types of requests made by patients. Moreover, interviews with owners of nursing homes about Hindus returning from the Gulf suggested that this group frequented nursing homes for general diagnostic tests far less than Muslims, although they did tend to have their wives deliver babies in nursing homes. The second possibility was that social status underlay the phenomenon. Attending a nursing home was a sign of prestige and accessing health care a form of symbolic capital. Considerable prestige was associated with placing one's wife or mother in a renowned nursing home where she would be attended to by a well-known doctor.

Ali's case suggested that the popularity of a stay in a nursing home was not merely linked to social status and conspicuous consumption of medical services. In the controlled environment of the nursing home, social relations were structured around support of a patient who did not have a pre-established sick role. While in the nursing home, such a role was assumed temporarily.[18] Patients were visited daily by family members who brought food and discussed the well-being of the patient in terms of diagnostic tests, which signified "all that could be done." Discussions in nursing homes between Gulf Syndrome patients and their relatives appeared to be infrequent. Arguments and heated discussions between family members were rarely observed by my research assistant over a six-month period while working as a nursing home attendant.

It has been pointed out by other researchers in India that a visit to a doctor or nursing home is treated as an outing by Muslim women (e.g. Jeffery 1979). For young men like Ali, it also constitutes a retreat. Daytime hours were spent visiting with relatives and evening hours visiting with his wife. The nursing home was one of the few places where Ali and his wife could find privacy and get a chance to be reacquainted without alienating other kin and creating tension. Overt displays of affection by a couple constitutes a threat to the integrity of a Muslim household and the power structure represented by the authority of elders.[19] Health, however, constitutes a domain where a married man can exercise some degree of autonomy and be attentive to his wife. The nursing home provided Ali with a space where he and his wife could be attentive to one another. My research assistant gave me greater insight into what was transpiring. During his time in the Gulf, Ali's feelings toward his wife had grown. At a distance, he imagined her in a way he had not done at home. My research assistant had had a similar experience and one evening both spoke to me about it outside the nursing home canteen. Letters from home while in a foreign environment, coupled with exposure to television and films portraying romantic love, had kindled feelings of longing for their wives that they had not experienced at home. Erotic body memories and a sense of anticipation entered their lives. As the time of their departure for home grew near, they experienced a growing desire for reunion with loved ones and for the tastes, sounds, and smells of home. Ali also spoke to me of having bad dreams where he vividly remembered the physical sensations of his kidney stones a year earlier, before his problem was diagnosed and he underwent a minor operation.[20] He had coined it within him as embodied memory of his hardships.

The nursing home was also a place where diagnostic tests and medicine use may be used to authenticate distress as well as communicate concern and affection.[21] Ali was able to communicate his concern for Fatima through diagnostic tests that affirmed her "weak state" followed by provision of medicines as tangible evidence of his attentiveness, support, and affection. By caring for his wife in this manner, her diminished status as well as weak state (bloodlessness, anemia) were being acknowledged and ameliorated. Fatima was moved by the concern that Ali displayed in requesting tests and asking for medicine. She told one of the nurses working in the nursing home that Ali was a "very good and understanding husband" and yet it is doubtful that she had directly communicated her feelings to him. Through his actions, Ali had acknowledged her hardships and expressed care and concern. Through her attentiveness to his food and health, and no doubt his sexual needs, Fatima had expressed intimacy.

Ali's tests constituted traces of his own hardships in the Gulf. The awareness of kin was raised without Ali having to talk of his difficulties in the Gulf, something most Gulf returnees chose not to do.[22] By having diagnostic tests, Ali mobilized a therapy management group. He flagged the possibility that something was not right without identifying a problem. Once mobilized, this group could not solve the problem (which was unknown), but only engage in social and moral support.[23] Diagnostic tests were more than a fetish for Ali, more than a status symbol. They provided a space for concern to be expressed and for healing to take place. Ali's test results appeared to me to be highly symbolic. I could not help but wonder whether Ali's relatives recognized any relationship between Ali's concern about his blood pressure and his feelings of social pressure to return to the Gulf, his complaints of pain in the abdomen and embodied memories of painful experiences in the Gulf, his concern about Fatima's anemia and her social situation in his absence. My research assistant made the first and third connections independent of me.[24]

The popularity and availability of diagnostic tests have been steadily increasing in India over the last decade. Doctors are employing more and more diagnostic tests for a number of reasons, ranging from medical to profit motives. By accommodating to consumer demand and market forces, practitioners have unintentionally provided those in the Indian population who can afford it new barometers of well being as well as a new means of communicating distress, care, and concern. Tests are not just instruments of surveillance in the sense of Foucault's (1980a, 1980b) notion of biopower. Tests provide a space within which social relations and agency may be articulated. Discourse on the need for tests and the meaning of test results enable members of one's therapy management group to interact in a variety of ways; they facilitate social practice. By calling attention to deviations from "normal values" appeals for and against change may be made. The interpretation and social relations of diagnostic testing are important to study as features of illness narratives, beyond the value of tests for "evidence-based medicine" (Boonmongkon et al. 2001). They are also worth studying as encounters that teach us something about the manner in which hybrid modernity is unfolding and science is being appropriated for social, political, and economic ends.

Conclusion

The two case studies may be compared. The first involves powerlessness, infectious disease, and the delicate balance between social and physical risk. In this case, the economic burden of treating Nora's aunt's disease in the private sector implicitly affected the actions of her therapy management group reflected in their silent acceptance of her choice to be noncompliant. The fact that they did not actively encourage her to purchase required medicines was not a reflection of a lack of concern. Quite the opposite, extended family members placed themselves at physical risk to maintain normal social relations with her as a measure of care. This continued even when Nora's child developed weak lungs. Responsibility for the child's illness was deflected away from Nora's aunt's presence in the house. When the child's illness was discussed, other risk factors were implicated, other truths produced. Attention was directed away from Nora's aunt by preventive health acts that were ritually performed by family members who maintained some level of recognition that the efficacy of these acts was limited.

Stigma is associated with TB in the Philippines. In this case we see that while stigma may exist in the community, it does not destabilize social relations within the family. By labeling Nora's aunt's illness as weak lungs, its stigma was reduced. Weak lungs is less threatening than TB and carries with it some degree of ambiguity (Nichter 1989). Feelings of sadness by therapy management group members unable to help her purchase medicine were mitigated through the passive acceptance of Nora's aunt's claim that the medication prescribed for weak lungs was incompatible with her body.

The second case involves potential illness signified by diagnostic tests and agency in the form of Ali's search for diagnosis and mobilization of a therapy management group for both himself and Fatima. Ali employed diagnostic tests to draw attention to his feelings of liminality and as a means of being attentive to his wife. While the doctor read laboratory values as texts indicating deviations from normal body functioning, for Ali they constituted traces of unspoken hardships.

Diagnostic tests and residence in the nursing home facilitated healing by fostering nurturance. A space was provided in which social relations were structured around support. In the nursing home Ali's problems remained to be discovered and, although undiagnosed, he was expected to recuperate. Family members and friends related to Ali as vulnerable, a condition requiring his emotional and physical well-being to be attended to with care. Ali's need for tests signaled to others, who wished to benefit from his Gulf contract, that the wealth he was able to accumulate was gained at a price. Tests reminded them that sacrifices had been made and taken their toll. Ali's attentiveness to Fatima during her stay in the nursing home set an example followed by visiting family members and helped normalize strained social relationships.

Both cases lead us to consider households as sites of cooperation as well as conflict. Illness mobilizes kin, neighbors, and practitioners into therapy management groups. It also places a strain on social relations in contexts of poverty when the relative needs of people must be weighed. This strain is compounded in contexts of social transformation where knowledge of potential medical interventions (tests, procedures, medicines) increases and entitlement is far from clear. Differences in perceptions of entitlement and possible course of action lead to critical appraisal of the quality of social relations.

In Nora's case, entitlement to her household's special remittance income became a personal issue when her child became ill with weak lungs. Not only was this money not offered to her, but household members continued to request loans of Nora whenever she gained access to cash income. Her child's long-term welfare was given less importance by household members than other immediate needs. Nora learned through experience that she was entitled to her household's resources only when her child was acutely ill.[25] An issue arose when Nora's interpretation of the health status of her child differed from that of other family members. Her perception was no doubt influenced by her participation in health-related research. After expressing concern to household members about her child and receiving little support in terms of resources, she responded to her family's lack of support personally.

Lack of support was interpreted by Nora as a sign of the overall poor quality of her relationships with household members. She critically evaluated these relationships during the course of constructing and revising a narrative marked by multiple voices.[26] One voice, that of the dutiful daughter, established a sense of her morality in accord with traditional values and norms. Another voice, that of Nora the victim, recalled a long history of neglect. A third voice, Nora the good mother, defended her right to expect more from her household than she was receiving. A fourth voice, Nora as transitional woman in today's world, sought approval for her desire (if not intention) to move away from a no-win situation represented by the hand-to-mouth existence of her family.

My presence influenced Nora's thinking. Nora sought approval from me as representative of an "other" who embodied western ideals of self sufficiency yet respected cultural values underscoring family relations. An implicit appeal was made to me above and beyond the periodic need for medicines for her child. This appeal entailed helping Nora find a position that would remove her physically from a context marked by the constant demands of her family, yet place her in a position to help them as she saw fit. The freedom Nora sought was to define her own level of interdependence with her family. In the process of redefining social relations, she related to me beyond that of empathetic witness. She sought active legitimization for her growing sense of entitlement in a changing world.

In the case of Ali, the issue of entitlement to resources also led to tension in the household. Upon his return from the Gulf, Ali was suddenly confronted by competing demands for material resources as measures of loyalty and markers of the quality of social relations. At stake was not only Ali's limited immediate wealth, but his future. Claims were being made on his future in terms of propositions to return to the Gulf for yet

another contract to finance joint business ventures. Competing propositions and jealousies among those people who constituted his support
network placed Ali in a no-win situation where he could not live up to
the expectations of all of those who made demands upon him. In the
nursing home situation where Ali's physical body was being evaluated, he
was able to re-evaluate the quality of his social relations and his plans for
the future. Ali's explicit request for tests was an implicit request for refuge.
Tests provided him with a legitimate refuge to which he was unques-
tionably entitled. Ali's doctor recognized that he was not mad. He was
not a case for a psychiatrist who diagnosed and treated individual
pathology as disease.

The social relations of therapy management are multidimensional and
difficult to access outside of detailed case studies. Cases such as the two
presented in this paper direct our attention to the social embeddedness
and microhistorical character of therapy management. They increase our
appreciation not only of choices made on behalf of the afflicted, but of
contexts such as poverty where choice is limited and members of a therapy
management group must cope with their powerlessness. The study of
therapy management entails not only what people do (and can do) and
reasons for actions taken, but what they are unable to do and what underlies apparent passivity, acceptance, or fatalism. Failure to appreciate this
side of therapy management contributes to simplistic impressions that
ignorance underlies "irrational health behavior" in contexts where other
factors are involved.

These cases also lead us to consider illness as a reflexive experience.
Illness challenges a sense of order in one's world and tests the integrity
of social relationships. Efforts extended as well as withheld lead to a
reevaluation of one's social capital and safety nets, especially in contexts
where economics place a strain on relationships. In such contexts, cultural
values are challenged and reciprocal relations are fragile.

Close consideration of therapy management, people's reflections about
entitlement, and the politics of responsibility (as it does and does not play
out), contribute to an anthropology of self. "Ethnographies of the particular" challenge simplistic notions of sociocentric (collectivist) vs
individualist selves critiqued by anthropologists and cross cultural psychologists (e.g., Spiro 1993, Triandis 1994, 1995), but still pervasive in the
literature.[27] All too often, cultural ideologies of self are mistaken for lived
selves due to the failure to recognize that "cultures and selves are internally differentiated into potentially conflicting domains of self interested
and group interested elements" (Gregg 2000). In today's world, globalization and increased migrant work opportunities have expanded horizons
of possibility and opened up new domains in which to experience and
imagine selves and social relationships.[28]

Cultural models based on collectivist principles, such as *utang na loob* in the Philippines, help explain the extent to which concerns about "social risk" eclipse concerns about physical risk. They help us understand Nora's reluctance to distance herself from her sick aunt. To a lesser degree, they help us appreciate Nora's emotional appraisal of her kin's actions when her child falls ill. What collectivist principles do not provide are insights into the other domains of Nora's life. They do not lead us to consider that tough life lessons have taught Nora to be independent and prioritize her child's health over household members demands for scarce resources. They also do not help us appreciate the significance of Nora's dreams of a different life distant from her family, her sense of personal ambition, and growing ambivalence toward family members. Her "moral identities" and "senses of self" have at once collectivist and individualist dimensions and voices.

A tension between collectivist principles and individualist inclinations is also apparent in Ali's case. Collectivist values and sensitivities guide Ali's demeanor in public and probably had much to do with his original decision to go to the Gulf as a migrant worker. They certainly had a lot to do with whom he married, but not the emotions he would experience for his wife after marriage while in the Gulf. Collectivist sentiments do not define Ali's experience of self. Ali skillfully negotiates multiple senses of self within domains of life where he has differing degrees of autonomy. Ali's health-care seeking behavior and pursuit of diagnostic tests affords him the space in which to engage in expressions of self that are distinctly not collectivist, yet do not undermine his social identity as a good son or brother. His stay in the nursing home was healing without the presence of a healer, and his story one for an anthropologist indeed.

The stories of Nora and Ali provide us with many lessons, lessons about therapy management and identity management, social relations and economic relations, the cultural work engaged in by kin as well as practitioners, and the value of specificity as well as ambiguity seen in the use of terms like weak lungs and in the interpretation of diagnostic test results. They lead us to appreciate what Leslie has argued throughout his writings: that more is at stake in the interpretation of illness than a set of medical practices, and that more is at stake in the practice of medicine than the treatment of disease, however diagnosed and defined. The stories also teach us the importance of studying the particular as a means of understanding how life is negotiated and circumstance as a means of seeing how priorities are (re-)established and social relationships revisited.

Notes

1 Leslie encouraged the study of "medical systems" as social systems, not as "systems of knowledge" in the sense critiqued by Hobart (1995), who takes anthropology to task for over systematizing healing traditions and not paying enough attention to ambiguity and the way knowledge is negotiated in context.

2 I use the term sickness here to signify the way in which illness and disease is socialized. Sickness is a social experience and as such involves roles and expectations. On medical anthropologists, the use of the terms illness, disease, and sickness, see Young (1980).

3 Both Straus's (1985) concept of the "works of illness" and Obeysekere's concept of the "work of culture" are useful heuristics. This does not mean I endorse the way each scholar has used them. Straus's writing on the "works of illness" are poorly developed theoretically and does not consider cultural or gender dynamics. Obeysekere's writing on how healing involves the reframing of repressed negative effect and guilt by transforming personal symbols into public symbols through subjectification and objectification is problematic. Culture comes to stand for public symbols located outside the person that the individual internalizes and uses to resolve traumatic experience in a culturally adaptive way. The opposition of private, public is problematic, the work of culture is overly psychologized and reductionistic, and too little attention is directed to the role of one's therapy management group in reframing, co-constructing, and sustaining meaning. More attention needs to be focused on the role of others in developing and sustaining scripts as cultural work. And as Hollan (1994) has noted more attention needs to be directed to distinguishing between life as lived, life as experienced, and life as narrated.

4 Beginning in the 1980s, the utility of structural definitions of the household began being questioned, and more activity-centered processual definitions proposed (Netting et al., 1984) as a means to facilitate research on specific issues, including the household production of health (Berman et al. 1988; Nichter 1995). Processual approaches viewed households less as physical structures (common hearths, etc.) and more as projects in the making inhabited by stakeholders having both common and diverse interests. Ethnographic studies in several different cultural contexts documented that (1) competition between household members co-existed with cultural institutions placing value on cooperation; (competition and cooperation both influenced decision-making); (2) subtle and not so subtle forms of bargaining and negotiation took place in households among stakeholders; (3) entitlement to household resources and the division of responsibilities were subject to gender, birth order, and intergenerational power dynamics; and (4) an individual's status, power, and entitlement to resources in the household altered throughout the course of life.

5 This research assistant had also worked in the Gulf for three years. At first I was surprised that he became Ali's confidant, because he was Hindu. I later came to understand that it was precisely because he was Hindu and not a member of Ali's caste and social network that this close personal relationship could develop at a safe social distance. A limitation of this ethnographic account is that neither I nor my research assistant was able to develop a close relationship with Fatina, Ali's wife. This would have required a female researcher. Information about her was gathered from Ali, Fatima's brother, a nurse with whom she became friends, and through observation of her interactions with Ali and her inlaws.

6 The term *kasundo* is a local equivalent of the term *hiyang* used in more formal Tagalog. On the use of this term to describe one's compatibility with medicine as well as to describe side-effects, see Tan (1989) and Hardon (1991).

7 As Appadurai (1991: 198) has noted, people in developing countries increasingly see their lives through "prisms of other possible lives offered by the media in all of its forms," through encounters with travelers and anthropologists and through the stories of migrant workers and mail-order brides. Fantasy

and fairy-tales of possible futures, like window shopping, are important social phenomena providing insights into social transformation and competing ideologies as well as romantic idealism and vicarious consumption.

8   Concern about offering a diagnosis to a patient or their patient's family that is stigmatizing leads health care providers to use more ambiguous language. For other examples, see Lock's (1998) study of Downs syndrome in Japan where a child is identified as slow or studies of cancer in Mexico where the diagnosis of cancer is not only thought to stigmatize the patient, but impact negatively on their condition. The difference in this case is that TB is highly contagious.

9   The concept of *utang na loob* is foundational to writings on Filipino Culture (Hollensteiner 1973, Ileto 1979, Kaut 1961, Lynch 1973, Rafael 1984). As it is described in the literature, *Utang na loob* indexes notions of gratitude, reciprocity, and indebtedness, which serve to connect one to others. In so doing, it structures social relations in the social body as well as the body politic. To have no *utang na loob* ties is to be excluded from a network of exchange, to be an outsider and subject to shame (*hiya*) of such magnitude that one is alienated. In life, one copes with a delimited amount of *hiya* associated with indebtedness as part of *utang na loob* relations, but fears being overwhelmed by an inability to repay kindness. This fear is not merely associated with guilt, but one's sense of person. According to some accounts, *loob* relations are responsible for one's sense of "inner self" (Ileto 1979: 331). A child (especially a girl) is socialized to believe that she always remains in a *loob* relationship with her mother. Hollensteiner (1973) notes that a child is told that nothing she can do during her lifetime will make up for the gift of life a mother has given. While this debt cannot be repaid in full, children are expected to offer token repayment in the form of gifts and respect. The principle of *utang na loob* relationship is extended to others who offer support of one kind or another. *Utang na loob* is an ideal type of expected behavior in the Philippines and has become a social fact. In reality, rhetoric on debts of gratitude often does not translate into practice and when it does, there are limits to its expression. Cross-cutting obligations exist in households such as the one being described. Responsibility is not clearly defined, often ambiguous, and negotiated in context. The ideal of "the Filipino family" as a harmonious "unit" is overemphasized in the literature. More research needs to be conducted on both how obligations are prioritized and acted upon in context as well as the ideology of *utang na loob* as hegemonic. *Utang na loob* renders the political patronage system in the Philippines ethical by using kinship to legitimate a patronage system internalized at the site of the family. A Gramscian analysis of *utang na loob* might prove very "productive" (Gramsci 1971).

10 This case illustrates the importance of the DOTS program later implemented in the Philippines, but it is still struggling to maintain an adequate medicine supply chain. What also needs to be established is trust in the medicines supplied by the government.

11 See Baru (1998) as well as Nichter and Van Sickle (2002) for a discussion of the growth of nursing homes in India and the rising availability and popularity of diagnostic tests employing sophisticated medical technology.

12 Improvement in his wife's hemoglobin was taken as a sign of improvement in her general well-being. This took on symbolic importance concordant with the meaning of blood as a medium within which the physical and psychosocial merged. Curiously, Ali secured both allopathic and ayurvedic tonics for his wife which were available at the nursing home. When I asked Ali why Fatima was taking both tonics, he replied that the allopathic tonic was for increasing the blood and the ayurvedic tonic for cleaning the blood. While I think the

act of giving a tonic supercedes the symbolism of tonic type, one might view one tonic as repairing the past and the other as building the future.

13 The Moplah caste located in North Malabar is largely matrilineal (D'Souza 1976) and as such follow the marumakkathayam system of "mother right" inheritance. By custom a husband often resides with his wife's family when they have property, but a fair amount of flexibility exists in residence when property does not exist or where the husband has self-acquired property. When a women resides at her maternal home she is entitled to a share of household resources, but more and more husbands maintain their wives and children irrespective of where they live. It is not uncommon for a husband who is earning to support both his wife and children and also his sisters and their children. This was true in Ali's case.

14 Leela Gulati (1988) has noted that psychological problems in migrant households on the Malabar coast constitute a source of expressed concern among health care providers. Articles in the popular press suggest that every other family having a relative in the Gulf suffers from some psychological problem. Groups at special risk identified by Gulati are women aged 15–25 who are recent brides of migrant workers left in the care of affines. Gulati further notes that remittances are a common source of conflict and distress.

15 Gulf-return workers have been exposed to modern diagnostic tests both during the course of medical treatment and as captured by the popular imagination. Descriptions of these tests merge with other forms of modern technology. In several countries in the Near East and Gulf, CAT scans are referred to as "Kambuter" and sonagrams as "telefizion" or "Sonar" (Beth Kangas, personal communication). There is little idea of what diseases the tests are for and there is confusion about what role they play in diagnosis and cure. In India, some nursing home doctors actually set up a separate screen so that the family members of patients can see the images created by ultrasound equipment. A neurosurgeon friend in Mangalore has complained to me on several occasions that patients walk into his office off the street seeking CAT scans for headaches and nervous conditions often associated with psychiatric problems and heart conditions.

16 Bank loans on an ultrasound machine, for example, might cover 75 per cent of the costs of the equipment (approximate cost rs. 200,000) at an interest rate of between 12–18 per cent. Depreciation on the machine is 22 per cent a year so that the equipment could be written off after four years while used for 15 years. A busy nursing home might use this machine 15 to 20 times a day charging rs. 200–300 per test.

17 In terms of cost, staying in a nursing home was about the same price as staying in a two-star hotel in Mangalore. Daily room rates were about rs. 50–75. A week's stay with a normal battery of tests would run up a bill of about rs. 1000–1500.

18 In this context, waiting for the results of diagnostic tests places one in an "at risk role," which overlaps with a "sick role" in the sense described by Parsons (1975). After receiving "suggestive" or "borderline" test results that are abnormal, but not abnormal enough to label a condition a disease by diagnostic criteria, a risk role may transform into a sick role if the person "at risk" begins to: (a) act as if they are actually experiencing the illness or (b) becomes hypervigilant to the point that concern about the disease organizes their everyday life. Whether or not this role is accepted as legitimate has a lot to do with the social relations of therapy management.

19 A son's infatuation with his wife is threatening to the extent that he neglects obligations to other family members. For this reason, love for one's wife is

supposed to be balanced against one's kin obligations and duties. Infatuation as a form of exclusive love is viewed as potentially destructive. This concern is also found among Hindus as well, especially those living in joint and extended families (Derne 1995). Romantic idealism is a feature of modernity that modern day youth in India are negotiating.

20 I find Cassey's (1987) distinction between pleasure/erotic body memory and traumatic body memory useful in understanding Ali's case. Ali's erotic and sensual body memories of Fatima, emplace him through dreams of reunion that have a future. Ali's traumatic body memories of kidney stones, on the other hand, evokes a sense of distress located within the landscape of his work environment in the Gulf. Ali associated these traumatic memories with a sense of poor fit between his body and the environment in which he worked. During one interview I asked him why he thought he had developed kidney stones (a common problem among Indian workers in the Gulf) at a young age. Ali stressed the poor fit between his body, this work environment, and the qualities of food and water available in the Gulf. Returning to the Gulf placed his health at risk, but it was a risk he was willing to take, he commented, should economic need arise. As Basso (1996) has noted, places come to be inhabited by memories. If memories dwell in places, for Ali the Gulf was inhabited by an embodied sense of trauma as much as fortune.

21 In instances such as this, the seeking of diagnostic tests sets in motion a somatic mode of attention (Csordas 1993) that may provide the afflicted with an idiom of distress (Nichter 1981). Encouragement to seek tests and discourse about tests may also be employed as an idiom for articulating concern, responsibility, and the like.

22 Workers returning from the Gulf rarely talk to relatives or friends about their hardships or the nature of their work in the Gulf. Upon returning home, friends in the Gulf rarely remind each other of the day-to-day reality they experienced.

23 I was unable to collect "diagnostic test stories" told by Ali's relatives. Stories about "modern tests" received by a patient constitute a distinct form of illness story in need of investigation. Such stories are told by relatives as well as the afflicted to legitimate courses of action, establish moral identity, index social status, and evoke concern.

24 This research assistant has conducted research with me for some years and it is likely that I have influenced the way he looks at the world. I raised this possibility with him following his comments to me about Ali's symptoms. His response was that Ali and Fatima were not acutely ill. Many people had high blood pressure and anemia. It was Ali's concern for these problems that would lead people to wonder about social relations in his household.

25 Entitlement is one of the least studied aspect of therapy management groups. When do household members and neighbors feel compelled to part with scare resources (take or offer loans etc.) to assist kin and members of important social networks? To what extent does this depend on the person afflicted and the acute, recurrent, or chronic nature of their illness, the age, birth order, and gender of the afflicted, competing emergencies? What impact have political policies such as structural adjustment had on the safety net function of social networks among the very poor and the mobilization of therapy management groups?

26 My use of the term voice corresponds most closely to Goffman's (1974) concept of figure in Frame Analysis. It is beyond the scope of this paper to examine Nora's retelling of her narrative. Suffice it to say that her narrative shifted in relation to audience (who was physically present and who was remembered)

and context. Once told and objectified, Nora commented upon and evaluated previous tellings of her story and new voices emerged.

27 According to this dichotomy, individualist selves and cultures give priority to personal goals over group goals. Collectivist selves and cultures give priority to in-group goals over personal goals. For an excellent critical review of the literature on this dichotomy in anthropology and psychology, see Gregg (2000). In the Indian context, a distinctive "dividual" concept of self has been described in the ethnographic literature. Described are permeable dividuals constantly being influenced by the substantial qualities of persons, things, places, and time (see for example Marriott 1989). Ethnographies of the particular have questioned the extent to which this sense of self guides actions. For an age specific, life stage perspective which attends to the difference between ideologies of self and actual behavior, and which calls attention to individuals as agents of their own destinies in India, see Mines (1988, 1994).

28 It is beyond the scope of this chapter to speak to the growing complexity of identity as a feature of globalization and the fact that people who appear to inhabit the same local world may have very different imaginaries, horizons of possibility and senses of identity.

References

Abu-Lughod, L. (1991). Writing Against Culture. In *Recapturing Anthropology: Working in the present*, edited by R.D. Fox, pp. 137–165. Santa Fe, NM: School of American Research Press.

Appadurai, A. (1991). Global Ethnoscapes: Notes and Queries for a Transnational Anthropology. In *Recapturing Anthropology: Working in the present*, edited by R.D. Fox, pp. 191–210. Santa Fe, NM: School of American Research Press.

Basso, K. (1996). Wisdom sits in places : Notes on a Western Apache Landscape. In *Senses of Place*, edited by Keith Basso and S. Fields, pp. 53–90. Santa Fe, NM: School of American Research Press.

Baru, R.V. (1998). *Private Health Care in India: Social Characteristics and Trends*. New Delhi: Sage Publications.

Berman, P., Kendall, C. and Bhattacharya, K. (1988). The Household Production of Health. Integrating Social Science Perspectives on Micro-Level Health Determinants. *Social Science and Medicine* 38(2): 205–215.

Boonmongkon, P., Nichter, M. and Pylypa, J. (2001). Women's mot luuk problems in Northeast Thailand: why women's own health concerns matter as much as disease rates. *Social Science and Medicine* 53: 223–236.

Bruce, J. (1989). Homes Divided. *World Development* 17(7): 979–991.

Cassey, E. (1987). *Remembering: a Phenomenological Study*. Bloomington, IN: Indiana University Press.

—— (1993). *Getting Back into Place: Toward a renewed understanding of Place – World*. Bloomington, IN: Indiana University Press.

Crandon, L. (1983). Why Susto? *Ethnology* XXII, 2: 153–167.

Csordas, T. (1993). Somatic Modes of Attention. *Cultural Anthropology* 8(2): 135–156.

Derne, S. (1995). *Culture in Action: Family Life, Emotion and Male Dominance in Barnes India*. State University Press of New York.

D'Souza, V. (1976). Kinship Organization and Marriage Customs among the Moplahs on the South-West Coast of India. In *Family, Kinship, and Marriage among Muslims in India*, edited by Imtiaz Ahmad, pp 141–68. New Delhi: Manohar Press.

Dwyer, D. and Bruce, J. (1988). *A Home Divided: Women and Income in the Third World*. Stanford: Stanford University Press.

Folbre, N. (1986a). Cleaning House: New Perspectives on Households and Economic Development. *Journal of Development Economics* 22: 5–40.

—— (1986b). Hearts and Spades: Paradigms of Households and Economics. *World Development* 14(2): 245–255.

Foucault, M. (1980a). *Power and Knowledge: Selected Interviews and other Writings*. Brighton, England: Harvester.

—— (1980b). *The History of Sexuality*: Vol.1. New York: Vintage.

Goffman, E. (1974). *Frame Analysis: An Essay on the Organization of Experience*. New York: Harper & Row.

Good, M., Bood, B.J., Schaffer, C. and Lind, S.E. (1990). American Oncology and the Discourse on Hope. *Culture, Medicine and Psychiatry* 14: 59–79.

Gramsci, A. (1971). *Selections from the Prison Notebooks*. New York: International Publishers.

Gregg, G. (2000). *Egocentric vs Sociocentric Selves: A wrong Idea Whose Time has Passed*. Unpublished paper presented at the American Anthropology Association Meeting, San Francisco Nov 19.

Gulati, L. (1988). Male Migration to the Middle East and the Impact on the Family: Some Evidence from Kerala. *Economic and Political Weekly*, Dec. 24, pp. 2217–2226.

Hardon, A. (1991). *Confronting Ill Health: Medicines, Self Care and the Poor in Manilla*. Quezon City: Health Action Information Network.

Hobart, M. (1995). As I lay laughing. In *Counterworks: Managing the Diversity of Knowledge*, edited by Richard Fardon, pp. 49–72. London: Routledge.

Hollan, D. (1994). Suffering and the Work of Culture: A Case of Magical Poisoning in Toraja. *American Ethnologist*, 21 (1): 74–87.

Hollensteiner, M. (1973). Reciprocity in the Lowland Philippines. In *Four Readings on Philippine Values*, edited by Frank Lynch and Alfonso de Guzman Institute of Philippine Culture Papers No. 2. Quezon City: Ateneo de Manila University Press.

Howard, M. (1994). Socio-economic Causes and Cultural Explanations of Childhood Malnutrition Among the Chagga of Tanzania. *Social Science and Medicine* 38(2): 239–251.

Ileto, R. (1979). *Payson and Revolution: Popular Movements in the Philippines 1840–1910*. Quezon City: Ateneo de Manila University Press.

Janzen, J. (1987). Therapy Management: Concept, Reality, Process. *Medical Anthropology Quarterly* 1(1): 68–84.

Janzen, J. (1978). *The Quest for Therapy: Medical Pluralism in Lower Zaire*. Berkley: University of California Press.

Jeffery, P. (1979). *Frogs in A well: Indian Women in Purdah*. Zed press: London.

Kaut, C. (1961). Utang na loob: A System of Contractual Obligation among Tagalogs. *Southwestern Journal of Anthropology* 17(3): 256–272.

Leslie, C. (1978). *Foreword to John Janzen's The Quest for Therapy: Medical Pluralism in Lower Zaire*. Berkley: University of California Press.

—— (1992). Interpretations of Illness: Syncretism in Modern Ayurveda. In *Paths to Asian Medical Knowledge*, edited by Charles Leslie and Allan Young, pp. 177–208. Berkley: University of California Press.

Lock, M. (1998). Perfecting society: reproductive technologies, genetic testing, and the planned family in Japan. In, *Pragmatic women and body politics*, edited by Margaret Lock and Patricia Kaufert, pp. 206–239. Cambridge: Cambridge University Press.

Lynch, F. (1964). Social Acceptance. In *Four Readings on Philippine Values.* Institute of Philippine Culture Papers No. 2, edited by F. Lynch. Quezon City: Ateneo de Manila University Press.

—— (1973). Social Acceptance Reconsidered. In *Four Readings on Philippine Values*, edited by Frank Lynch and Alfonso de Guzman. Institute of Philippine Culture Papers No. 2. Quezon City, Philippines, Ateneo de Manila University Press.

Marriott, M. (1989). Constructing an Indian Ethnosociology, *Contributions to Indian Sociology.* 23 : 1–39.

Mines, M. (1987). Conceptualizing the Person: Hierarchical Society and Individual Autonomy in India. *American Anthropologist* 90(3): 568–578.

—— (1994). Public Faces, Private Voices: Community and Individuality in South India. Berkley: University of California Press.

Nations, M. and Rebhun, L. (1988). Angels with Wet Wings Won't Fly: Maternal Sentiment in Brazil and the Image of Neglect. *Culture, Medicine, and Psychiatry* 12: 141–200.

Netting, R., Wilk, R. and Arnould, E. (1984). *Households: Comparative and Historical Studies of the Domestic Group.* Berkeley: University of California Press.

Nichter, M. (1995). Rethinking Household and Community in the Context of International Health. Invited paper, American Anthropological Association Annual Meeting, November, Washington, D.C. [files of author.]

—— (1994). Illness Semantics and International Health: The Weak Lungs/TB Complex in the Philippines. *Social Science and Medicine* 38(5): 649–663.

—— (1989). *Anthropology and International Health: South Asian Case Studies.* Dordrecht, Netherlands: Kluwer Press.

—— (1981). Idioms of distress: Alternatives in the expression of psychosocial distress: A case study from South India. *Culture, Medicine, and Psychiatry* 5: 379–408.

Nichter, M. and Nichter, M. (1994). Acute Respiratory Illness: Popular Health Culture and Mothers Knowledge in the Philippines. *Medical Anthropology* 15: 1–23.

Nichter, M. and Van Sickle, D. (2002). The Challenges Of India's Health and Health Care Transition. In *India Briefing*, edited by Alysia Ayres and Philipp Oldenbeurg. New York : M.E. Sharpe.

Parsons, T. (1975). The Sick Role and the Role of the Physician Reconsidered. *Health Society* 53: 257–278.

Rafael, V. (1984). *Contracting Christianity: Conversion and Translations in Early Tagalog Colonial Society.* Doctoral dissertation, Cornell University. Ann Arbor: University Microfilms.

Sen, A.K. (1990). Gender and Cooperative Conflicts. In *Persistent Inequalities: Women and World Development*, edited by Irene Tinke, pp. 123–149. New York: Oxford University Press.

Scheper-Hughes, N. (1985). Culture, Scarcity, and Maternal Thinking: Maternal Detachment and Infant Survival in a Brazilian Shantytown. *Ethos* 13(4): 291–317.
—— (1992). *Death Without Weeping: The Violence of Everyday Life in Brazil.* Berkeley: University of California Press.
Spiro, M. (1993). Is the Western conception of the self "peculiar" within the context of the world cultures? *Ethos* 21(2): 107–153.
Straus, A. (1985). *The Social Organization of Medical Work.* Chicago: University of Chicago Press.
Tan, M. (1989). Traditional or Transitional Medical Systems? *Social Science and Medicine* 29(3): 301–307.
Triandis, H. (1994). Theoretical and methodological approaches to the study of collectivism and individualism. In *Individualism and Collectivism: Theory, method, and applications*, edited by U. Kim, H. Triandis, C. Kagitcibasi, S. Choi, and G. Yoon, pp. 41–51. Thousand Oaks, CA: Sage Publications.
—— (1995). *Individualism & Collectivism.* Boulder: Westview Press.

Chapter 5

Making sense out of modernity

Marina Roseman

A banner year for medical anthropology, 1976 heralded the publication of two seminal volumes dedicated to the study of the medical systems of complex Asian societies. Charles Leslie's edited volume *Asian Medical Systems*, fruit of a 1971 conference sponsored by the Wenner-Gren Foundation, articulated a fresh and distinctly anthropological approach to the study of illness and health. In his introduction, Leslie (1976b) set forth a series of basic tenets that would become paradigmatic for subsequent scholarship in medical anthropology. Leslie's introduction argued and volume articles demonstrated that, like medical systems elsewhere, each Asian medical system "consists of beliefs and practices connected by an underlying logic and each is underpinned by a coherent network of assumptions about pathophysiology, therapeutics, and so forth" (Leslie and Young 1992: 4). Asian medical practices, recognized as logically integrated systems, were grounded in the specificity of local practices, historically situated, and dynamically evolving.

Western "cosmopolitan medicine" or "biomedicine," then, was shown to be one system among many. The second landmark volume to be published in 1976 emerged from the Fogarty International Center conference on "Medicine in Chinese Cultures." Informed by theoretical developments in interpretive and symbolic anthropology, Arthur Kleinman (Kleinman et al., eds. 1976) designated the medical system a "cultural system." Here and elsewhere (Kleinman 1973) he demonstrated how culture serves as a symbolic bridge between intersubjective meanings and the human body, shaping clinical interactions in Asian and biomedical settings.

Both these individuals and their works were early inspirations as I developed my own orientation toward the anthropological study of the knowledge and practices, the physical, social, and historical force-fields constituting illness and health. At the conclusion of his introduction to *Asian Medical Systems,* Leslie made a statement I took to heart, and pass along here: "Our work will have been well done if others find in it both something to correct and something to build upon" (Leslie 1976b: 12). While his own work focused on the medical practices of complex, literate Asian societies, Leslie equally supported the investigation of what he termed "ritual curing" (Leslie and Young 1992: 7). As senior editor of *Social Science and Medicine,* he encouraged my first publication on that subject (Roseman 1988) in a special volume of the journal dedicated to "Techniques of Healing in Southeast Asia" guest-edited by Carol Laderman and Penny van Esterik. Building upon the epistemological insights gained by designating medical practices a logically integrated system, I began, in that article, the process of refining the concept of a "medical system" by focusing upon the ethnographic and historical particulars of how that system is operationalized.

Trained in the cultural analysis of sound and motion in performance, I explored the everyday and ritual practices and sensory experiences through which the Temiars of peninsular Malaysia constitute their particular reality of living, interacting, suffering and alleviating suffering. My work benefited from the influence of phenomenology, practice, and performance theories. These have helped move interpretive anthropology beyond the interpretation of symbolic *forms*, directing it instead toward what Good (1994: 169) terms the "interpretive practices" or "*formative activities*' through which illness is constituted, made the object of knowledge and control, embedded in experience and social life, and transformed through therapies and the 'work of culture'" (italics added).

The study of health care systems, thus conceived, problematizes the relationship of illness and culture. A medical system, in this vein, is not viewed merely as that logically interconnected system of "beliefs and practices" through which members of a culture respond to illness or disease, conceived of as a predetermined biological domain. Rather, interpretive practices and the institutional frameworks they inform are examined as they shape, in fundamental ways, the illnesses members of a culture suffer, the strategies they follow to alleviate that suffering, and the forms of "health" they strive to ensure. "Reality in this view," Good (1994: 176) continues, "is not that which precedes interpretation. It is rather that which rises amidst the interactions or relationship among the physical body, the lived body, and the interpretive activities of the sufferer, healers, and others in the social world." His argument finds its correlate in performative approaches to the relationship between sex and gender. Judith Butler (1990: 7) argues, for example, "gender is not to culture as sex is to nature; gender is also the discursive/cultural means by which 'sexed nature' or a 'natural sex' is produced and established as 'prediscursive,' prior to culture, a politically neutral surface on which culture acts."

A primary task for the anthropological analysis of medical systems becomes the identification of such "interpretive" or "formative" practices, the exploration of how they mediate the experience of illness, and the investigation of the networks of association through which medical practices are intimately interconnected with other cultural domains. Interpretive studies in medical anthropology draw upon theories of narrative construction and reader-interaction (Good 1994), performance theory (Laderman and Roseman 1996), the paradigm of embodiment (Scheper-Hughes and Lock 1987; Csordas 1990), and sensorial anthropology (Howes 1991; Stoller 1989) to investigate the experiential grounds of illness and health. Conjoined, they provide a powerful theoretical apparatus for investigating the experiences and actions through which illness and health are culturally, historically, and individually constituted.

The "paradigm of embodiment" articulated by Csordas (1990, 1994a, 1994b) understands ritual healing as a "rhetorical means of ordering experience and directing attention," a way of evoking particular "somatic modes of attention" through which the self is transformed in accordance with such psychocultural themes (ibid: 22). A synergistic confluence of Merleau-Ponty's phenomenology of experience and Bourdieu's practice theory, this paradigm grounds culture and self in the phenomenology of the body. "Self" is defined as "neither substance nor entity, but an indeterminate capacity to engage or become oriented in the world, characterized by effort and reflexivity" (Csordas 1994a: 5), while the body is the "existential ground of the self" (Csordas 1994b). Therapeutic specificity in a medical system can be identified in the ethnographic specificity of "self processes," orientational processes in which aspects of the world are thematized in accordance with salient values of a particular cultural milieu (Csordas 1994a: 15). The task of comprehending a particular medical system involves determining the ontological themes and qualities of effort whereby the sufferer is reflexively engaged and reoriented in the world by healing practices.

Our ability to discern how medical practices are inscribed in the curves of the body and language of the senses owes much, as well, to feminist theory and ethnography. Feminist anthropology transformed both the language and the scope of ethnographic theory and method. In concert with postmodern recalculations of identity and subjectivity, and postcolonial sensitivity to the politically motivated history of the ethnographic gaze, feminist ethnography supported the growing recognition that living within the "body politic" indeed entailed disciplining the body. Attention toward traditional ethnological realms such as "kinship" was progressively refocused and rephrased in a move from structural toward experiential terms: first as gender, then sex, person/self/emotion, and finally, embodiment and the senses.

A given worldview is made "emotionally acceptable" by an ethos, and an ethos is made "intellectually reasonable" by a worldview, Clifford Geertz argues in one of his most influential examples of the "cultural system" approach, "Religion as a Cultural System" (1973: 87 ff). "Thought-provoking as this suggestion may be," sensorial anthropologist David Howes (1991: 13) responds, "it completely ignores the 'sensory dimension of symbolic perception'" (see also Ohnuki-Tierney 1981: 8, 17). A more penetrating analysis, in his view, is Steven Feld's (1990, 1991) analysis of Kaluli drumming in Papua New Guinea, "for it shows how idea and affect, cosmology and ethos, are integrated, in the Kaluli case, through the medium of sound." The senses, rather than the emotions, are the locus for networks of associations that operationalize the transformative capacities of therapeutic practices.

Where Csordas directs us toward the body and self processes in order to ground cultural systems in lived experience, Howes directs our attention to the senses. Cultures are "ways of sensing the world," and cultures vary in terms of the "distinctive patterns to the interplay of the senses they present" (Howes 1991: 8). Yet, whether promulgating formative practices, performance, self processes, embodiment, or sensory dimensions, these various approaches share an orientation toward the experiential and performative activities through which participants co-construct illness and health, and formulate responses to misfortune. In this article, I examine the ways in which sounds, motions, and sensations are configured and experienced as "formative practices" which constitute illness and enable its treatment. Under the rubrics *rhythm, rapture, and rupture,* I explore how specific sounds and motions, manipulated within healing ceremonies, constellate particular experiential states and transformative self-processes. I show how these sounds, motions, and sensations synthesize networks of associations, integrating idea and affect, cosmology and ethos toward the promotion of health.

Leslie emphasized the "logical integration" of Asian medical systems in deliberate rhetorical response to analyses which evaluated (and devalued) non-Western medical systems according to their relative rationality (or irrationality) *vis-à-vis* Western science and biomedicine. Postmodern and postcolonial theories, as well as the historical experience of globalization, have led us to view biomedical science as less than purely rational, and cultural logic as less of a well-integrated "seamless web" and more of a patchwork, a heterophonic overlay of multiple, hybridized, and disjunct voices. I will argue below that a Temiar sensibility and performance of healthy "integration," for both person and community, is more akin to the interactive overlap and dynamic interpenetration of call and response. Also termed heterophony or "echo polyphony" (Keil and Feld 1994), this musical form, seminal to Temiar ritual curing, preserves multiplicity even as voices conjoin. As such, performance practices surrounding illness and healing provide Temiars with fertile ground on which to confront and dynamically reconfigure the "disjunctures and differences" (Appadurai 1999: 27ff) posed by increasingly intrusive colonial, national, and global forces.

Contending that medical systems are historically situated, locally practiced, and dynamically changing, Leslie was intrigued by the interplay and
negotiations among "traditional" and "modern," or "endogenous" and
"exogenous" ideologies, practices, and sectors in contemporary Asian
medical systems. Like those of many anthropologists and historians
working in the maritime and overland crossroads of Asia, his observations about competing medical paradigms interfacing within particular
medical systems prefigured later developments in critical studies, world
systems theories, and colonial and postcolonial studies. These theoretical
orientations expanded the purview of interpretive analyses by reincorporating into ethnographic research the global, historical, political, and
economic frameworks informing local clinical interactions.

My research enters this trajectory within medical anthropology by
asking, in particular, how and why indigenous peoples who are grappling
with the physical, psychological, and social consequences of nation-state
formation call upon technologies of healing engaging the spirit world.[1]
While I indicate the ways in which Temiar "ritual curing" is directed
toward individual healings, I focus in this article upon the ways in which
the transformative effects of "ritual curing" are directed toward mitigating
the effects of colonialism and postcolonialism experienced by Temiars.

The shocks of modernity

Preparing to depart after my first two years in the rainforest of peninsular Malaysia nearly twenty years ago, I was called before major spirit
mediums from each village. The river I followed, the Nenggiri and its trib-
utaries, flowed from highland Temiar villages to lowland peasant Malay
dwellings, then on into the towns and cities of Kelantan before emptying
into the oceans of Malaysia's east coast. For Temiars, this trajectory, from
upstream jungle (beek) to downstream market (kəday), links two ends of
a continuum within which they carve their homelands (deek).

In village after village, mediums blew into my head soul and heart soul,
shaping that miniature image of the self that dwells somewhat unsteadily
(in semi-sedentary hunter-horticulturalist fashion, perhaps?) in the fontan-
elle. "I tend it like we pat and shape the earth around a young plant
shoot," one medium explained his gentle manipulations, "and blow in the
spirit's cooling liquid to strengthen you for the assaults to come." "You've
changed now," another commented, "you've tranced and danced with
us, and it's dangerous, rumbling and roaring, out there." Careful hosts
they'd been throughout my stay, they were preparing me for the next set
of unexpected dangers into which I, naïve and exploratory neophyte, was
about to careen. I set on downstream toward the shocks of the ever-closer
marketplace.

As I moved downstream, I left the domain of the "forest peoples"

(sɛnʔɔɔy sɛnrok) and entered that of "those from beyond the forest" (gɔb).
Temiar horticulturalists and hunter-gatherers have long interacted with
those from beyond the forest, particularly gɔb *melayu*, the people now
known as Malays, the dominant population of the Malaysian nation-state,
who began arriving on the coasts and moving inland about 2,000 years
ago. Through networks of exchange, the various influences criss-crossing
Southeast Asia from India, China, the Middle East in the first though four-
teenth centuries A.D. reached into and flowed from the forests. Yet even
through the early colonial period, Temiars could withdraw farther into their
refuge in the forest, cultivating certain interactions while fleeing others.

In the 1930s, however, Temiar lands finally entered the colonial records
of the gɔb puteh, the "white foreigners," as the highland forest was
inscribed on British colonial administrator H. D. Noone's map of the
Perak-Kelantan watershed. Temiars engaged and mourned the encroach-
ment of both lowland Malay peasants and British administrators on their
forests and ricefields in the song genre cincɛm.[2] Land "ownership," newly
circumscribed in British land maps and deeds, was contested by Temiars,
who inscribed their own dream song maps in performance.

Temiar headman and spirit medium Tok Ngah Bintang dreamt a
marauding elephant robbed his rice fields.[3] "Why do you steal the fruits
of my muscle's labor?" Ngah Bintang pleaded. "Well, then, I shall stop,
and give you a song instead, as a sign of our relationship," the elephant
replied. The elephant, followed in another dream by Ngah Bintang's
recently deceased younger sister, gave him the genre *cincɛm*, with a specific
melodic contour, style of vocal delivery, dance steps, leaf ornaments, and
fragrances. *Cincɛm* is known for song phrases in which vocables are melis-
matically elongated across a descending melodic contour, iconic with a
wail: of loss of land and its ecologically interdependent social universe.
The genre *cincɛm* and practices associated with it sparked a revitalization movement of sorts that helped Temiars maintain their cultural
integrity as they strove to "make sense" out of and adapt to geopolitical
and socioeconomic changes.

In Temiar history, the quintessential mark of a new "life"-style period
began with the Japanese Occupation of Malaysia during World War II
and the subsequent Emergency of 1948–1965. Contemporary Temiars peri-
odize world history in two segments. "The old days", "the peaceful times"
(manaʔ ʔanin) precede the rupture of 1941, when their jungle refuge
suddenly became the scene of flights, fights, and bombs. At great cost to
life and livelihood, these bombs, too, have been encompassed within the
rhythm of life in Temiar ceremonies. In a dream song received from an
airplane spirit, Busu Ngah sings: "I alight/bomb, bomb, bomb [trailing
behind] me/ ... Flying across from the country of Japan/ ... In which
houses shall I descend?/ ... I am a Siamese boss/I am a Japanese boss/We
ask your blessings/Bomb, bomb, bomb, to me here/. ..."[4]

The Austroasiatic-speaking Temiars, now numbering approximately 13,000, are one cultural and linguistic group among the 60,000 Orang Asli or "aboriginal peoples" of peninsular Malaysia. The Orang Asli constitute a miniscule proportion, less than one per cent, of Malaysia's population of 17.9 million, of whom 55 per cent are Malays, 33 per cent Chinese, and 10 per cent Indians, primarily Tamils. When such indigenous peoples are incorporated into colony, nation-state, and global economy, their "economic integration" – the term preferred by Malaysian government policy-makers – usually means dislocation and deterritorialization.

If, as sensorial anthropology, medical anthropology, and dance ethnology suggest, cultural meanings are encoded, embodied, and negotiated through sensory experience and techniques of the body, then sociocultural changes must also be. What, then, of the radical changes experienced by indigenous peoples from the colonial period onward? Ecological disruption, resource loss, changes in health status and medical protocol, commodity imports, mechanization, and urbanization assault and excite the senses of aboriginal peoples like the Orang Asli of Malaysia who, increasingly, have limited economic options or geographic terrain in which to take refuge.[5] Here, I examine how modernity is experienced at the site of the body. What does it mean to transcend different spaces and climates and rhythms of life? What can medical and sensorial anthropology contribute to our understandings of social change, culture contact, and globalization? Might sensorial and medical anthropology provide knowledge bases to support critical and political interventions by indigenous activists?

To address these questions, I investigate how Temiars strategically apply ethnotheories of sensory adaptation and response, illness prevention, and therapeutic intervention to negotiate the shifting landscape of modernity.[6] Temiars recognize multiple, detachable, and permeable soul substance in all entities. While these qualities are operative in daily life, they are capitalized upon during ceremonies. This ontological structuring of experience, the ground bass upon which everyday and ceremonial life are played out, is extended to their interactions with the peoples and things arriving into their world from "beyond the forest." In my inquiry, I move through a series of contexts that comprise not a continuum, but rather an interactive overlap of experiential realms. They range from those heightened presentations of self and society Milton Singer (1991) terms "cultural performance" (and Temiars, pɛhnɔɔh, "singing and trance-dancing ceremonies") to the equally rich, historically sedimented, customary activities of daily life that Bourdieu terms "habitus," and Temiars, ʔɛs-ʔis (everyday).

As we explore the phenomenology of experience through which Temiars negotiate sociocultural change, three rubrics help us enter the Temiars' sensory world: *rhythm, rapture, and rupture*.

Rhythm

What we might gloss the "rhythm of life" is embodied in the bamboo-tube stampers beating a continuous ostinato during Temiar singing and trance-dancing ceremonies. Like life's capricious flow, the rhythm of the bamboo tubes is hardly bland as it repeats: though organized in duple rhythmic units (divisible by two), it is nuanced in tempo, rhythmic configuration, and textural density, stopping and starting as dancers faint, suspended in the momentary "death" (kɛsbʉs) of trance. These night-time, house-bound events, ranging from two to ten hours long, usually begin about an hour after sundown and can continue until an hour after sunrise.

Singing and trance-dancing ceremonies are held for various purposes, including healing, preparation for or return from substantial travels, initiating or concluding the rice harvest, ending a mourning period, introducing a newly-received dream song, or merely celebrating and negotiating relations among human and spirit realms. Most members of a settlement, traditionally numbering about twenty to seventy-five people, participate in some fashion.[7] A predominantly female chorus responds to phrases sung by an initial singer, male or female, who has received a song from a spirit during dreams. Each chorus member holds two bamboo tubes, one short, one long, which she beats against a wooden post laid on the floor before the group (Figure 1).

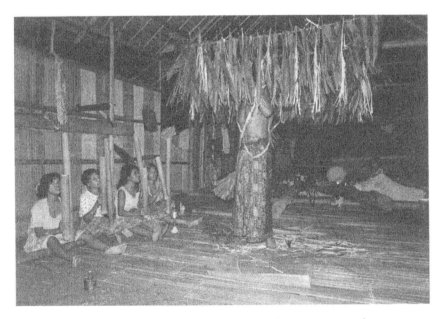

Figure 1 Women play pairs of bamboo-tube stampers during a singing and trance-dancing ceremony, while a medium sings and dances, surrounded by fragrant, shimmering leaf ornaments

Chorus members sit next to one another in a somewhat informal, haphazard fashion, legs alternately outstretched or curled up, children playing tubes while seated in their mothers' laps. The tube-players produce a duple rhythm, accentuated by drum and/or gong, alternating *HIGH-low, HIGH-low* in various rhythmic configurations and tempos. Translated into admittedly limited Western notational terms for purposes of scholarly communication, we might hear a rhythmic configuration of two high- and two low-pitched quarter notes, or two eighth-note highs and a quarter-note low, or two eighth-note highs and an eighth and two sixteenths low ... but always a duple rhythm.

The tube rhythm is both affected and effective, responding to and compelling changes in the dancers' level of trance intensity. As the trance deepens, the tube-players subdivide their rhythmic configurations and speed up the tempo. The resulting rhythmic intensification and densification is described spatio-temporally as having become "crowded." Temiars compare this rhythm – alternating high and low, changeable in pattern and tempo yet continuous – to rhythms of heartbeat and breath inhalation/exhalation. Heart and breath are categorically distinct at some levels, but conceptually conjoined as bodily "points of contact" with the world in their characteristic rhythmic alternations, and in the immediacy of their responsiveness to changing circumstances and emotions. Both are conjoined in the Temiar heart soul, seat of memory and stored emotion, one of four multiple and permeable components of self including head, shadow, and odor souls.[8]

The longer tube, producing the lower pitch, is engendered "male," and the shorter, higher-pitched tube "female." Steadily laboring to jointly produce the alternating rhythm, the bamboo-tubes' high and low pitches metaphorically link instrument construction and musical sound with gendered division of labor and geographic range. Explaining their musical terminology, Temiars point out that men, predominant in hunting, are said to go long distances, whereas women, predominant in gathering and hearth activities, travel shorter distances. The alternating sounds of the long, low-pitched tubes and the short, high-pitched tubes, linked in a system of distinctions, contrast yet interrelate male:female, expansiveness:constraint, and projective:concentric with the reciprocal division of labor. Symbolic economy at its best.

Men, traveling long distances through forested terrain, are thus said to have more access to those experiences that might generate spirit-guide relationships. Yet in typical Temiar play with stating and undermining difference during ceremony, a male singer during ritual performance is now constrained, "stuck-on-the-ground," needing the expansive perspective of a female spirit guide singing to and through him, and vice versa. So too, the duple rhythm that guides daily and ceremonial life receives pitch-differentiated but temporally equal contributions from "male" and "female" sound sources.

The steadily alternating *HIGH-low, HIGH-low* of the tube percussion creates, for Temiars, a sense of strolling along a path. Terms describing body motion in daily and ceremonial life, as well as internal sensations of alternated motion (the proprioceptive sensations of heart and breath pulse) reinforce this link. Several dance movements are compared to "strolling in place." As trance-dancing begins, a "sway" or gentle oscillation develops in dance movement, tube percussion, and motions of leaf ornaments worn and held as whisks by the dancers. Linguistic expressives[9] describing "sway" display, in themselves, reduplicative, oscillatory sound play: loŋɛt-loŋat, ləlaŋɔɔy, rəlawɛd.

The synesthetic realignment of sensory realms through the device of sonic, kinetic, and proprioceptive oscillation is best displayed by the movement of the bamboo floor during singing and trance-dancing ceremonies. Constructed from bamboo slats lashed together and suspended eight to ten feet above the ground, the floor oscillates with dancers' duple-rhythmed steps and hops. The sonic clack and motionary "give" of the bamboo slats bring even seemingly stationary, seated participants into the shared rhythmic oscillation of bamboo-tube percussion and swaying dancers' steps.

This iconicity across sensory realms leads us to ask whether synesthesia is the sensory correlate of metaphor. The associative series continues into the proprioceptive realm through symbolic and loosely biological entrainment. "It moves with my heart," a trancer comments on the commensuration of bamboo-tube percussion, swaying dance movements, sounds and movements of leaf whisks and body ornaments, clack and give of the bamboo floor.[10] "Exterior" object and "interior" sensation are increasingly experienced in dynamic interrelation as trancers move from rhythm toward *rapture*. But before we address "rapture," let us turn to the relationship between tube rhythm and song melody. For this, we must return to the path.

With its visual, sonic, kinetic, and olfactory density, the forest emits a complex and multilayered sensory presence. The path (nɔŋ), and travel upon it, becomes a potent image for a forest people. The concept – cognitive, sensory, emotional – of the path becomes an organizing principle as one orients oneself within the density of experience. Structuring the experience linguistic metaphors then render concrete with verbal labels, the process of negotiating paths through the dense forest generates what Lakoff and Johnson (1980) would call a "conceptual metaphor."

Health and well being involve knowing one's position along a path, whether during daily or ceremonial performance. This involves maintaining a temporally appropriate modicum of permeability and detachability during ceremonial performance: in short, being able to find one's way "home" at the conclusion of a ceremony. Illness is experienced as an enduring disintegration: being lost, disconnected, and displaced. This can be experienced as the displacement of an integral soul component, as when a patient's head soul becomes disengaged from the body, off somewhere in the jungle. Alternately, displacement can involve being entered by an intrusive entity, as when a person becomes ill by inadvertently picking up the trace of someone else's odor left behind. Health is regained through reorientation along the path and re-situation of disengaged or intrusive soul components during musical healing ceremonies.

Song itself is termed a "path", and choral response, "following the path". The alternating pitches of the bamboo tubes and the strolling footsteps of the dancers enact the rhythms – continual yet quixotic – of travel back and forward along a path. The singers' melody moves through three-dimensional space in the vertical, diagonal, and sagittal planes: up, down, and around. Temiars call on linguistic descriptors for traveling along footpaths and rivers – leveling, climbing, falling, winding, slipping out of visible range, angling across a hillside – to talk about melodic contour and vocal interaction. The melody, reflecting in stylistic parameters its spirit-guide source, describes the "shape" of the particular path as it leads up, down, around. The melody grafts the strangeness of encounter with new places and shapes onto the familiar alternation of the rhythmic stroll.[11]

The tubes set *and follow* the pace of experience. Rhythmic configurations, continuously duple in pitch and rhythm, change tempo and pattern in response to variations in genre, which in turn vary by spirit source chosen by the dream song singer. They respond, as well, to "rapture level:" what effort-shape[12] would analytically term the energy or effort motivating the dancers' movements. This, in turn, correlates with the current intensity of the relation between human body and spirit source.

And here, the possibility for *rapture* (lɛslããs "transformation") occurs. This is the realm of shimmer, shudder, and swirl.

Rapture

Shamanistic discourse and practice entangle the empirically observable with the magically real in a world of temporal, sensorial, and experiential overlap. Offering Temiars a space for the exploration of hybridity and multiplicity, trance and healing ceremonies interpolate self and alter, human and spirit. This experiential quality of shamanistic experience may explain its involvement, throughout the world, in situations where indigenous peoples are mediating the simultaneous yet differentiated, overlapped, and overlaid world of transnational communication and global economies.[13] Indeed, in Temiar dreams and trance, animated spirits of forest things like trees, rivers, flowers, tigers, as well as non-forester others – Malays, British, airplanes, canned sardines – participate. As spirit guides, they sing through the voices of mediums and dance with trancers.

"Shimmering" in the visual, kinetic, tactile, and auditory channels activates and consecrates these moments during ceremonial performances.

The glimmer of hearthfire lights on shredded leaves of ritual ornaments, in its quick-shifting presence and absence, disassembles the visual field. Shimmering things, combining movement and light, exist at the fuzzy boundary between the visual and the kinetic, disassembling distinct sensory fields, as well. Temiars say they don't just "see" the leaves shimmer, they *experience* a sympathetic shivering in their hearts.[14] They verbalize about this sensation, again using the reduplicative sonic play of "expressives:" pɛpəsõõy, sɛrsudɛɛr.

Sway and shudder "shimmer" in the kinetic realm. Recall the North American popular dance of the 1930s, the shimmy, resurging in 1960s rhythm n' blues: the 1930s flapper's dress fringe accentuated the shaking of the upper torso. So too, Temiar ceremonial leaf ornaments – worn as bandoliers and head wreaths, held as leaf whisks, or suspended from the building's rafters – accentuate sway and shudder. Beneath the shimmering leaves, dancers' movements progress from gentle sway into periodic shudders. The quickening and destablization of "shudder" (kɛnroʔ), marks the onset of deepened trance. "Whoa, she's transformed, gone into trance!"[15] onlookers grinningly observe to one another.

Dancers progress from sway to shudder, from graceful bending and strolling to a double-time, light-footed hopping in place. Female chorus members watch for dancers' shudders, speeding up their tempo and sub-dividing the tube-beat. Their stark, clear alternating duple rhythms *HIGH-low, HIGH-low*, become increasingly dense (bə-ʔasil "crowded"), fuzzing the boundaries between sound and silence *HIGH-HIGH low-low, HIGH-HIGH low-low* in acoustic sympathy with the visual shimmer, kinetic shudder, and experiential shiver. Oscillatory sway quickens to a wobble in these climactic moments of ritual performance.

Trance-dancers and mediums report they move from a position of relatively distinct subject-object relations into an experience they describe as a dizzying sensation of internal (and often, through intensified bending and swaying movements, external) "swirling." In movement, sound, and inner sensation, they move ever more deeply into a world beyond binary opposition. Later, slowly reawakening to the world of distinctions, dancers or mediums are said to return to their "true eyes" or to "think again."[16] As dancers sit, resting, at the edge of the dance space, fellow participants welcome them back "home" with hand-rolled tobacco cigarettes and a chuckle or light banter. Trance-dancers progress through such cycles of increasing then decreasing intensity throughout the night, though climactic moments tend to be concentrated in the second third of the event.

Temiars employ a variety of sensate tools that "beg the difference" between binary oppositions to support this experiential progression. The densified bamboo-tube rhythm begs the difference between sound and silence. Vocally, tremolo, or vibrato, blurs distinctions between one tone and another. Melismatic treatments of song syllables, as well as melodic contours, wind and tug like a river or swirl like a whirlpool. The glint of shredded leaves and flickering firelight beg the difference between light and darkness, while trancers tremble between one bodily position and another.

An ambient, continual, duple pulsation of cicadas, barbets, and tree frogs fills the forest with palpable presence, varying in composition and intensity throughout the day and night. This is the sound most audible immediately prior to ceremonial performance; and when the musicians set down their tubes and the dancers cease, the pulsation of the forest rises again to audible awareness. This sound shape is iconically replicated in the bamboo-tube rhythms. As a musical sign produced during ceremonies, it becomes the connective tissue interweaving body rhythms with forest environment through the medium of spirit energy. "Internal" heartbeat and "external" forest sounds are linked in the pulse of the bamboo tubes. In ceremony, Temiars participate in their "musecological" (Keil and Feld 1994) biosphere through the agency of this pulsation, mirrored in the bamboo tube rhythm, recoiling in dance sways and strolls, refracted in the heightened sensory awareness of pulsing heartbeat and breath.[17] Body motions and rhythms are experienced as commensurate with rhythmic forest sounds. Boundaries between inner and outer, self and alter, human and enspirited environment interpolate.

The human realm conjoins with that of forest (and other) spirits, male with female, exterior with interior, self with alter, in a space beyond opposition. Victor Turner (1969) might have deemed this the antistructural ritual moment of "communitas." Yet, unlike his melded vision of communitas, this is not, for Temiars, a realm of homogeneity, nor static harmony. Rather, its dynamism resembles the interactive overlap of lead singer and choral response in song, or the alternating, continual yet quixotic rhythm of the bamboo tubes. Here, in a relatively safe moment ritually bounded in place and time, the cosmos is recognized at its most detachable and porous, multiple yet integrated.

The continual rhythm of the bamboo tubes is intriguing here, for it sets up the possibility for both repetition and *différance*, in the Derridean sense of both "different" and "deferred," that is, with a time-lag (Derrida 1968/1982). In another theoretical language, repetition and *différance* are read as mimesis and alterity (see W. Benjamin 1968a, 1968b; Taussig1993; Stoller 1994). Whichever theoretical language is used, the dynamic tension between original and duplicate destabilizes the firmament upholding the making of meaning or "sense." The repetition of the original can never be identical with, yet seems so similar to the original; the slippage created in the act of repetition produces a destabilizing "lack" in the integrity of the original and the authenticity of the duplicate, even while their presence is being reiterated. In repetition, crucible of similarity and difference, Benjamin bemoans the loss of "aura" through modernity's mechanical reproduction, Taussig explores the magical tension of colonizers' reduplications of the colonized, Freud examines the power of repression and its expression, while shamans and mediums mine a technology for moving spirit through the world.[18]

As each duple pair of beats follows another, the tubes move forward in time, and the footpath traveler/dancer, in space. Each repeated beat defers to (and differs from) that which preceded it, while deferring to that which will follow (Figure 2). Temiars musically create what Bhabha identifies as the "future anterior" (or "projective past"): the time-lag in which past, present, and future are interlayered (1994a: 254). Bhabha commends this tense as a temporal metaphor for our globally interlayered times (. . . spaces, places, and peoples). Hybridization, Bhabha posits, results from the rearticulation of ideas, narratives, theories – or, we might add, of sounds, sights, odors, presences – in a different context. He identifies this temporal mode of repetition and reinscription , this "*aporetic coexistence*, within the cultural history of the *modern* imagined community, of both the dynastic, hierarchical, prefigurative "medieval" traditions (the past), and the secular, homogeneous, synchronous cross-time of modernity," as the hybridity of the colonial space (1994a: 250).

Interestingly, even Bhabha recognizes the spirit world as a place where past, present, and future coil in sensible insensibility. He finds his clearest

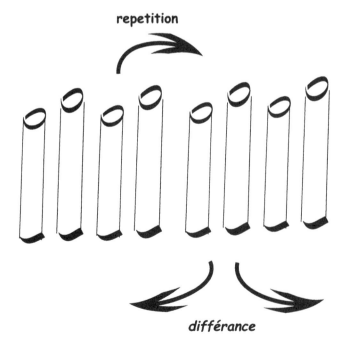

Figure 2 Repetition and *différance* in the bamboo-tube stampers

example of the future anterior in Toni Morrison's (1987) *Beloved* child borne in slavery, sacrificed in infanticide, who becomes a spirit presence guiding her mother's life: unborn-child-as-ancestor, what might have been come to be. This is the projective past, the time-lag overlay of the future anterior.

The act of repeating or mirroring highlights the disjuncture between what is shared (mimesis) and what differs (alterity). The sense of sameness yet *différance*, embodied in the repetition and alteration of the continual tube beats, sets the stage sensorily for heightened relationships between familiarity and strangeness. These are established as the song "path" moves through old (repeatedly visited) yet new (always encountered differently) territory. This space is performatively constructed not only through the tube-beats' relationships to one another, but through the relationship between constantly duple-rhythmed percussion, on one hand, and changing melodies, on the other. It is here, in this interlayered space-time of the "spirit" world, of energies reconfigured, that Temiars comingle with their alters, whether forest, settlement, or foreign, from beyond-the-forest.

Diasporic "time out of place" (Senders and Stewart 1999) finds its correlate in the skewed temporalities of religious experience. As Marjorie Balzer (1999b: 1–2) reminds us, "One of the hallmarks of . . . shamanic thinking is the confounding of space and time." Studying the cultural manipulations of ritual media such as sound, light, and movement, as we do by exploring Temiar sensibilities, helps us understand how space and time are structurally ordered and strategically confounded in healing and other rituals.

In order to understand how ritual language contributed to that confusion, Malinowski (1935/1978, Vol. 2: 218–223) explored the strategic application of "nonsense," which he called the "coefficient of weirdness" in the language of Trobriand garden magic. Briggs (1996) extends this linguistic analysis of the "sense of nonsense" in his study of vocables chanted during Warao curative spirit seances in Venezuela's Amazon. He carefully analyzes dramatic cues interspersed throughout the ritual in the form of *dynamic*, *timbral*, and *tempo* changes in rattle sounds and vocalizations. By widening the parameters of his study to include these qualities of sound, Briggs illuminates the "sense" within the "nonsense."

The power of sound, light, and movement to *create and confuse* order clarifies how and why such media are called into play, whether by Temiar healers or MTV videographers, to grapple with the "time out of place" of (neo)colonialism and postmodernity. Temiar ontology and epistemology exhibit a level of recognition and comfort with the space beyond binary opposition that I find fascinating, especially given the time it has taken EuroAmerican philosophers of meaning and experience to evolve comparably suitable constructs. Barthes intuits this space with his discussion of that which is "outside" (but always contextualizing our reading of) the sentence. For Barthes, it is the brushing up of that which is outside with that which is inside the sentence that constitutes the moment of bliss or rapture in the text. Spivak searches for this space in her catachrestic elaboration of Derrida's *tout autre* (the "wholly Other"), while Bhabha locates it in the concepts of "future anterior" and hybridity.[19] For Temiars, it is the moment when the singing medium's heart moves "elsewhere", "to the other side" (hʉp ʔɛh tuuy), while the animated spirit of the Other sings through the medium. Embodying that which is beyond the body, Temiars' theories of interpolated difference compel us to incorporate non-Eurocentric paradigms not just as grist for the ethnographic mill, but as conceptual models that can be "good to theorize with."[20]

Rupture

But danger lurks in the swirl and whoosh of the river. Within rapture resides the possibility for ***rupture***. Experienced as "shock" or "startle," Temiar rupture is that moment when meanings become unbridgeably disjunct from those entities that anchor them in the "real" world. Head-souls separate from the body – not in the momentary safety of trance or dreams, but lost without return: illness as dis-integration. That slippage, Derridean theories of meaning so poignantly remind us, looms constantly, thinly shrouded by fruitless attempts to comfort ourselves with the reality of our categorical distinctions.

Rupture is experienced in daily life in several ways. First, as excessively blurred distinctions: the dizzying swirl (lɛŋwĩĩŋ), as when clothes during washing are grabbed by the river current and whisked (bar-wɛ̃jwɛ̃j) beyond sight or touch. In ceremony, this is the moment when spirit becomes embodied within self. Swirling's excessive danger is enshrined in the song genre *səlombaŋ*, received during peninsular Malaysia's floods of 1926 from the Temiar version of the Indic *naga*, the waterserpent who whips up whirlpools and storms.[21]

Secondly, as excessively vivid distinctions: rupture arrives in the spatio-temporal sensation of abrupt and unexpected differentiation. The torsion created by interrupted rhythm is expressed and sensed visually, acoustically, kinetically, and/or spatio-temporally. In the visual-kinetic realm, Temiars sense shimmer's danger in its wavering which, ungoverned, might set the cosmos in motion at inappropriate times or places. Flashing and glittering items like mirrors, trees with white trunks, or the anthropologist's glossy paper are handled carefully during potentially dangerous periods such as illness, prior to ceremonies, or when working in clearings where refracting light might attract the attention of the thunder deities.[22]

Shock or startle, so important throughout Southeast Asia, is heavily researched in the "culture-bound" syndrome of *latah* among Malays (Simons 1980). For Temiars, it is experienced as the suddenly strange uncushioned by the familiarity of the continuous, a break in the continuity of heartbeat, breath, motion. The sudden change from silence to sound, dark to light, soft to loud, sway to lurch, far to close, odorless or fragrantly pungent to smelly, pungent, or rancid. The flash of lightning, the clap of thunder, the dog's sudden bark during a trancing ritual. The tiger's pounce, the snake bite, the boat overturned. A gun shot intensified by surrounding hills; a bumpy jeep ride on a rutted logging road. A loud angry voice; the jerky motions of anger; the disruption of sound, space, and social cohesion that anger constitutes for Temiars. Threshing rice like those (according to Temiars) "violent" slave-raiding, land-grabbing lowland Malays, who beat the stalks to separate grain from shaft rather than separating grain from shaft by a subtler, sinuous, continuous twisting motion of the feet, as Temiars do.[23] To experience any of these might precipitate "startle," frightening soul-components to eject from the body, causing illness. However, preventative measures, as well as therapeutic responses, exist.

It is here, in "startle," that we can begin to comprehend some of the ways Temiars have grafted the experience of modernity onto an indigenous cosmology and into a cultural logic or embodied in their system of sensory modalities, i.e., their sensorium. Though they recognize the potential for "startle" in their natural and social world, Temiars often expressed their amazement at "marketplace" or urban culture, which seems, to them, to be set on startle, like one might set a radio on a particular station. Reveling in the blaze and glory, living amidst neon flashing, music barking from radio speakers, cars rumbling and jumbling their inhabitants, out-foresters seem, to Temiars, to be hooked on startle.[24]

Enter, then, modernity, with a crunch and a roar. Temiars draft both everyday and ceremonial techniques to engage the shocks of modernity. You can see it in the shaping and strengthening of a traveler's head and heart-soul as he departs for the city, or even for just a ride from one village to another on a rumbling Land Rover. And in the purification with smoke of goods brought home, whether from marketplace or jungle. Through such acts, Temiars prepare their multiple self-components for the onslaught of startle, or cleanse themselves from intrusive disembodied soul-components travelers might have carried home.

Temiars employ their elaborate sensorium, with its preventive and therapeutic mechanisms for negotiating bodily points of contact with and immersion within its surroundings, like a cultural shield. And in those self-consciously heightened artifacts (or social facts) of cultural performance, Temiars contrive their dance of survival, choreographing "startle", then smoothing the break. Indeed, the "break-beat" in rap and breakdance, hallmark of an urban African-American music and dance form, would epitomize, for Temiars, the moment of shock or startle. Tricia Rose (1994: 38–39, 62–74), Cheryl Keyes (1996: 236–241), and others have written insightfully on the development of musical, technological, and choreographic "breaks" in hip hop as a performative and expressive response to the ruptures daily bridged by urban improvisational lifestyles in the inner city.

In Temiar ceremonies, this is the moment of kɛnrok, when trancers "shudder" as tube players intensify their rhythms. At this point, in genres such as the Annual Fruit Tree, a trancer may suddenly faint, falling to the floor near tube-players who scurry backwards to safety, momentarily disrupting both beat and choral response. Moving forward again, giggling, wise-cracking, complaining, they re-establish the rhythm of life and the responsive dialogue of song, resuming their tube-playing and choral response.[25]

It should come as no surprise, then, that spirit mediums and dream song singers – masters of realms of rhythm, rapture, and rupture – become conduits for mediating (post)modern social transformations. Nor should it be surprising that landscape spirits, compass points for a people dislocated, are often the compositional sources for songs that both anchor and transport Temiars. As Temiar singing and trance-dancing ceremonies progress from evenly pulsing rhythm to the swirl of rapture through the shock of rupture to rhythm restored, a patient is brought forward to be moved from illness to health. If strong enough, the sufferer is invited to sit or lie beneath the central hanging leaf ornament (tənamu? < Malay, *tamu* "guest"), where spirits first alight upon entry into the human realm. Here, in this space of difference stated and undermined, a medium sings and ministrates to a patient, withdrawing an intrusive component or returning a lost head-soul, infusing the patient with the cool, strengthening liquid that flows from spirits along with their songs. Other participants benefit from what also constitutes a Temiar version of preventive medicine. "If I go too long without a ceremony," Balɛh Biba of Belau observes, "I don't feel right. I must sing, dance, greet the spirits. And then I come home."

Healing the wounds of modernity

Through rupture, as it relates to rhythm and rapture, Temiars actively "make sense" out of schisms in everyday forest and community life. Increasingly, they use this space to manipulate the effects of forces of modernity and postmodernity, even as crushingly hegemonic as they manifest in today's fast-disappearing rainforest refuges.

Nineteenth-century Romantic painters, poets, and composers in Europe responded through their arts as they sought to come to terms with industrialization and urbanization: the noise, air, and water pollution; rural migration into densely populated urban spaces; the radically reorganized social and geographic landscapes. So too, in dream songs and spirit ceremonies, Temiars artfully craft both preventive medicine and therapeutic response. Singing and trance-dancing sessions constitute a place where the drama of permeability, porosity, and boundaries – multiplicity, disintegration, and reintegration – is enacted and social commentary phrased. Where better to grapple with the shocking impacts of colonial and neocolonial incursions?

Dancing on the edge of the gap where distinctions swirl, Temiars encounter and mediate the disembodied spirits of people, things, and places that surround them. I use "mediate" here deliberately, both in terms of communicative conduit and broadcast transmittal. For spirit mediums are the public broadcast networks of their communities. Negotiators of public policy and community interaction, they also mediate by bringing disparate factions into communication, both human and nonhuman. Like lightning rods, spirit mediums conduct and ground potentially startling energies. Songs received from the Motorboat Spirit, the Canned Sardine spirit, the Wristwatch Spirit, join with those from the spirits of the annual fruiting trees, the riverbend, the Cempakah flower, to bring knowledge and healing power into the community. Spiritualizing entities of both forest and marketplace, in a paradox of adaptation and resistance, Temiar mediums and dream song singers expropriate power and knowledge from the commodities that simultaneously link them ever more securely into the lowest social classes of mercantile and postindustrial capitalism.

Writing in the early decades of the twentieth century, Walter Benjamin saw both tragic decay and celebratory potential in the literary shift from epic storyteller to modern novel. This change, he posited, was paralleled in the differences between the private, segmented architecture of the Germanic home, on the one hand, and, on the other, the strange urban structures presaged in the city of Naples. The turn toward modernity was typified, he believed, in the architecture and social geography of the glass and steel Paris Arcade, with its sudden twists and turns, involutions and evolutions, cul-de-sacs that become vistas, home to the voyeuristic consumer, the strolling *flaneur*.[26] For Benjamin, these new structures, porous and multifaceted, packed the "shock" of modernity in all its horror and its glory.

Temiars, too, appreciate the horror and the glories of the new: the female medium Lopa Along refuses to ride in a Land Rover, though her sons regularly trek from Kelantan highlands to lowland frontier towns on motorcycles, in four-wheel drives, and on logging trucks. Yet, with trepidation – that shudder, of dread? of excitement? – Lopa Along's sons still request a spirit medium's ministrations to strengthen their head and heart-souls, in and out of ceremony, before, during, or after travel. A trepidation we can, perhaps, appreciate, standing at the edge of a new millennium.

Temiars use sensorial processes to get a grip on social life and change. But we must not forget that a sensorium, an embodied cultural disposition experienced through sensory modalities, is imperfectly shared by a social group. It is shared enough to be implicitly co-recognized, among those who identify themselves as Temiars, as part of what *makes* them

Temiars. Yet it is differentiated by the *heterogeneity* that also constitutes culture: by differences in age-grade, gender, class, personal-biographical experience, or sensory "intelligence level." These differences in social and individual responsivity apply both to sensory stimuli and interpretive schema. To rephrase Bakhtin, "each sensing is half my own:" we share some measure of sensory experience and sensibility as members of a society in communication, but we each have our own particular "take" on the intersubjective communicative exchange.

Recall Lopa Along, who will not ride in a motor vehicle, and her sons, who make their livelihoods doing so. Skilled negotiators of muddy footpaths, Temiars transfer their sensory knowledge and skills to driving motorcycles, Land Rovers, and trucks, responding with exquisite dexterity and timing to mud-caked ruts in weatherbeaten logging roads, their hands computing information from tires to feet to brake to tires at lightning speeds. Transnational slaves to the dictates of logging-road builders, Temiar men have become masters of road travel. But lest such nimble aesthetic and sensory adaptations deployed by young Temiar men be employed by policy makers, as they most certainly will be, to legitimize Temiar disenfranchisement and deterritorialization – since, in international-and-government-policy-speak, "The Temiar [sic] will of course adapt and survive as they always have" – let me reiterate here that the choices and definitions of what constitutes loss or gain, or whether roads should even exist there to be adapted to, should ultimately be theirs. These are real people, facing real life changes and hardships.

Ethnohistory, medical anthropology, and sensory anthropology can supply a corrective for those approaches that, while reincorporating so-called marginalized peoples into the world system, render them passively adrift in the wake of colonial and neocolonial hegemony.[27] Yet, real global forces with vested interests are moving indigenous peoples out of their homes and cutting down their forests at a speed no hunter-gatherer or horticulturalist ever imagined possible. We must not lose our grounding in the exigencies of global labor and the social consequences of material forces, even as we tip the theoretical balance to recognize the material effects of representational practices.

Attention to sensorial processes helps us keep it real: the effects of industrialization and modernization are felt in the body, both individual and body politic, as Marx himself noted and the histories of capitalist, socialist, and communist social formations have shown.[28] Medical anthropology struggles to theoretically situate relationships between human agency and biological imperatives in the constitution of illness. So too, historical anthropology and postcolonial studies strive toward a theoretical approach that will dissolve "the division between synchrony and diachrony, ethnography and historiography; that refuses to separate cultural from political economy, insisting instead on the simultaneity of the meaningful and the material in all things; that acknowledges – no stresses – the brute realities of colonialism and its aftermath without assuming that they have robbed [indigenous] peoples of their capacity to act on the world" (Comaroff and Comaroff 1993: xiv). The anthropology of the senses and the body, medical anthropology, and performance studies enable us to move into microanalytical realms of study. But they become powerful critical apparatuses for us only if we do not ignore the macrosocial forces that real people mediate.

Making sense out of injustice is not easy. Nor is making sense out of misfortune. The consequences of both are deeply experienced in the physical, social, and lived body: as lives and livelihoods lost, pain and disability, lands and resources expropriated, social relations disrupted, expectations unfulfilled, intentions thwarted. Medical and religious systems – taking shape at the nexus where humans grapple with their capacity to confront the resistance of the world – marshal the empirical and imaginative resources of a people toward surviving, mitigating, or at least comprehending such powerful forces in their lives. Temiars, faced with the shocks of an ever more persistent presence of modernity in their lives, craft their dance of survival in the context of spirit rituals that have often been called into play when human agency, alone, seems insufficient to mediate among self, society, and cosmos.

"How is illness inserted into life," Good (1994: 167) queries, "and why does it so often serve as the source of a society's reflections about the ultimate nature of reality and about what matters most in life?" The Temiar world is one in which the constituting of self and community is based on a never-ending dialectical incorporation of that which is outside, be it spirits, other humans, neighboring forest peoples, non-foresters, or colonials. This process of dialectical incorporation, negotiated in sound and motion, destablizes and decenters as much as it controls and contains.[29] Here – during dreams and healing rituals when that which is Other is brought, through song and movement, into the realm of human sensibility and agency – Temiars deal with the disintegrations of both "illness" and "sociocultural change," both experienced dramatically at the site of the body. Submerging us in the specificities of Temiar ritual curing – in rhythm, rapture, and rupture; shimmer, shudder, and swirl – I suggest an avenue for investigating how Temiars craft a distinctive alternate modernity as they negotiate the junctures and disjunctures of self and other, forest and foreigner.

Acknowledgments

Research among the Temiars has benefitted from support by the Social Science Research Foundation (1981–82, 1994–95); Asian Cultural Council (1995, 1997–99); Wenner Gren Foundation for Anthropological Research

(1981, Grant No. 4064); National Science Foundation (1981, BNS81–02784); Research Foundation of the University of Pennsylvania (1991, 1992); Dean's Faculty Research Fellowship, School of Arts and Sciences, University of Pennsylvania (1994–95); with additional travel funds provided by Universiti Sains Malaysia and Malaysian Air Lines (1991). Analysis and writing were furthered by a Guggenheim Foundation Fellowship (1996–97), Professional-in-Residence Fellowship from the Annenberg School for Communications at the University of Pennsylvania (1996–97), and a Research Fellowship from the National Endowment for the Humanities (2000). My gratitude to these organizations; to my sponsors at Universiti Malaya, Cultural Centre; Universiti Kebangsaan Malaysia; and Muzium Negara (National Museum, Kuala Lumpur); and to my numerous Temiar and Malay hosts and colleagues.

This paper was first presented at the panel, "Sensorial Anthropology: Ontological and Epistemological Inquiries," organized by Kathryn Linn Geurts and Ernst Long for the 98th Annual Meetings of the American Anthropological Association (Chicago, 1999). Discussions with panelists furthered its development, as did conversations with graduate students in my seminar on Postcolonialism and Ethnomusicology, University of Maryland, College Park, Fall 1999.

Notes

1 I employ "technologies" here as used by Teresa de Lauretis (in her discussion of technologies of gender), to encompass the multiply intersecting ideologies and practices, histories and performances, within which particular interpretations and acts of healing are embedded.

2 Roseman 1998 details the history of this period; see also Roseman 1996, Geoffrey Benjamin 1996.

3 Tok Ngah Bintang's settlement in Perak, at that time, was in Simpak along the Kɛrbuu? (Malay, Korbu) and Kuwah rivers. The settlement later moved to Jalong, Lasah, Perak (Alang Uda, son of Ngah Bintang, personal communication, 1995).

4 For a transcription of this song, see Roseman 1996.

5 Dentan (1992) and Dentan and Williams-Hunt (1999) explore the consequences of loss of forest refuge as a buffer between forest peoples and those from "beyond the forest."

6 Medical anthropology has long addressed the history of change in medical systems (Porkert 1976; Unschuld 1985); negotiations between "traditional" and "modern" health care ideologies, practices, and sectors (Leslie 1976a; Jaspan 1976; Kleinman 1980; Leslie and Young 1992; Connor and Samuel 2000); (post)modernity and medicalization (Lock 1992); and the interface between political economy and epidemiology in industrialization, urbanization, modernization, and "development" (Nichter 1987, Packard 1989, Freund and McGuire 1999). In this article, attention to sensory experience (Howes 1991), performance and aesthetics (Roseman 1990, Good 1994: 166ff), and the culturally specific imagery and experience of embodiment (Csordas 1994) combine with analyses of the history and political economy of colonial and nation-state interaction with indigenous peoples of Malaysia (Benjamin, G. 1985; Dentan 1992;

Dentan et al. 1997; Roseman 1998; Nicholas 2000) to enrich this enterprise.

7 With ever-decreasing land areas reserved for their use in Malaysian Government Regroupment Programs (Rancangan Perkumpulan Semula), Temiars are unable to continue traditional population density control measures. Historically, these included a pattern of fissioning and re-fusing into new settlements. Currently, therefore, the number of inhabitants in a settlement may increase to between one hundred and five hundred. Temiars attempt to replicate their earlier settlement groupings, on far less land, as subsets within larger Government Regroupment Program designs. These "village" groupings constitute the mainstay of ceremonial gatherings. For further discussion of the history and consequences of government-sponsored resettlement programs and government appropriation of land and resources, see Dentan et al. 1997 and Nicholas 2000.

8 The terms for heart (hup) and breath (hinum) are both used to refer to the heart soul. See Roseman 1990 for further discussion of the four "souls" and their impact on Temiar constructions of emotion, self, and ritual performance.

9 See Diffloth (1976) on expressives in Austroasiatic languages.

10 In one recording I've collected, a Temiar jaws-harp player adds another layer of meta-communicative commentary in his solo composition replicating "floor sounds during ceremonies."

11 For culturally specific examples of visual-spatial-kinetic metaphors describing melody and other musical parameters, see Robertson (1976, 1979) on Mapuche *tayil*; Keil (1979: 181ff) on the Tiv; Feld (1981) on the Kaluli; Vander (1988: 68–69,78–81,128–129) on the Shoshone; Kemler (1999) on EuroAmerican concert music; and Ness (1992) on dance.

12 Effort-shape analysis developed within Laban notation to illustrate how the mover concentrates exertion or *effort* and how that effort takes *shape* as the body changes its relationship among its parts and to the surrounding space (Dell 1977).

13 See, for example, Ong 1987; Comaroff and Comaroff 1993; Mageo and Howard 1996; Kendall 1996; Roseman 1996; Proschan 1998; Balzer 1999a; Buenconsejo 1999; Laderman 2000.

14 The Temiar term for "shimmer" (bɛgyʉg, biyʉgp) identifies the color "white"; its extension to the quality of shimmer is through the reflective glare and glint Temiars sense in the color white.

15 Temiar, "Yah, hoj na-lããs!"

16 "True eyes" (Temiar, mad mʉn); to "think again" (Temiar, na-nim wɛl).

17 For a detailed analysis of the relationship between forest sounds and sounds of the bamboo tubes, see spectral analyses and discussion in Roseman 1990 and 1991: 168ff.

18 Freud (1914/1949) discusses repetition in the context of repression, its expression in repeated acts or symptoms, and the achievement of the goal of remembrance through the "conjuring into existence of a piece of real life" (ibid: 371) during analytic treatment. His comments are intriguing in the context of the alternation between "forgetting" (wɛlwəl) and "remembering" (na-nim) that are characteristic of Temiar trance, and the role of the bamboo-tube percussion's continual pulse in the trance experience (see also Roseman 1991: 151ff).

19 "Thus," Barthes writes, "what I enjoy in a narrative is not directly its content or even its structure, but rather the abrasions I impose upon the fine surface: I read on, I skip, I look up, I dip in again" (1975: 11). While Barthes poses an absolute distinction between the sentence and the "non-sentence," that which is "eternally, splendidly, outside the sentence" (ibid: 49), Bhabha (1994b: 180–182) develops Barthes' concept of the space "outside the sentence" into

a third term positioned in-between the sentence and the non-sentence. This space is, in one sense, outside the sentence, but it is also necessarily *inside* the sentence. In turn, Spivak employs Derrida's concept of the "wholly other" to suggest a position – beyond that of either the subject *or* the "self-consolidating other" – from whence the subaltern subject, perchance, might speak (1988/1994: 89). In a language oddly reminiscent of that in which Temiars verbalize about spirit mediums singing through them, she suggests that "Derrida does not invoke 'letting the other(s) speak for himself' but rather invokes an 'appeal' to or 'call' to the 'quite-other' (*tout-autre* as opposed to a self-consolidating other), of 'rendering *delirious* that interior voice that is the voice of the other in us'" (ibid.).

20 Gayatri Spivak's recent attempt to move beyond the Western theoretical language of English literary theory and Judeo-Christian philosophy to use the Hindu concept of *dharma*, Indic texts, and "Indic popular ethical performance" as a foundation for critical analysis and an "instrument of philosophizing" is a case in point. Hers is a politically and ethically, as well as theoretically, motivated choice (Danius and Jonsson 1993: 33–34; see also Moore-Gilbert 1997: 98).

21 On the Temiar spirit song genre səlombay, see Roseman 1991: 103–105. Bosch (1960) traces the role of the waterserpent *naga* (Temiar, daŋgah) in Indic theology and art; Sumet Chumsai (1988) charts the naga's influence in Southeast Asia.

22 The repercussions following the glint off a white log carried past a house where healing ceremonies were being held is recounted in Roseman 1991: 42–45.

23 Practices for cushioning the rice spirit against startle abound among the Malay peoples across Southeast Asia and among the ethnic minorities practicing shifting cultivation on the mainland (Endicott 1970: 23–24, 146ff, 167; Laderman 1991: 42; Tanaka 1991).

24 Temiars' perceptions concerning the city-dweller's seeming appetite for a high level of "startle" find concordance in chronicles of modern life such as James Gleick's (1999) *Faster: The Acceleration of Just About Everything*. Gleick interprets this prediliction toward what Temiars would term "startle" as the over-stimulated urban dweller's need for ever-higher levels of stimulation to initiate the pleasure of an adrenalin rush. The upsurge in tendencies to diagnose and chemically treat attention deficit disorder among urban school children and preschoolers is traced, in some quarters, to relationships between urban life, contemporary mediated forms, and long-term heightening of adrenalin levels. This brings increased urgency, so to speak, to the discussion of issues concerning post(neo)colonialism (or what Dentan, 1992, calls "internal colonialism" of the modern nation-state), indigenous peoples, violence, and adaptation (see Taussig 1992).

25 Rouget (1980) observes that syncopation, a momentary contradiction of the prevailing meter or pulse, is one of the musical characteristics often emphasized in that portion of a culture's musical repertoire used to prompt and accompany trance states. Such valued musical forms, he suggests, do not so much mechanically precipitate but rather "socialise trance" (1977), tapping into socially cued proclivities, marking contexts and moments appropriate for participating in trance behavior.

26 See Walter Benjamin (1968c) for his exploration of the consequences derived from storytelling's changing technologies. His reflections on the architecture in "Naples" (1996: 414–421) and "One Way Street" (1996: 444–448) prefigure his thirteen-year project on the Paris Arcades (1999).

27 In his "world system" study of the cosmologies of capitalism in the trans-Pacific sector, Sahlins (1994) urges a shift in Western orientations concerning the writing of history and the attribution of agency; see also Frank (1998).

28 See Marx 1903: 227ff, 391ff; also Scheper-Hughes and Lock 1987; Kleinman, Das, and Lock 1997.

29 Piot (1999: 23) argues similarly for the Kabre of Northern Togo. Noting that spirit communication is fraught with ambiguity and uncertainty, he contends that so-called "traditional" Kabre "villagers" are cosmopolitan, "if by cosmopolitanism we mean that people partake in a social life characterized by flux, uncertainty, encounters with difference, and the experience of processes of transculturation."

References

Appadurai, A. (1999). *Modernity at Large: Cultural Dimensions of Globalization.* Minneapolis: University of Minnesota Press.

Balzer, M.M. (1999a). *The Tenacity of Ethnicity: A Siberian Saga in Global Perspective.* Princeton: Princeton University Press.

—— (1999b). Bending Mind and Space: Shamanic Concepts of Time, Paper presented at the 98th Annual Meetings of the American Anthropological Association, Chicago, November 17–21, 1999.

Barthes, R. (1975). *The Pleasure of the Text.* New York: Farrar, Straus, & Giroux.

Benjamin, G. (1995). In the Long Term: Three Themes in Malayan Cultural Ecology. In *Cultural Values and Human Ecology in Southeast Asia*, edited by Karl L. Hutterer, A. Terry Rambo, and George Lovelace, pp. 219–278. Ann Arbor: Center for South and Southeast Asian Studies.

—— (1996). Rationalisation and Re-enchantment in Malaysia: Temiar Religion 1964–1995. Department of Sociology Working Papers No. 130. Singapore: Department of Sociology, National University of Singapore.

Benjamin, W. (1968a). The Task of the Translator: An Introduction to the Translation of Baudelaire's *Tableaux parisiens*. In *Illuminations: Walter Benjamin*, edited by Hannah Arendt; Harry Zohn, trans., pp. 69–82. New York: Schocken.

—— (1968b). The Work of Art in the Age of Mechanical Reproduction. In *Illuminations: Walter Benjamin*, edited by Hannah Arendt; Harry Zohn, transl., pp. 217–252. New York: Schocken.

—— (1968c). The Storyteller: Reflections on the Works of Nikolai Leskov. In *Illuminations: Walter Benjamin*, edited by Hannah Arendt; Harry Zohn, trans., pp. 83–110. New York: Schocken.

—— (1996). *Selected Writings, Volume 1: 1913–1926*, edited by Marcus Bullock and M.W. Jennings. Cambridge, MA: The Belknap Press of Harvard University Press.

—— (1999). *The Arcades Project*, edited by Rolf Tiedemann; Howard Eiland and Kevin McLaughlin, trans. Cambridge, Mass.: The Belknap Press of Harvard University Press.

Bhabha, H.K. (1994a). Conclusion: "Race", Time and the Revision of Modernity. In *The Location of Culture,* edited by Homi K. Bhabha, pp. 236–256. New York: Routledge.

—— (1994b). The Postcolonial and the Postmodern. In *The Location of Culture,* by Homi K. Bhabha, pp. 171–197. New York: Routledge.

Bosch, F., Kan, D. (1960). *The Golden Germ: An Introduction to Indian Symbolism.* 's Gravenhage, Netherlands: Mouton de Gruyter.

Briggs, C.L. (1996). The Meaning of Nonsense, the Poetics of Embodiment, and the Production of Power in Warao Healing. In *The Performance of Healing,* edited by Carol Laderman and Marina Roseman, pp. 185–232. New York: Routledge.

Buenconsejo, J.S. (1999). *Songs and Gifts at the Colonial Frontier: The Aesthetics of Agusan Manobo Spirit-Possession Ritual, Philippines.* Doctoral dissertation, University of Pennsylvania. Ann Arbor: University Microfilms.

Butler, J. (1990). *Gender Trouble.* New York: Routledge.

Comaroff, J. and Comaroff, J. (editors) (1993). *Modernity and its Malcontents: Ritual and Power in Postcolonial Africa.* Chicago: University of Chicago Press.

Connor, L.H. and Samuel, G. (editors) (2000). *Healing Powers and Modernity: Traditional Medicine, Shamanism, and Science in Asian Societies.* Westport, Connecticut: Greenwood Publishing Group.

Csordas, T.J. (1994a). *The Sacred Self: A Cultural Phenomenology of Charismatic Healing.* Berkeley, Los Angeles: University of California Press.

—— (1994b). Introduction: the body as representation and being-in-the-world. In *Embodiment and Experience: The Existential Ground of Culture and Self,* edited by Thomas Csordas, pp. 1–24. Cambridge: Cambridge University Press.

Danius, S. and Jonsson, S. (2000). An Interview with Gayatri Chakravorty Spivak. *boundary 2* 20(2): 24–50.

de Lauretis, T. (1987). *Technologies of Gender.* Bloomington, Indiana: Indiana University Press.

Dell, C. (1977). *A Primer for Movement Description: Using Effort-Shape and Supplementary Concepts.* New York: Dance Notation Bureau Press.

Dentan, R.K. (1992). The Rise, Maintenance, and Destruction of a Peaceable Polity: A Preliminary Essay in Political Ecology. In *Aggression and Peacefulness in Humans and Other Primates,* edited by J. Silverberg and J.P. Gray, pp. 214–270. New York and Oxford: Oxford University Press.

Dentan, R.K. and Williams-Hunt, Bah A. (1999). Untransfiguring Death: A Case Study of Rape, Drunkenness, Development and Homicide in an Apprehensive Void. *rima (Review of Indonesian and Malaysian Affairs)* 33(1): 17–65.

Dentan, R.K., Endicott, K., Gomes, A. and Hooker, M.B. (1997). *Malaysia and the "Original People": a Case Study of the Impact of Development on Indigenous Peoples.* Boston: Allyn & Bacon.

Derrida, J. (1968/1982). Différance. In *Margins of Philosophy* by J. Derrida, pp. 1–27. Alan Bass, trans. Chicago: University of Chicago Press.

Diffloth, G. (1976). Expressives in Semai. In *Austroasiatic Studies,* pt. 1, edited by Phillip N. Jenner et al., pp. 249–264. Honolulu: University of Hawaii Press.

Endicott, K. (1970). *An Analysis of Malay Magic.* New York, London: Oxford University Press.

Feld, S. (1981). "Flow like a Waterfall": the Metaphors of Kaluli Musical Theory. *Yearbook for Traditional Music* 13: 22–47.

——— (1990). *Sound and Sentiment: Birds, Weeping, Poetics, and Song in Kaluli Expression.* Philadelphia: University of Pennsylvania Press.

——— (1991). Sound as a Symbolic System: The Kaluli Drum. In *The Varieties of Sensory Experience: A Sourcebook in the Anthropology of the Senses*, edited by David Howes, pp. 79–99. Toronto: University of Toronto Press.

Frank, A.G. (1998). *ReOrient: Global Economy in the Asian Age.* Berkeley: Univeristy of California Press.

Freud, S. (1914/1949). Further Recommendations in the Technique of Psycho-Analysis: Recollection, Repetition and Working Through. In *Collected Papers*, by Sigmund Freud, vol. 2., pp. 366–376. Joan Riviere, trans. London: The Hogarth Press and the Institute of Psycho-Analysis.

Freund, P.E. and McGuire, M.B. (1999). *Health, Illness, and the Social Body: A Critical Sociology.* Upper Saddle River, New Jersey: Prentice Hall.

Geertz, C. (1973). *The Interpretation of Cultures.* New York: Basic Books.

Gleick, J. (1999). *Faster: The Acceleration of Just About Everything.* New York: Pantheon.

Good, B.J. (1994). *Medicine, rationality, and experience: an anthropological perspective.* Cambridge: Cambridge University Press.

Howes, D. (editor) (1991). *The Varieties of Sensory Experience: A Sourcebook in the Anthropology of the Senses.* Toronto: University of Toronto Press.

Jaspan, M. A. (1976). The Social Organization of Indigenous and Modern Medical Practices in Southwest Sumatra. In *Asian Medical Systems: A Comparative Study*, edited by Charles Leslie, pp. 227–242. Berkeley, Los Angeles: University of California Press.

Keil, C. (1979). *Tiv Song: The Sociology of Art in a Classless Society.* Chicago: University of Chicago Press.

Keil, C. and Feld, S. (1994). *Music Grooves.* Chicago: University of Chicago Press.

Kemler, D. (1999). A Play or a Feelingful Immersion? Dual Musical Event Structure Metaphors. Unpublished paper presented at the Conference on Musical Imagery, Oslo, Norway.

Kendall, L. (1996). Korean Shamans and the Spirit of Capitalism. *American Anthropologist.* 98(3): 512–527.

Keyes, C. (1996). At the Crossroads: Rap Music and Its African Nexus. *Ethnomusicology* 40(2): 223–248.

Kleinman, A. (1973). Medicine's Symbolic Reality: On the Central Problem in the Philosophy of Medicine. *Inquiry* 16: 206–213.

——— (1980). *Patients and Healers in the Context of Culture: an Exploration of the Borderland between Anthropology, Medicine, and Psychiatry.* Berkeley: University of California Press.

Kleinman, A., Kunstadter, P., Alexander, E. and Gale, J. (editors) (1976). *Medicine in Chinese Cultures: Comparative Studies of Health Care in Chinese and Other Societies.* Washington, DC: U.S. Government Printing Office for Fogerty International Center, National Institute of Health.

Kleinman, A., Das, V. and Lock, M. (editors) (1997). *Social Suffering.* Berkeley: University of California Press.

Laderman, C. (1991). *Taming the Wind of Desire: Psychology, Medicine, and Aesthetics in Malay Shamanistic Performance.* Berkeley: University of California Press.

—— (2000). Tradition and Change in Malay Healing. In *Healing Powers and Modernity: Traditional Medicine, Shamanism, and Science in Asian Societies*, edited by Linda H. Connor and Geoffrey Samuel, pp. 42–63. Westport, Connecticut: Greenwood Publishing Group.

Laderman, C. and van Esterik, P. (editors) (1988). *Techniques of Healing in Southeast Asia*. Special volume of *Social Science and Medicine* 27(7).

Laderman, C. and Roseman, M. (editors)(1996). *The Performance of Healing*. New York: Routledge.

Lakoff, G. and Johnson, M. (1980). *Metaphors We Live By*. Chicago: University of Chicago Press.

Leslie, C. (1976a). The Ambiguities of Medical Revivalism in Modern India. In *Asian Medical Systems: A Comparative Study*, edited by Charles Leslie, pp. 356–367. Berkeley, Los Angeles: University of California Press.

—— (1976b). Introduction. In *Asian Medical Systems: A Comparative Study*, edited by Charles Leslie, pp. 1–12. Berkeley, Los Angeles: University of California Press.

—— (1992). Interpretations of Illness: Syncretism in Modern Ayurveda. In *Paths to Asian Medical Knowledge*, edited by Charles Leslie and Allan Young, pp. 177–208. Berkeley: University of California Press.

Leslie, C. and Young, A. (1992). Introduction. In *Paths to Asian Medical Knowledge*, edited by Charles Leslie and Allan Young, pp. 1–18. Berkeley, Los Angeles: University of California Press.

Lock, M. (1992). The Fragile Japanese Family: Narratives about Individualism and the Postmodern State. In *Paths to Asian Medical Knowledge*, edited by Charles Leslie and Allan Young, pp. 98–125. Berkeley: University of California Press.

Mageo, J.M. and Howard, A. (editors) (1996). *Spirits in Culture, History, and Mind*. New York: Routledge.

Malinowski, B. (1935/1978). *Coral Gardens and their Magic: A Study of the Methods of Tilling the Soil and of Agricultural Rites in the Trobriand Islands* (In Two Volumes Bound as One). New York: Dover.

Marx, K. (1903). *Capital: A Critical Analysis of Capitalist Production*. London: Swan, Sonnenschein & Co.

Moore-Gilbert, B. (1997). *Postcolonial Theory: Contexts, Practices, Politics*. London: Verso.

Morrison, T. (1987). *Beloved: a novel*. New York: Knopf.

Ness, S.A. (1992). *Body, Movement, and Culture: Kinesthetic and Visual Symbolism in a Philippine Community*. Philadelphia: University of Pennsylvania.

Nicholas, C. (2000). *The Orang Asli and the Contest for Resources: Indigenous Politics, Development and Identity in Peninsular Malaysia*. Copenhagen, Denmark: International Work Group for Indigenous Affairs.

Nichter, M. (1987). Kyasanur Forest Disease: An Ethnography of a Disease of Development. *Medical Anthropology* 1 new series (4): 406–423.

Ohnuki-Tierney, E. (1981). *Illness and Healing among the Sakhalin Ainu: A Symbolic Interpretation*. London and New York: Cambridge University Press.

Ong, A. (1987). *Spirits of Resistance and Capitalist Discipline: Factory Women in Malaysia*. Albany: State University of New York Press.

Packard, R.M. (1989). *White Plague, Black Labor: Tuberculosis and the Political Economy of Health and Disease in South Africa.* Berkeley, Los Angeles: University of California Press.

Piot, C. (1999). *Remotely Global: Village Modernity in West Africa.* Chicago: University of Chicago Press.

Porkert, M. (1976). The Intellectual and Social Impulses Behind the Evolution of Traditional Chinese Medicine. In *Asian Medical Systems: A Comparative Study,* edited by Charles Leslie, pp. 63–76. Berkeley: University of California Press.

Proschan, F. (1998). Cheuang in Kmhmu Folklore, History, and Memory. In *Tamnan keokap thao hung thao chuang: miti thang prawattisat lae wattanatham [Proceedings of the First International Conference on the Literary, Historical, and Cultural Aspects of Thao Hung Thao Cheuang],* edited by Sumitr Pitiphat, pp. 174–209. Bangkok: Thammasat University, Thai Khadai Research Institute.

Robertson, C. (1976). *Tayil* as Category and Communication among the Argentine Mapuche. *Yearbook of the International Folk Music Council* (Now entitled *Yearbook for Traditional Music*) 8: 35–52.

—— (1979). "Pulling the Ancestors": Performance Practice and Praxis in Mapuche Ordering. *Ethnomusicology* 23(3): 395–416.

Rose, T. (1994). *Black Noise: Rap Music and Black Culture in Contemporary America.* Hanover, Connecticut: Wesleyan University Press.

Roseman, M. (1988). The Pragmatics of Aesthetics: The Performance of Healing among Senoi Temiar. *Social Science and Medicine* (guest editors, Carol Laderman and Peggy van Esterik) 27(7): 811–818.

—— (1990). Head, Heart, Odor and Shadow: The Structure of the Self, Ritual Performance and the Emotional World. *Ethos* 18(3): 227–250. [Reprinted in *The Meanings of Madness,* edited by Richard J. Castillo, pp. 45–55. Pacific Grove, California: Brookes/Cole, 1997.]

—— (1991). *Healing Sounds from the Malaysian Rainforest: Temiar Music and Medicine.* Los Angeles, Berkeley: University of California Press.

—— (1996). "Pure Products Go Crazy": Rainforest Healing in a Nation-state. In *The Performance of Healing,* edited by Carol Laderman and Marina Roseman, pp. 233–269. New York: Routledge.

—— (1998). Temiar Singers of the Landscape: Song, History, and Property Rights in the Malaysian Rainforest. *American Anthropologist* 100(1): 106–121.

Rouget, G. (1977). Music and Possession Trance. In *The Anthropology of the Body,* edited by John Blacking, pp. 233–239. ASA Monograph No. 15. London: Academic Press.

—— (1980). *Music and Trance.* Chicago: University of Chicago Press.

Sahlins, M. (1994). Cosmologies of Capitalism: The Trans-Pacific Sector of "The World System". In *Culture/Power/History,* edited by Nicholas Dirks et al., pp. 412–455. New York: Routledge.

Scheper-Hughes, N. and Lock, M. (1987). The Mindful Body: A Prolegomenon to Future Work in Medical Anthropology. *Medical Anthropology Quarterly* 1 n.s. (1): 6–41.

Senders, S. and Stewart, C. (1999). Time Out of Place: The Temporalities of Diaspora. Panel organized for the 98th Annual Meetings of the American Anthropological Association, Chicago, November 20.

140 Marina Roseman

Simons, R.C. (1980). The Resolution of the *Latah* Paradox. *Journal of Nervous and Mental Disease* 168: 195–206.

Singer, M. (1991). *Semiotics of Cities, Selves, and Cultures : Explorations in Semiotic Anthropology*. New York: Mouton de Gruyter.

Spivak, G.C. (1998/1994). Can the Subaltern Speak? In *Colonial Discourse and Post-Colonial Theory: A Reader*, edited by Patrick Williams and Laura Chrisman, pp. 66–111. New York: Columbia University Press.

Stoller, P. (1989). *The Taste of Ethnographic Things: The Senses in Anthropology*. Philadelphia: University of Pennsylvania Press.

—— (1994). *Embodying Colonial Memories: Spirit Possession, Power, and the Hauka in West Africa*. New York: Routledge.

Sumet, C. (1988). *Naga: Cultural Origins in Siam and the West Pacific*. With contributions by R. Buckminster Fuller. Singapore: Oxford University Press.

Tanaka, K. (1991). The Malayan-Type Rice Culture and its Distribution. *Southeast Asian Studies* 29(3): 306–382.

Taussig, M. (1992). *The Nervous System*. New York: Routledge.

—— (1993). *Mimesis and Alterity: A Particular History of the Senses*. New York: Routledge.

Turner, V. (1969). *The Ritual Process: Sturcture and Anti-Structure*. Ithaca, New York: Cornell University Press.

Unschuld, P. (1985). *Medicine in China: a History of Ideas*. Berkeley: University of California Press.

Vander, J. (1988). *Songprints: The Musical Experience of Five Shoshone Women*. Urbana: University of Illinois Press.

Chapter 6

A return to scientific racism in medical social sciences

The case of sexuality and the AIDS epidemic in Africa

Gilles Bibeau and Duncan Pedersen

In 1990, during his tenure as Medical Anthropology Editor for the journal *Social Science & Medicine*, Charles Leslie wrote, in the journal, of his outrage at a controversial article entitled "Population Differences in Susceptibility to AIDS: An Evolutionary Analysis" written by J. P. Rushton and A. F. Bogaert (1989). Leslie manifested his deep concern as to how a *faux pas* in scientific thinking, which carried obvious racist overtones, could possibly be published in this renowned and peer-reviewed international journal.[1]

Beyond the heated discussion and arguments that followed this publication, Leslie raised a more fundamental point: if such ambiguity and confusion of thought could actually prevail among medical and social scientists, then nothing could be challenged on scientific grounds. He further asked whether we, as a community of scientists, collectively subscribed to the naïve idea that direct linkages existed between social organization, sexual behavior, physical characteristics, and genetic programing. Leslie's main concern was why scientists involved in the peer-review process failed to recognize the inherently racist premises of the Rushton and Bogaert paper: "What appealed to these social scientists so that garbled biology and sociology appeared to be 'sufficiently respectable to merit publication,' and racism appeared to be 'reasoned argument'?" (Leslie 1990: 892). At various points in his rebuttal, Leslie seemed to agonize in trying to deconstruct the central issues step by step, a process he likened to ". . . trying to shovel manure from the barn with a teaspoon." He further stated: "Like the fundamentalists who clothe their religious cosmology in a scientific vocabulary, Rushton's agenda lies outside the work itself" (Leslie 1990: 894).[2]

In this essay we follow the path of deconstruction of the central issues that Leslie raises. We explore the connection between sexuality and culture and discuss different scientific approaches used to explain why certain sexually transmitted diseases, such as AIDS, seem more prevalent in Africa than on other latitudes and continents. We aim to uncover the ideological substratum and implicit assumptions that structure the scientific discourses held not only by scholars and scientists in the past, but also by contemporary scientists who have sought to explain the epidemiological patterns and dramatic spread of the AIDS epidemic in Africa.[3] What imaginary place do Africa and its peoples occupy in the explanatory models produced by contemporary Western scholars (epidemiologists, demographers, social psychologists, medical social scientists, for instance), when analyzing differential rates of AIDS among regions of the world?

We try to demonstrate that often Western scholars hold "scientific views" that are deeply flawed: first, they often rely on a body of insufficient or inadequate data – either unverifiable, biased or simply untrue – when dealing with sexual practices of Africans; and second, their analyses are usually situated in an interpretive frame largely inspired by the works of the Comte de Buffon and other eighteenth-century scientists (see below), which are subsequently rephrased in rather trivial sociobiological schemata.

In order to answer these questions, we choose to deconstruct two paradigmatic examples: the sociobiological arguments defended by J. Philippe Rushton (from the University of Western Ontario, Canada) and the behaviorist model of African sexuality as presented by John and Pat Caldwell (from the Australian National University, Canberra). These modern scientists, though from different perspectives, have tried to explain why African populations are more susceptible than other human groups to sexually transmitted diseases and to HIV infection. In our view, however, they incarnate a Western Africanist discourse in its worst and most dangerous version: it is due time that such false science is deconstructed.

Homo Africanus: Dapper and the long life of Comte de Buffon's model

> The Negro makes little ado in conducting his amorous affairs; the extreme liberty the girls enjoy provides ample opportunity to make their acquaintance, and for this reason they do not remain virgins for long. Polygamy is permitted, adultery is no less fashionable and gentlemen especially are given to excesses of immodesty. Wives very much submit to their husband's will, but their fidelity is nonetheless questionable.
>
> O. Dapper, (1686: 304)

In the late seventeenth century, Olfert Dapper (c. 1635–1689), a physician and geographer from Amsterdam wrote a book about Africa in which he attempted to synthesize the body of knowledge Europeans had collected about the continent up to that time.[4] Dapper never had occasion to visit personally any of the African countries he described, sometimes with great accuracy, in his book. He nevertheless reconstituted, as an honest armchair ethnographer, the "customs" of African peoples on the basis of secondary sources he consulted in his hometown: books, reports, narratives, and documents produced by explorers, inland travelers, sailors, traders, and missionaries. He may have also interviewed Dutch merchants who were regularly involved in trading along the African coasts as well as captains of ships engaged in the trade of slaves who were sold as workers in the New World plantations.

Dapper's *Description of Africa* (1686)[5] is organized along a fairly methodical table of contents, predating the entries of the *Ethnographic Survey of Africa*, which served, during colonial times, as a blueprint for describing African peoples. Contemporary ethnographic bibliographies produced about African cultures largely repeat the same organization of the subject matter, with large sections successively dedicated to the description of nature (i.e., land, rivers, villages), individuals (physical, intellectual, and moral characteristics), and peoples and society (religion, economic activities, politics, kinship organization, family structure, rules governing marriage, sexual practices, and so on).

When Dapper talks about marriage, family life, and sexuality among Africans, he eloquently evokes the themes of adultery, polygamy, pregnancy, and delivery, and describes the conditions of women's lives within and outside the wedlock system. The Dutch doctor-turned-ethnographer insists that young men and women are sexual libertines and notes that in Africa, very few women are still virgins by the time marriage is consummated. According to him, polygamy is widespread, women are subordinated before marriage to their father, and after, to their husband; men's adultery is easily forgiven whereas the social order severely punishes the unfaithful woman (Dapper 1686: 304–320).

What is most interesting in Dapper's book is that his interpretation of ethnographic data is based on the ecologically oriented humoral theory that still dominated medicine in the late seventeenth century. In conformity with the Hippocratic tradition, Dapper and his fellow physicians assumed that strong links existed between characteristics of the physical milieu (hot-cold; dry-humid), particular biological features, temperaments of individuals, and prevalent diseases. For example, he attributed the high prevalence of sterility among Gold Coast women[6] to an excess of heat and humidity in their temperament.[7] Freedom in sexual practices, polygamy, adultery and sterility were ultimately seen by Dapper as the direct result of the impact of actual environmental conditions on the temperaments ("hot blood") of African people, both men and women. It was taken for granted, even by an honest scholar such as Dapper, that the dominant humoral theory commonly held by scientists of his time was the best or perhaps even the "only" theory that really made sense of the collected data. Dapper thus simply adopted the prevailing scientific explanation of his time in identifying environmental conditions as the key explanatory factor in understanding both the "excesses" of sexuality and sterility among Africans.

Racial discrimination and racism always imply negative views of others. The slow emergence of comparative anthropobiological science in the eighteenth century provides a case study to sharply illustrate the close connection between ideology, politics, moral issues, and scientific ideas. Science in the Age of Enlightenment served as a basis for legitimizing the hierarchical structure of society, with certain races placed at the top and other groups displaced to the margins or the very bottom of the social ladder.

In his *Systema Naturae* (1735), the biologist Karl von Linné affirmed that all biological species (plants and animals) had been created at the same moment and in their present form; he wrote that this was also the case for human beings, who formed altogether only one species divided into four varieties: Homo Europaeus, Homo Asiaticus, Homo Afer, and Homo Americanus. Von Linné attributed distinctive characteristics to each of the four varieties without imposing, this should be noted, a hierarchy between these varieties. At the time, Voltaire argued in accord with the School of Anatomists (Malpighi in particular) that humanity was divided in singular fixed racial groups, either red, white, or black, with multiple nuances and alterations produced by interbreeding among these groups. Such views were commonly held in the mid-eighteenth century.

The enlightened European thinkers shared a remarkably similar view about the human races:

1   the natural condition of humanity is that of *whiteness* that some groups may have lost because of degeneracy or environmental conditions;
2   each racial group is attributed distinctive qualities of mentality, character, and behavior;
3   the intellectual and emotional capabilities of the black and red groups are quite different from those of white Europeans; and finally,
4   certain human groups (although they look human) might be a separate species, closer to non-human groups. In using anthropometry as a method, researchers trying to find evidence of the differences between human groups often focused on two main features:
    (a) skull size (and its connection with intelligence in different races), and
    (b) the racial differences in primary (size of genitalia) and secondary sexual characteristics.

The Comte de Buffon is a prime example of European thinking at the time, when he contrasted, in his well-known *Histoire naturelle* (1753), the differences between the European (white), Amerindian (red), and negro (black) male genitals:

In the savage, the organs of generation are small and feeble. He has no hair, no beard, no ardour for the female. Though nimbler than the European, because more accustomed to running, his strength is not so great. His sensations are less acute. . . .

(Buffon 1753)

Cornelius de Pauw was soon to follow these ideas in how he referred to the "natural parts" among different human races, including the Amerindians:

On top of a complete lack of beard/facial hair, Amerindians all show no signs of any hair on the epidermis and their natural parts, which distinguishes them from all other nations of this earth. From this, one can draw some conclusions about the weakness and distortion of those natural parts, that we haven't noticed to be extraordinary or irregular in any way, except for the smallness of the organ and the length of the scrotum, excessive in some.

(Pauw 1774: 30)

In 1792, Peter Camper, a Dutch scientist who followed Buffon's model, published his theory about the connection between the "facial angle" and the level of intelligence: the greater the prognathism of the human face, the lesser the level of intelligence. He stated:

When I placed the heads of a European and a monkey next to the heads of a Negro and a Calmuque, I noticed a difference in their respective physiognomies by observing the line from the forehead to the upper lip in each one – this revealed a marked similarity between the head of the Negro and the head of the monkey (Camper 1792: 12). . . . Nature has not created anything uglier than the physiognomy of the Calmuques, particularly if you compare it to ours, and, especially, to the beautiful classical faces of antiquity (p. 19). . . . I freely agree with de Buffon (1753) that all the inhabitants of the North, of Mongolia and Persia, as well as Armenians, Turks, Georgians, Mingrelians and Circassians, and all the peoples of Europe are not only the whitest but also the most beautiful and best proportioned in the world. (p. 21)

In *An account of the regular gradation in man and in different animals and vegetables* (1799), Charles White, an Englishman, made public his theory of the cranial volume by which he attempted to establish a linkage between the size of the skull and the degree of intelligence. His concerns were typically confined to racial differences between skull measures and degree of "bruteness," size of genitalia, and the quality of certain senses, including memory, which, according to him, was superior in blacks when compared with white Europeans:

> I did not carry my inquiries into provincial or national varieties or features, but confined them chiefly to the extremes of the human race: to the European, on the one hand, and, on the other, to the African, who seems to approach nearer to the brute creation than any other of the human species (White 1799: 42). That the penis of an African is larger than that of an European, has, I believe, been shown in every anatomical school in London (p. 48) ... The circumference of the Negro skull, ascertained by a cord passing horizontally over the eyebrows and the upper margin of the os temporum, is considerably less ... [than that of the European skull]. (p. 159)[8]

In all these accounts, blacks are either distinguished for the small or large size of genitalia or situated at the very bottom of the scale for intelligence. We do think that contemporary scientific racism, expressed by modern medical social scientists, finds its roots largely in the racial prejudices and principles that were put forward by eighteenth-century biologists. While the rhetoric contemporary scholars use is actually quite different from the idioms of de Buffon, de Pauw, Camper, and White, the ideological substratum remains the same, despite great advances in evolution studies (Durham 1990) and, more globally, in the ways biological anthropologists look at human races today.

The approach to the politics of racism we put forward in this essay challenges the idea that there exists such a thing as a "racial essence" expressed either in specific moral qualities, in distinctive intellectual capabilities, or in a particular set of behaviors. We see racism as the ideological formation that provides the foundation for the establishment of a science of racial difference. We acknowledge that our own thinking has been framed by the genealogy of racialism and racism proposed by the Ghanean-born philosopher A. Kwame Appiah, who firmly established a close connection between "the invention of Africa" and the emergence of the racialist doctrine among European scholars.

> Unlike most Western-educated people, I believe that racialism is false, but by itself, it seems to be a cognitive rather than a moral problem. The issue is how the world is, not how we would want it to be. Racialism is, however, a presupposition of other doctrines that have been called "racism," and these doctrines have been, in the last few centuries, the basis of a great deal of human suffering and the source of great deal of moral error.
>
> (Appiah 1992: 13)

Despite efforts to eradicate past derogatory positions, racism is still today a typical ideological product that accompanies human history (see also Benoist 1995). This old banner of Africanism appears to be as deeply rooted as Orientalism – a representational system of the Orient constructed by and existing only in relation to Western culture.

"Homo Sexualis Africanus" according to Rushton and Bogaert and to the Caldwells

Rushton and Bogaert (1989: 1214) affirm explicitly that the patterns of racial differences in sexual behavior are correlated with certain features of an organism's life history, using the evolutionary theory of r/K reproductive strategies. We borrow the following definition of the r/K selection theory from our colleague Jerome H. Barkow, from Dalhousie University (Halifax, Nova Scotia). "In biological terminology," writes Barkow (1989: 317), "we react to resources by becoming more K- and less r-selected. A K-selected species is marked by few and relatively infrequent offspring but by low infant mortality rates and by heavy investment in each offspring. Elephants are K-selected, as are human beings. Rabbits are relatively r-selected, as are (to take an extreme example) frogs." Barkow (1989: 328) further gives a clear synthesis of Lovejoy's (see below) position: "Lovejoy emphasizes that the Old World monkeys and apes have moved in the direction of increasing 'K selection.' That is, they have moved in the direction of providing increasingly heavy parental investment to each of fewer, more dependent, but longer-lived offspring. At the extremes of this movement are the chimpanzee and ourselves." In Rushton and Bogaert's view, African (Negroid) populations, when compared to others (Caucasoids and Mongoloids), are genetically and socially programmed along a gradient of r/K reproductive strategies associated with some specific traits. They attempt to prove what they contend by ranking three racially distinct world groups, Mongoloids, Caucasoids, and Negroids, according to certain attributes grouped in five categories of data: brain weight and intelligence (cranial capacity, brain weight, million of "excess neurons," and IQ test scores); maturation rate (i.e., gestation time, age of first intercourse, and early pregnancy, etc.); personality and temperament (i.e., aggressiveness, impulsivity, etc.); reproductive effort (i.e., size of genitalia, intercourse frequency, sexually permissive attitudes, androgen levels, etc.); and levels of social organization (law abidingness, marital stability, and mental health) (Rushton and Bogaert 1989: 1216).

By reducing the "r/K selection" theory that Lovejoy (1981) proposed to explain how hominoids separated themselves from simians (apes), and simplifying Wilson's (1975) thinking, Rushton and Bogaert arrived at the conclusion that the Negroids constitute, with respect to reproductive strategies, the less advanced group of human primates. Lovejoy had theorized that pongid evolution entailed progressive growth in "K selection:" in this evolutionary movement, the chimpanzees and humans would represent the most advanced forms. Pongid parents would have accorded more attachment to their offspring, because the offspring were less mobile and more dependent for a longer period of time. Lovejoy would without doubt have thought that monogamy constituted one of the central mechanisms in that evolution: the strategy of monogamous couples (or at least a stable partner) would have been more adapted than polygamous reproductive strategies in permitting greater assurance of the biological paternity, an enhanced protection for females, and the better care of children. Bipedalism and the use of the hands would have also developed within the context of increasing monogamy: the vertical posture and the freeing of the hands conferred males with greater ease in transporting food and females with the ability to carry their young, so they must have theoretically been the first to stand on their legs!

Monogamy, as a reproductive strategy, would have led, in turn, to certain modifications in the family (fewer children, wider intervals between births, and better parental investment), in individual characteristics (slower physical maturation, later sexual reproduction, more intelligence), in the modalities of exploiting the natural resources (progressive sedentarization, for example), as well as in the organization of social life (altruism and cooperation). Rushton and Bogaert (1989: 1215) write in this context:

> At the "K" end of the continuum organisms produce very few offspring but invest a large amount of care in each. At the "r" end (opposite pole), organisms produce a large number of offspring but provide little or no parental care. ... As a species, humans are at the "K" end of the continuum, although some people are postulated to be more K than others. The more K a person is, the more likely he or she is expected to come from an intact family, with more intensive parental care, with fewer and more widely spaced offspring, and with a lower incidence of multiple birthing and infant mortality. ... Moreover, the K person is inclined to be more intelligent, altruistic, law-abiding, and behaviourally restrained.[9]

The argument presented by Rushton and Bogaert (1989) in this article is too well-known to repeat it here in much detail. In essence, its authors argue for a ranking of populations on r/K attributes (p. 1216), where the Negroids are represented by less-K individuals (p. 1217) and therefore are more "pro-sexual." In short, these racial differences are based in a genetic program that, combined with higher androgen levels, in a way "determines" certain sexual behaviors (i.e., uninhibited sexuality, higher rape figures) and that in turn leads to a higher prevalence of STDs and AIDS. Moreover, Rushton and Bogaert further postulate that lower levels of intelligence attributed to blacks should also be considered a "risk factor" for STDs and AIDS (p. 1217).

They list most, if not all, attributes along a gradient that presents Negroids at the worst end of the scale, when compared with Mongoloids, whereas Caucasoids show average or "medium" figures. They suggest that Africans would more likely be victims of sexually transmitted diseases, including AIDS, because substantive racial differences exist in brain weight, intelligence, size of genitalia, and sexual behavior. These differential rates of STDs and HIV infection lie in the following "ranking order": Mongoloids<Caucasoids<Negroids. The authors claim that "racial differences in sexual behavior translate into consequences," such as teenage fertility rates and related psychological phenomena (Rushton and Bogaert 1989: 1215).

One may find a few loose ends in their reconstructed genealogy of the epidemic, but Rushton and Bogaert are most probably right when they refer to documented HIV cases as far back as the late 1960s.[10] Many theories and conjectures have strived to explain the origins of AIDS, and although most theories locate the origins of the HIV virus in Central Africa, no one yet seems to know exactly what happened and why this happened when it happened.[11]

Explanatory models have included AIDS as "an act of God," a punishment on humanity for its sins; a virus that came from outer space or that has "escaped" from germ warfare labs in the US or the former Soviet Union. An unorthodox theory postulates that the HIV virus passed from primates to humans during the development of oral polio vaccines through field trials conducted by Belgian authorities in the late 1950s and involving about one million Africans in Burundi, Congo, and Rwanda, (Epstein 1999). So-called "AIDS dissidents" believe that the virus was accidentally spread through contaminated needles, tainted blood transfusions, or massive vaccination campaigns, or worse, that scientists "are part of a vast conspiracy cooked up by the pharmaceutical industry to justify the market in anti-AIDS drugs ... worth billions of dollars a year" (Epstein 2000). Since the 1980s, the "natural transfer" theory has gained some acceptance, though skeptics challenge this theory on a number of grounds. According to the theory of "natural transfer," the viruses' original habitat was confined to forest-dwelling communities, where HIV had been passed from monkeys and apes to men (possibly hunters became infected subduing or butchering their prey). After the African wars of independence, the growth of African cities, the construction of highways, and the successive changes in the social landscape (i.e. tribal wars, trucking, mining, prostitution, etc.) brought large numbers of people (mostly men), some of whom were HIV-infected, to the cities. Heterosexual encounters, multiple sexual partners, and commercial sex were the main routes for HIV transmission and the spread of AIDS.

Unlike these other theoreticians, aside from pointing to Africa as the origin of AIDS, Rushton and Bogaert do not venture to explain what remains to be explained: what happened exactly and why did AIDS develop first in Central Africa and not elsewhere? Their conclusion is simple: due to human evolution and genetics, certain "races," such as the Negroid, present an inherited configuration of sexual traits (less K and therefore more "pro-sexual") that render them much more likely than white Caucasians or Asian Mongoloids to succumb to the actual AIDS epidemic. One of the most deplorable statements comes when Rushton and Bogaert (1989: 1216), paraphrasing Freedman (1979) and their own work, assert that:

> ... people create norms and environments maximally compatible with their genotypes. This would explain why in China and Japan clothing styles have often been chosen to flatten the breast and buttocks in an explicit attempt "to deanimalize," with an opposite clothing style often chosen in Africa. Moreover, in Africa dances have been invented which emphasize undulating rhythms and mock copulation.

What renders Africans more likely to be infected by HIV is situated, therefore, in their genotype, which then leaves them no other recourse but to rerun the course of evolutionary history in order to genetically reprogram themselves. All of the sexual behaviors found in Africa would be genetically inherited in such a way that their maneuverability remains extremely limited: most Africans would think of sex every day, whereas only half of English university students and scarcely one per cent of Japanese students would dare to think of it (the statistics are obviously those of Rushton and Bogaert). Black Africans are doomed to have AIDS, which seems not to be the case for Caucasoids and Mongoloids.[12] Finally, their smaller brains and low level of intelligence would forever prevent them from appreciating the dangers of engaging in high-risk sexual relationships or dangerous practices such as scarification, tattooing, circumcision, and exchanging blood in friendship pacts (Rushton and Bogaert 1989: 1217).

Their argument is straightforward: evolution has equipped Africans with a genetic program that predisposes black peoples to an absence of sexual restraint, to polygyny, to higher exposure to sexually transmitted diseases, and thus to AIDS. Moreover, their interpretation is often expressed in behavioral terms loaded with racial stereotypes: blacks have developed sexual cultures characterized by overall sexual permissiveness, multiple sexual partners, greater female extramarital sexual activity, and so on, which make them "vulnerable to attack by all coital-related disorders" (Caldwell, Caldwell and Quiggin 1989: 187). In short, such positions suggest that Africa is "ontologically" plagued by the AIDS epidemics and little, if anything, can be done to control HIV transmission on this continent. This view strongly suggests that Africanism is still alive in certain academic circles.

It is not unusual to find a growing number of references made, in papers published in the late 1980s and early 1990s, to a "deviant" African sexuality, ranging from "bulimic" sexual appetites to "pathological" cultures of sexuality. Few articles have made more explicit this distorted view of African sexuality than the one written by John Caldwell, a demographer, Pat Caldwell, an anthropologist, and their colleague Pat Quiggin, in the *Population and Development Review*.[13] They argue in this well-known paper, that ". . . there is a distinct and internally coherent African pattern embracing sexuality, marriage and much else" (Caldwell et al. 1989: 187) and that this African model is structurally different from the "Eurasian system," a term derived from "Eurasian society" and proposed by the British anthropologist Jack Goody (1976).

The Caldwells and Quiggin claimed to have identified the key elements that make up the "African system of sexuality":

> The following are typical characteristics of the African system: great emphasis on the importance of ancestry and descent, usually accompanied by a belief in ancestral spirit intervention in the affairs of the living; a related social system which, in its most complex form, the lineage, places greater importance on intergenerational links than on conjugal ones and that gives great respect and power to the old; an inheritance system whereby property, which is usually communal, remains within the lineage or clan and normally passes between members of the same sex (. . .) The marriage bond is typically weak, with spouses retaining strong lineage links; (. . .) polygyny exists on a scale not found in the Eurasian system and consequently the basic family unit is a mother and her children; husbands are usually much older than wives; divorce is fairly common among most ethnic groups; and women, at least in the past, abstained from sexual relations after giving birth. . . .
>
> (Caldwell et al. 1989: 188)

Although many Africanist anthropologists would tend to concur that a number of these features are characteristic in various African groups, most would strongly disagree either with the methods used by the Caldwells (their research was largely based on materials extracted from the Human Relations Areas Files) or with the interpretation they give to the data in what they call the "African system" of sexuality.[14]

Let's take a closer look at the interpretation of African sexuality by the Caldwells and Quiggin. They conclude their list of characteristic features of the African system of sexuality by noting that all the identified elements are "logically related to one another" and that they form an integrated behavioral system which has a long history (since the early Neolithic period) and has been resistant to change over the millennia. We mention here only three elements, central in the reconstituted model of African sexuality, that they abstracted from the ethnographic literature:

1   in talking about sexuality in sub-Saharan Africa, they claim: "The evidence is that Africans neither placed aspects of sexual behavior at the center of their moral and social systems nor sanctified chastity ...." (Caldwell et al. 1989: 194);

2   the fact that "the weak conjugal bond follows from the strong lineage one, but it also allows the lineage to retain its strength." (p. 189); and

3   the existence of a great tolerance concerning sexuality of women: "with a fair degree of permissiveness toward premarital relations that are not too blatantly public, and a degree of acceptance that surreptitious extramarital relations are not the high point of sin and usually should not be severely punished." (p. 197).

According to the Caldwells and Quiggin (1989: 197), "the touchstone of the contrast between Eurasia and Africa is not male but female sexuality." To construct their so-called "African sexual system," these authors gathered more than 200 quotations, borrowed from statements mostly made by ethnographers, and pasted them together in a large patchwork piece. In this article, readers are led to discover a collection of sexual customs and sexually related stories in different African tribal societies, with an accent being placed on promiscuous sexual life, adultery, age at the time of first sexual encounter, lack of guilt and sexual permissiveness of women, loss of virginity and pre-marital sex, and the absence of moral and institutional rules in the control of their sexuality (pp. 189–222). It is interesting to note that their overview appeared in mid-1989 and that Rushton and Bogaert were most likely unaware of its existence at the time they published their controversial article. For their part, the Caldwells do not explicitly see the African sexual model as a product of evolution, but it is pretty clear that the article by Rushton and Bogaert provides the biological substratum that fits fairly well the behavioral model described by the Australian scholars.

   In our view, far from providing an in-depth analysis of values and diversity of practices associated with sexuality in African societies, the Caldwells have relied on a descriptive voyeuristic sightseeing tour of African sexuality, based on a highly selective (and biased) reading of the existing literature. They are a prime example of AIDS' experts playing "anthropologist," while labeling Africans as "promiscuous," using "an archaic Victorian standard of morality for Africa, largely discarded in the West" (Feldman 1991: 784).

It should be noted that this is not the first time such criticisms have been aimed at the Caldwells. In 1991, two anthropologists and a demographer from the University of Montreal argued in the *Population and Development Review* that the Caldwells' "use of anthropological evidence is fraught with serious methodological flaws" and that "they have omitted many ethnographic sources that would undermine their argument" (Le Blanc, Meintel and Piché 1991: 497). In their reply to the Montreal-based scholars, the Caldwells took an anti-anthropological stance in stating that the "methodological flaws identified by Le Blanc et al. represent an attack on all anthropological research rather than on our essay" (p. 512). We may be wrong – argued the Australian scholars – in our assessment of the African sexual culture, but the ones responsible for that are the anthropologists themselves, because we just repeated the information provided in their ethnographies. The Caldwells' argument speaks against itself: "just repeating" information out of context often results – whether deliberately or not – in poor science (or poor journalism). To simply "repeat" information elicited by others (with other aims) can lead to distortion and further misinterpretation of the facts.

In 1994, in an essay published in *Africa* entitled "Is there a distinct African sexuality? A critical response to Caldwell," Beth M. Ahlberg states that the Caldwells' and Quiggin's (1989: 194) thesis on permissive African sexuality is undermined by wrong assumptions (such as sexual activity in Africa being free and devoid of moral value) and she points at three major shortcomings of their article. They neglect, first, to acknowledge the problems and limitations of research into sexual behavior that inevitably influence the quality of the data; second, to place moral and religious values in context; and third, to bring a historical perspective to bear in the analysis. Recent studies among the Kikuyu conducted by Ahlberg (1991) seem to indicate that "the openness with which sexuality is expressed does not necessarily mean that sexual activity is indiscriminate," the problem arising, in fact, when African sexuality is analyzed using "foreign moral formulations" (Ahlberg 1991: 226). These criticisms are consistent with the ones we have delineated in our essay.

In short, the Caldwells provide a modern, socially oriented version of Africanism while complementing the genetic-evolutionary model put forward by Rushton and Bogaert. In our view, scientific racism, as defined by Charles Leslie (1990), still prevails among medical social scientists, particularly among those who pretend to have established direct links between the low-K selective basis of African sexual culture and its permissiveness and resistance to change as determinant factors in the spread of AIDS on the African continent.

Cultura Sexualis Africana: toward a more ethnographically based version

Statistical projections about the spread of the AIDS epidemic in Africa often paint a dramatic picture. In 1991, Way and Stanecki, from the US Census Bureau, calculated that by the year 2015 about 70 million Africans (out of a total of 940 million) would be HIV-positive. The rate of infection would reach 16 per cent in the cities and 5 per cent in rural areas and more than one-third of all annual deaths (all causes) would be related to AIDS (Way and Stanecki 1991). Medical social scientists have for their part predicted that the family system will soon be unable to absorb the increasing number of AIDS' orphans, health care services will be over-burdened or simply paralyzed by the excessive demands imposed by AIDS patients, and young adults will flee the cities because these will be seen as hopeless "large cemeteries." (It is estimated that AIDS deaths number approximately 6,000 a day in Africa today (UNAIDS 2000).) In addition, most of them conclude that, in spite of prevention campaigns, African men will go on resisting condom use and people will die in their age of greatest productivity, causing a vicious circle of economic chaos. Such an apocalyptic scenario is often presented as inescapable by many international AIDS experts who, blaming the victim, claim that unless Africans urgently undertake radical changes in their sexual values, attitudes, and practices, they will be confronted with extinction.[15]

In one of the first socio-cultural studies dealing specifically with AIDS in Africa, Nathan Clumeck et al. (1984: 496) wrote, with a great deal of caution, in the *New England Journal of Medicine*:

> It is not known how the agent of AIDS is transmitted in the African population. The occurrence of the syndrome in young to middle-aged men and women suggests that heterosexual contact may be a mode of transmission.

Only three years later, in an interview given to *Le Monde*, the same Clumek talks about ". . . the unrestrained sexuality of Africans," comparing their sexual glut to "a population of obese bulimics" (Nau 1987).

The issue of the "sexual promiscuity" of Africans was already well consolidated in the mind of many medical social scientists by the mid-1980s, as can be seen in two papers published in *The Lancet* by Van de Perre et al. (1985) and Serwadda et al. (1985), and one paper by Douglas A. Feldman (1986) in *Medical Anthropology Quarterly*. These three articles make explicit reference to the "heterosexual promiscuity" of Africans.[16] Despite the absence of solid information about sexual practices in Africa, the hypothesis of "sexual promiscuity" rapidly became dogma, widely disseminated by major scientific journals, and adopted as such by medical social scientists across disciplines, while alternative hypotheses were abandoned, in particular those explanations dealing with the political context and socio-economic conditions in which Africans live.

Packard and Epstein (1991: 781) were among the first to notice that the increasing demand for studies focusing almost exclusively on the sexual practices of Africans was going to obliterate all other alternative approaches to explain the AIDS epidemic in Africa. They wrote in a 1991 issue of *Social Science & Medicine*:

> This narrowing of research in turn discouraged serious consideration of the role of alternative avenues of transmission, such as injections, or the role of possible co-factors, such as high background levels of infection and malnutrition and associated problems of poverty and maldevelopment which may be as important in the heterosexual transmission of HIV as the frequency of sexual contacts.

Our objective in this essay is not to introduce corrections to the biased views held by the Caldwells, Rushton and Bogaert, or similar thinkers. We are instead openly opposed to their "hypothetical" views and propose ethnographic evidence that reveals their positions to be erroneous on three main grounds:

First, we do think that such positions, which still shape large sectors of public health in the area of STDs, have little ethnographic relevance and largely ignore the social and cultural patterns that shape the actual organization of sexuality, family, and kinship within African societies. For ethnographers, social and cultural facts make sense only when they are reported within the global configuration of representations and practices that prevail in one particular group. To grasp the African structures of sexuality, anthropologists think there is no other reliable way than entering the specific universe of representations, identifying key elements around which local sexual cultures are organized, and reconstructing, via the comparative method, the multiple sexual systems developed by human groups.

Today, one finds an increasing number of medical social scientists and anthropologists who have worked in Africa making significant contributions and comprehensive descriptions of sexuality among the various African cultures, such as Françoise Héritier (1984), Norman Miller and Richard Rockwell (1988), and Didier Fassin (1999) among others. We have chosen the study carried out by Héritier among the Samo, in Burkina Faso, to illustrate the validity of the ethnographic method. Building on a solid ethnographic knowledge of the Samo kinship system, Héritier posits a fundamental principle around what she calls "the symbolic anthropology of the body": fecundity and sterility, femininity and masculinity, filiation and lineage, as well as matrimonial prohibitions and prescriptions, the relations between corporeal fluids (blood, semen, and milk) and the sharing of food and other elements, all form "fields of signification," within which certain concepts act as mediating mechanisms, allowing the passage from one domain to the next: from the biological body (sexual practices) to the social space (relations between lineage, the production of descendants and the control of sexuality) to the reproduction of cultural values (the ancestors as guardians of the social order). A strong associative chain links the fecundity of the body and the dynamics of lineage to such a point that the sexuality of individuals is imprisoned in a network of obligations that is at the very core of the ideology of fertility, marriage, and filiation. What seems important for Africans is to produce children and at the same time maintain connections with parents and ancestors, in such a way that ascendance and filiation remain indissoluble (Héritier 1984).

In-depth monographs of this kind provide a more appropriate ethnographic frame for understanding African cultures of sexuality. The labeling of sexual behaviors as "promiscuous" or "aberrant" reveals a moralistic view of an ethnographic reality. In the African case, sexual practices should be read against the background of multiple connections between lineage and the corpus of values and rules controlling relations between the sexes. This type of ethnography presupposes a solid knowledge of particular societies, which is far more useful than using a collection of isolated fragmentary descriptions of sexual behaviors in different cultures to build a Pan-African cultural model of sexuality, as proposed by the Caldwells. We are not advocating against a culturalist approach to sexuality and AIDS in Africa, as long as the cultural elements are rigorously studied in connection with specific societies.

Second, we think that the behaviorist frame, such as the one sketched by the Caldwells (it is the same in the case of Rushton and Bogaert's sociobiological model), remains invalid because it decontextualizes AIDS and African sexuality, ignoring the daily conditions in which people live. It is trivial and much too general to simply associate the high prevalence rate of AIDS in Africa either to a genetic program inherited by Africans or to the so-called "African system of sexuality" (Caldwell et al. 1989).

In a more recent paper published in *Scientific American*, the Caldwells remind readers that they "have been working [in Nigeria] over a 30-year period, studying the very traditions and sexual behavior that might affect AIDS transmission" (Caldwell and Caldwell 1996: 66). In association with a Nigerian colleague, I. O. Orubuloye, the Caldwells conducted, among other studies, field research in the early 1990s on the sexual practices among the Yoruba (Caldwell, Orubuloye, and Caldwell 1991). Their study, entitled "The destabilization of the traditional Yoruba sexual system," was built up around the notions of "sexual networking" and "high-risk behaviors." Research results seemed to confirm the inaccurate hypothesis put forward in their 1989 overview: that in Africa greater sexual tolerance exists, characterized by a permissive attitude toward extra-conjugal relations; an absence of culpability in relation to sexuality; and greater sexual freedom among African women than in their Western counterparts. Although the Caldwells reiterate here their claim of a "promiscuous African culture of sexuality," they also attempt to show that the existing AIDS belt in Central, East, and Southeast Africa corresponds largely to geographical "areas of Africa with large numbers of uncircumcised men" (1996: 67). The absence of male circumcision was thus added to the list as another key element in the "risk model" for AIDS, along with "promiscuous men and women." Consequently, it is suggested that in sub-Saharan Africa ". . . circumcision could be offered as a reinforcement of other protective measures" (1996: 68).

Recent epidemiological surveys have shown that young women, particularly those under 30 years of age, are proportionally more infected than older women; that age of HIV infection is much higher in men than among women; that urban people have higher HIV rates than people from rural areas; and that the prevalence rate of HIV seropositivity varies greatly from region to region, with dramatic figures as high as 30 per cent in certain towns of post-apartheid South Africa to rates as low as 2 per cent for the whole of Senegal (Fassin 2000). If all Africans inherited the same genetic susceptibility to AIDS or if they are part of the same African (cultural) system of sexuality, how can one explain all the variations epidemiologists have amply documented in contemporary Africa? We do think that any reliable explanation of the differences found between countries and cultures in Africa should take into account the historical as well as the social, political, and economic context in which the AIDS epidemic evolves.

Third, anyone who wants to understand the variables associated with the spread of AIDS in Africa better needs to take a closer look at the particular situation of African women living in large cities. The vast majority of HIV-infected women have a low socioeconomic status and take part in one or many sexual networks on which they rely as a sort of economic support system. We do not imply here that these women are prostitutes (it is known that prostitutes are at much higher risk than other women) or that they do not marry and have sex at random with multiple partners. It is rather the dynamic functioning of sexual networks in the daily life of men and women that should be understood if one wants to explain the differential prevalence rates between rural and urban populations. For example, the facts that infected African men are most often older men, that they usually have a higher socioeconomic status, and that they are sexually engaged with multiple partners should lead us to a context-sensitive interpretation that diverges from the narrow structural views of sexuality of the Caldwells' or the deterministic genetic framework put forward by Rushton.

The social determinants of AIDS

AIDS is above all an urban epidemic, a reality that forces researchers to take into account the social and economic context in which Africans live their sexuality in the cities of the continent. The traditional sexual culture has gone through radical changes in African urban settings: women are more liberated *vis-à-vis* their lineage; young women are leaving their villages at a young age and migrating to the cities in large numbers; the number of households with women acting as family heads is increasing; the control exercised by elders and parents on the selection of marital partners has markedly decreased; the past polygamic structure is currently being replaced by a system based on "bureaux" (literally "offices"), a term commonly used in Francophone Africa to refer to women with whom a man maintains extramarital sexual relations on a regular basis. Patterns of family organization and sexual lifestyles appear to be undergoing a profound restructuring process within African urban settings, a process that is taking place in the context of globalization and the introduction of a market economy, which is accentuating existing economic and social inequalities among urban residents in Africa.

The various strategies of economic survival used by urban Africans today can begin to explain why African cities are so massively plagued by the AIDS epidemic. The high level of unemployment and the deterioration of the overall economy do not allow women to achieve the financial independence to which they aspired when leaving their villages. In the absence of stable revenues provided by a regular job, many young women are forced to rely on the informal economy, as street ambulant vendors for example, and sometimes to become the second or the third "bureau" of older men or "sugar daddies," who are ready to exchange modest financial or material support for sexual favors. The survival strategies of women are generally well accepted by men, because they allow them to preserve their position of power, to avoid engaging in village-style polygynic alliances, which remain highly codified, and to limit their involvement in negotiating sex for money. New urban forms of sexual behaviors and family organization (a matrifocal style) imply the participation of multiple partners within loosely articulated networks, which function as structures of economic support. The existing urban culture of sexuality seems to be nothing else than an epiphenomenon emerging from the redefinition of gender roles and relations and from the effort, largely aborted, to create alternative family structures adjusted to modern urban life. The problem is amplified many times by the fact that this social experimentation is actually performed in a precarious economic context that leads people to pay with their lives for their effort to adjust from the rural cultures of sexuality to life in the cities (Goze and Séri 1991).

We think it is more worthwhile to look for an explanation to the dramatic rise of AIDS in African cities by taking into account the impact of daily conditions of life on individuals, instead of postulating the existence either of a structural permissiveness of sexual relations (as in the case of the Caldwells) or of an inescapable genetically driven sexual behavior (as in the case of Rushton). We reiterate that the magnitude of prostitution in African cities has much less to do with the assumed sexual "promiscuity" than with the prevailing economic and social conditions in which women live.[17] For that reason, we must urgently reintroduce the social, political, and economic dimensions in interpreting sexuality and the AIDS epidemic in Africa, since it has been too heavily biased on the side of biology or culture. The example of African-Americans living in Harlem, New York that we briefly discuss below lends support to the socioeconomic and contextual approach we are proposing to explain the spread of AIDS.

In 1990, McCord and Freeman, two American researchers, showed that the life expectancy of 40 year-old Black men living in Harlem was lower than that of Bangladeshi peasants. Prior to this study, it was already known that the mortality rate among the 25–44 year-olds of Harlem was six times higher for men and five times higher for women compared to the white American population. McCord and Freeman's new data shocked the North American public health community: the death rate from cirrhosis was ten times higher in African-Americans living in Harlem than in Caucasian Americans. Similarly, homicides were 14 times more likely to occur among blacks and drug-related death rates were 300 times higher in this group when compared with whites. Moreover, African-Americans in Harlem were also battling a substantially higher rate of cardio-vascular-related illnesses and cancer than their Caucasian counterparts. Complementary studies revealed that such disparities were much the same in New York neighborhoods in which there was a majority of Hispanics or African-Americans (54 out of 342).

Critical public health specialists have shown that a direct, one-to-one relation cannot be established between, on the one hand, the marginal position of an individual, a person's economic insecurity within a frail social network and an eroded value system (all these being variables of an individuals' past) and on the other, the better or worse quality of life of this person, the levels of alcohol or drug abuse, the prevailing violence and crime rates around them, and their overall psychological and phys-ical health. There is no doubt that these elements are all interrelated, but they are linked through an extremely complex network of mediations, interactions, and processes. Public health professionals and medical social scientists need to rethink social determinants and health in ways that are radically different from how they have explained these relations in the past. It seems to us that it is time to take the social, political, and economic conditions of people's lives as a starting point to engage in a more fruitful debate.

In summary, our position can be stated as follows: the issue at the center of our argument calls for the identification of the mediating mechanisms through which the internal contradictions of daily life impact on people and for an explanation of how the collective order hinges on the personal order. To take on such a challenge, medical social scientists must reexamine their understanding of social theory and develop new interpretative frameworks closer to the reality of people's lives.

Back to the Rushton-Leslie controversy

Theories and "models" advocated by scholars such as the Caldwells and Rushton are so manifestly biased, distilling their crypto-racism in scientific jargon borrowed from human genetics, modern evolutionary theories, or ethnographic studies, that they could only set off an explosion or incite a general incensed outcry from the ranks of social scientists, particularly ethnologists and physical anthropologists. In fact, to date, very few voices have been heard, with the exception of Charles Leslie's.[18]

Leslie's critique takes aim at Rushton's perversion of the distinction between K-selection and r-selection. Rushton distorts ". . . the concept of Hominid r-selection for birth spacing by identifying it with an alleged racial pattern of psychological and social traits that he [Rushton] associated with small brain and large genital phenotype." A second part of Leslie's critique evolves around the implicit analogy of Rushton's thesis with the anthropocentric notions of the origins of races, as depicted in the "Family tree of the primates" and the "Family tree of man," two illustrations from an anthropological textbook published in 1947 by E. A. Hooton, *Up from the Ape*. In these drawings, the "basic white" race is shown as the main stem of evolution, and the "Ancestral Negroids" and the "Mongoloids" are shown as "primary races" branching out from the main stem.

Finally, Leslie analyzes the demise of the race concept in American physical anthropology textbooks published between 1932 and 1979. At the time, the social science mainstream either rejected or did not mention "race" in its discussions or claimed that "race" as a concept should be abandoned in dealing with human variation. At the end of the 1970s, few texts would argue that races were "real" notions. Leslie closes his discussion by reflecting on the fairness and validity of the peer-review process. He rightly refers to the peer-review process as the "most neglected topic in the sociology of science," and argues about the abuses and inconsistencies that at times materialize in the peer-review system.

It is obvious that few scholars have dared to publish in a prestigious scientific journal positions that are manifestly based on racist foundations and on a deviation in the thinking currently held in the primatology and paleontology milieux. The Rushton and Bogaert article has the style to satisfy the requirements of contemporary positivist mentality: maps and tables attesting to a judgment based on statistics; multiple references to specialists in evolutionary theory; and the use of a technical vocabulary conferring an apparent stamp of scientific authenticity to disguise a fundamentally racist ideology. We thought it important to identify the major flaws in Rushton and Bogaert's venture, not because similar positions may be commonly held in the scientific community (see Durham 1990 for further evidence), but because certain versions manifestly belittle actual evolutionary theories, cloaking themselves in a scientific jargon of alleged science and insinuating themselves into the writings of medical social scientists. It is obvious that their "scientific" interpretations are made within a strictly deterministic and reductionistic schema. From a scientific point of view, it seems to us that these authors erred (voluntarily or not) with respect to, in our view, four essential requirements of all scientific discourse.

First of all, we regret that thinking in such a limited frame led them to confound the orders of causality and correlation (Gould 1983) in attributing all contemporary human behaviors to the evolutionary history of humans, to their hormone levels, or to a single genetic program, as if animals had survived under a human guise. It matters little whether the evolution scenario, borrowed from Lovejoy and then revisited by other authors, is true or false. We think it is a largely speculative scenario, which one could easily counter with facts and more particularly the universally repeated observation of the existence of polygyny in many human groups. Instead, the real problem seems to be the exclusive recourse to the genetic and biological or to the oversimplification of sexuality to explain the complex behavior of people living today in highly diversified sociocultural and physical environments. Why must scientists privilege explanations based solely on a genetic program or a sexual cultural system when more straightforward hypotheses can account for people's behaviors? Why choose complex and convoluted explanations when there are others more immediately obvious? The reason can be found in the fact that our scientific culture considers an explanation appealing to the biological structures or neuro-endocrine mechanisms as invested with more explanatory power than the social, political or economic arguments, by which human behaviors are interpreted as complex dynamic responses or a constructed social product within particular contexts.

In reality, it is a biosocial model and a context-sensitive frame that is needed, if one does not want to play biology against the social sciences, structure against history, and vice versa *ad infinitum*. And, it is with respect to this second point that both teams of researchers, Rushton and Bogaert, and the Caldwells and Quiggin, gravely fail. These authors seem to ignore the contemporary orientations of biological anthropology, human ecology, and medical anthropology (see, among others, Durham 1990), where the relationships between a population and its environment are always mediated by cultural and social elements. The dominant model of reference is neo-Darwinian and researchers today tend to speak of biological gradients to contrast populations rather than pit races against each other based on a distribution of separate genetic traits, as scholars did two centuries ago. Today's biological anthropology forces us to take note of the variations among human groups at the heart of a dynamic schema that interrelates biology, the sociocultural, and the natural environment: human beings are defined as polymorphic, that is, capable of producing multiple cultures adapted to different contexts and historical particulars.[19]

Third, we would like to ask Rushton and Bogaert to tell us which genes determine higher levels of social organization in Caucasians and Mongoloids (as measured by law-abidingness, marital stability, and mental health) when compared to Negroids (Rushton and Bogaert 1989: 1216)? Moreover, which racial genetic makeup (blacks or less-K populations) "generate decentralized organizations with weak power structures" (p. 1217)? There might be several genetic interactions that give rise to such variation in social structures, but even if that is the case, why must "social variation" be the simple manifestation of "genotype variation"? Would there not exist, even minimally, certain degrees of cultural creativity, which would be deployed in the midst of imposing constraints (that is, the environment or the history of contact with other human groups)? In raising these questions, we want to suggest that Rushton and Bogaert's model is essentially an animal one and that they have unduly imposed it on human populations.

Finally, their last *faux pas* lies in making typological use of the notion of race. Rushton and Bogaert put a few million (or even billion) individuals in the same box as if no differences exist between them, assign hierarchies between them and the other categories, and end up "biologizing" their social and behavioral differences. It has been almost fifty years since Montagu (1964) and Lévi-Strauss (1952) proposed that the concept of "race" for explaining variations between humans be abandoned from the scientific repertoire, since it did not exist as a biological reality and popular usage had negatively branded the notion. However, scientists have been unable to refer neutrally to the term "race" and in most cases their position has led to the return of scientific racism and the politicization of science, judging by the distinctly racist assertions still prevailing in the medical social sciences literature today.

Contemporary communicable disease experts and AIDS specialists in Africa could have avoided falling into the same trap as their predecessors when trying to explain the origins and increased frequency of tuberculosis and syphilis in Africa. Nevertheless, as with the case of AIDS today, the existence of individual behaviors particular to Africans was invoked to explain their vulnerability to these diseases, neglecting the determining factors of context and environment. The historical studies led by Packard (1989) on the evolution of tuberculosis in Africa demonstrated that Africans are not in themselves more susceptible than others to Koch's bacillus, but that the interactions between diverse co-factors (like state of general health and nutrition) and environmental conditions create a greater vulnerability within certain specific groups of people.

Likewise, the historian Dawson (1983) told us that the pattern of the syphilis epidemic in East Africa could have rendered the African AIDS specialists more cautious. At the beginning of the twentieth century, he writes, several district doctors in Africa argued that 50 to 90 per cent of the population at the district level were syphilitic, and concluded that entire populations would soon see themselves wiped off the map. Furthermore, they attributed the massive contamination to "sexual promiscuity and immorality." It is now known that the epidemic also encompassed an endemic form of non-venereal syphilis, also caused by a *Treponema* but not requiring sexual contact for transmission, just as in the case of yaws (*Treponema pertenue*), or another treponematosis called "pinta" (*Treponema carateum*). There were, of course, some epidemics of venereal syphilis in East Africa but their presence is probably not explained strictly by the high prevalence rates that one finds there. The inappropriate nature of the response furnished by medical science and conventional (Western-based) epidemiology, with regard to the tuberculosis and syphilis epidemics, calls for an exploration of other explanatory scenarios not centered exclusively on the question of sexual practices (Gilman 1985).

Concluding remarks

Historically, stereotypes, clichés, and prejudiced concepts have shaped both lay discourses as well as scientific theories held by Western scholars about Africans and African cultures. Medical social scientists seem unable to shake off these pejorative images, and these are conjured up, even today, in their positions on sexuality and AIDS in Africa. Despite the lack of reliable data, they insist in placing the origin of the virus in the heart of Africa. Some go so far as to say that a genetic code predisposes African populations to polygyny, to loose sexual mores, and therefore places them at greater risk for AIDS. This critical essay has revealed some of the limits of certain conceptual models that disguise plain racism under the cloak of scientific discourse.

As a conclusion we want to evoke other approaches that might be pursued in order to better understand why contemporary scientists are still practicing "scientific racism." Let us turn to colonial literature: In *The Heart of Darkness* (1898), Joseph Conrad narrates the upstream travel of Marlow along the Congo (now Zaire) river, on his way to the company station where Kurtz – the Belgian trader Marlow finds at Stanley Falls –

is an agonizing, dehumanized man, who survives by killing elephants and Africans, a man turned crazy, swallowed by the darkness of the "Black" continent. In Conrad's novel, as well as in many contemporary scientific works, Africa appears to serve as a mirror against which the white writers project the dark side of their humanity (Jacquemin 1991). We do feel this is the case for contemporary scientists like Rushton and Bogaert and the Caldwells, among others.

This derogatory attitude toward Africans is paradigmatic: on the one hand, they "invent" an ethnography of African sexuality based on misguided interpretations far from what has been consistently reported by ethnographers over the past decades; and on other hand, they imagine Africa as a place of unrestrained sexuality, largely due to biological (genetic) drives inexorably pushing African peoples to more and more permissive sexual practices. We have argued that these contemporary scientists "invent" an Africa that they see as an obscure, savage, and primitive continent around which they repeat, under a new scientific guise, the same old stereotypes, clichés, and false images based on a biased selective reading of the literature, which is even less nuanced than the accounts of Olfert Dapper and others from centuries ago.

It might also be enlightening to analyze the papers we discussed in this essay from a deconstructionist approach. In his book *The Invention of Africa* (1988), the Zaire-born American scholar V. Y. Mudimbe writes that Western scholars have invented two contradictory myths in connection with Africa, namely:

> ... the Hobbesian picture of a pre-European Africa, in which there was no account of Time; no Arts; no Letters; no Society; and which is worst of all, continued fear, and danger of violent death; and the Rousseauian picture of an African golden age of perfect liberty, equality and fraternity.
>
> (Mudimbe 1988: 1)

Mudimbe demonstrates that the Western discourses of African life and thought have introduced major distortions not only for Westerners but also for Africans who try to understand themselves using Western interpretive models. One may also wish to read the papers discussed in this essay using the concepts and theories provided by philosophers of science, such as Bruno Latour (1999) and Ian Hacking (1999), who demonstrate that knowledge is fundamentally a social product that often incorporates ideological elements.

Charles Leslie is one among few contemporary scholars who has led the way to this assertion and further demonstrated that scientific theories infiltrate quite naturally the practice of scientists and that such views are generally supported by hidden ideologies, rarely made explicit.

Acknowledgements

We are grateful to Kendra McKnight for the translation of some French passages into English and the arduous task of editing our English drafts. We are also thankful to Jean-Michel Billette, who compiled the quotations presented in the first part of this essay and to Mark Nichter and anonymous reviewers who contributed with their constructive criticisms to this final version.

Notes

1 The article in question was published in 1989 in *Social Science & Medicine* 28(12): 1211–1220.

2 See *Social Science & Medicine* 31(8): 891–912, 1990; for Leslie's original rebuttal (pp. 891–905), followed in the same issue with comments by J. Philippe Rushton (pp. 905–909), C. Owen Lovejoy (pp. 909–910), Glen D. Wilson (pp. 910–911), Peter J. M. McEwan, founder and Editor-in-Chief of the journal (at the time) (pp. 911–912), and a final rejoinder by Charles Leslie (p. 912).

3 It is common epidemiological knowledge that about two-thirds of AIDS cases in the world live today in sub-Saharan Africa and that the disease may have been present on the continent since the late 1950s.

4 Dapper devoted most of his life to geographical and ethnographic research, which resulted in the publication of a series of large illustrated in-folio books (over 500 pages each) describing various regions around the world: his home-town Amsterdam (1663), China (1670), North India, Persia and Georgia (1672), Palestine and Syria (1677), Arabia (1680), and Greece (1688). His most popular book has been the *Description of Africa* (920 pp.), which was first published in 1668 and reprinted in 1676; the French edition here quoted (and translated into English by us) was published in Amsterdam in 1686. Readers should be reminded that the Netherlands were in those days at the peak of their maritime expansion and commercial stations were established in North America (the Hudson valley, New Amsterdam/New York), Asia (Sri Lanka), South America (Surinam), and different parts of Africa. When Dapper wrote his book, the famous Dutch Company of the Western Indies had over twenty permanent agents based in West and Central Africa. Amsterdam was also the center of important editorial and publishing activities during the second part of the seventeenth century.

5 In his bibliography, Dapper mentions over a hundred publications in Latin, Dutch, Spanish, English, French, Italian, and other languages, on a wide variety of subjects: geography, botany, zoology, linguistics, history, ethnography, economy, politics, medicine, and physical anthropology. Most likely these sources were accessed in private collections rather than public libraries, which were rare and ill-equipped in those days. The ethnographic style of Dapper should also be acknowledged: he refused to make generalizations about Africans and preferred describing each society separately, with minimal ethno-centric connotations. For example, he described African ritual practices as cults and not as superstitions; he stressed the aesthetic qualities of material culture; and he mentioned the reliability of oral traditions for the reconstruction of the history of African societies.

6 The epigraph of this section, taken from Dapper's *Description of Africa*, refers to sexual practices in this region (now Ghana).

7 It seems more plausible that sterility among Gold Coast women was actually related to sexually transmitted diseases (particularly gonorrhea and syphilis) most likely introduced by European navigators and travelers who had been roving along these coasts for more than 150 years at the time Dapper was writing.

8 White (1799: 77) further writes: "From which it appears that in those particulars wherein mankind excels brutes, the European excels the African. It remains yet to notice that in those particular respects in which the brutes excel mankind, the African excels the European: these are chiefly the senses of seeing, hearing, and smelling; the faculty of memory, and the power of mastication." (p. 77). Although attributing Africans with a mnemonic capacity superior to Europeans, White (p. 82) justifies his assertion in the following terms: "It is said that Negroes excel Europeans in memory; but those domestic animals with which we are best acquainted, as the horse and the dog, excel the human species in this faculty."

9 We will not be surprised if one or another sociobiologist will sooner or later argue that the return to conjugal fidelity in postmodern couples of the late twentieth century constitutes an adaptive response inscribed in the genetic material of humans. Monogamy, they will probably write, has developed in the context of the pandemic of sexually transmitted diseases, where couples formed as exclusive partners had a greater tendency to survive.

10 An analysis conducted in 1976 by Getchell et al. (1987) in serum samples of 454 individuals from the Abumonbazi region, in Zaire, revealed that 5% were testing HIV-positive (Bibeau 1991: 128).

11 In a recent overview of this issue, De Cock (1996) states that although we may not know exactly when humans were initially infected with HIV, tests carried out in blood serum banks suggest that HIV-1 may have been present in Central Africa as early as 1959 and that HIV-2 has been in Western Africa since the 1960s. He adds that descriptions of a clinical illness in Central Africa suggestive of AIDS were published in the mid-1970s and maybe even earlier and that similarly, in Western Africa, cases of AIDS have been reported in people who were likely infected in the 1960s or 1970s. These various data sets suggest, according to him, that HIV-1 and HIV-2 were present in Central and Western Africa for some time, and the AIDS epidemic developed in the mid- to late 1970s (De Cock 1996).

12 This contention made in 1989 by Rushton and Bogaert about low rates of HIV infection among Mongoloids proved not to be true: though AIDS was slower to emerge in Asia, WHO estimates there are currently more than 5.5 million people infected with HIV in South-East Asia only (including India, Thailand, and Myanmar), which represents 18% of the global total number of cases (WHO 1999: 26).

13 In 1987 Daniel Hrdy had also published, in the *Review of Infectious Diseases*, an overview of the ethnographic information, which had great impact, particularly among microbiologists and public health specialists, for the promotion of a behaviorist approach to AIDS. Hrdy examined "sexual behaviours," "ritual practices," and customs from the point of view of their potential as a "risk factor" for HIV transmission and sketched, mainly on the basis of the "Human Relations Area Files," an "ethnic cartography" of the level of risk according to the local ritual and sexual practices.

14 As most junior anthropologists would know, there are many limitations in using the fragmented and narrow data set offered by the Human Relations Area Files, and authors should remain cautious in drawing conclusions

and making generalizations from this source. In short, we do not see much difference between the strategy followed by Caldwell et al. in assembling data for their paper and Dapper's famous *Description of Africa* (1686), except that the latter presents a more balanced picture of the diversity found in African cultures at the time.

15 According to Sander Gilman (quoted by Packard and Epstein 1991), the tendency to link African sexuality with communicable diseases, such as tuberculosis and syphilis, has a long history in Western thought (Gilman 1985).

16 We must acknowledge that, in the last few years, Feldman retreated to a less sexually driven explanation of HIV transmission and became more critical of Western approaches linking sexuality to the AIDS epidemic in Africa.

17 The critical perspective advocating the importance of the political and economic context for the study of health problems is steadily developing among medical anthropologists. Didier Fassin (1996, 1997) in France and Paul Farmer (1992, 1999) in the U.S. are actively engaged in promoting politico-economic approaches as a way to counterbalance the dominant culturalist frame in medical anthropology.

18 Among the few scholars who have contradicted Rushton's views in recent years we think it important to highlight an excellent overview and critical analysis of racism as an ideological construct made by Margaret Lock (1993), as well as the work of Peter Rigby (1996). More recently, Peter N. Peregrine et al. (2000) published a piece in the *Anthropology News*, a monthly publication of the American Anthropological Association (AAA), urging colleagues to critically examine Rushton's scientific claims, by "... forcefully demonstrating the flaws in logic, theory and substance upon which his work is based" (p. 29). Peregrine and colleagues from the Human Relations Area Files were upset by the fact that members of the AAA, the American Psychological Association and the American Sociological Association received "... an unsolicited copy of J. Philippe Rushton's 'Special Abridged Edition' (1999) of *Race, Evolution, and Behavior*."

19 In his response to the Rushton and Bogaert paper, Charles Leslie (1990) has skillfully described the biosocial models upon which biological anthropology is now structured.

References

Ahlberg, B.M. (1991). *Women, Sexuality and the Changing Social Order: the impact of government policies on reproductive behaviour in Kenya*. New York: Gordon & Breach.

—— (1994). Is there a distinct African sexuality? A critical response to Caldwell. *Africa* 64(2): 220–242.

Appiah, K.A. (1992). *In My Father's House. Africa in the Philosophy of Culture*. New York: Oxford University Press.

Barkow, J.H. (1989). *Darwin, Sex, and Status. Biological Approaches to Mind and Culture*. Toronto: University of Toronto Press.

Benoist, J. (1995). Races et racisme: à propos de quelques entrechats de la science et de l'idéologie. In P. Blanchard (ed.) *L'autre et nous*. Paris: Syros, pp. 21–28.

Bibeau, G. (1991). L'Afrique, terre imaginaire du sida. La subversion du discours scientifique par le jeu des fantasmes. *Anthropologie et sociétés* 15(2–3): 126–146.

Buffon, G.-L.L. (1753). *Histoire naturelle, générale et particulière*. Paris: Syros.

Bygbjerg, I.C. (1983). AIDS in a Danish Surgeon (Zaire, 1976). *Lancet* 1(8330): 925.

Caldwell, J.C. and Caldwell, P. (1996). The African AIDS epidemic. *Scientific American* 274(3): 62–68.

Caldwell, J.C., Caldwell, P. and Quiggin, P. (1989). Disaster in an Alternative Civilization. The Social Dimension of AIDS in Sub-Saharan Africa. *Population and Development Review* 15(2): 185–234.

Caldwell, J.C., Orubuloye, I.O. and Caldwell, P. (1991). The destabilization of the traditional Yoruba sexual system. *Population and Development Review* 17(2): 229–262.

Camper, P. (1792). *Dissertation sur les variétés naturelles qui caractérisent la physionomie des hommes des divers climats et des différents ages.* Paris: Francart.

Clumeck, N., Sonnet, J., Taelman, H., Mascart-Lemone, F., De Bruyere, M., Vandeperre, P., Dasnoy, J., Marcelis, L., Lamy, M., Jonas, C. (1984). Acquired immunodeficiency syndrome in African patients. *New England Journal of Medicine* 310(8): 492–497.

Conrad, J. (1995) (1898). *Heart of Darkness.* Peterborough, Ontario: Broadview Press.

Dapper, O. (1686). *Description de l'Afrique.* Amsterdam: Wolfgang, Waesberge, Boom and van Someren. (Original Dutch edition: 1668).

Dawson, M. (1983). *Socio-Economic and Epidemiological Change in Kenya: 1880–1925.* Doctoral dissertation, University of Wisconsin at Madison.

De Cock, K.M. (1984). AIDS: An Old Disease from Africa? *British Medical Journal* 289: 306–308.

—— (1996). The emergence of HIV/AIDS in Africa. *Revue d'épidémiologie et de santé publique* 44: 511–518.

Durham, W.H. (1990). Advances in Evolutionary Culture Theory. *Annual Review of Anthropology* 19: 187–210.

Epstein, H. (1999). "Something Happened," a review of Edward Hooper "The River: A Journey to the Source of HIV and AIDS" in *The New York Review of Books* 46(19): 14–18.

—— (2000). "The Mystery of AIDS in South Africa." *The New York Review of Books* 47(12): 50–55.

Essex, M. and Kanky, P.J. (1988). The origins of the AIDS virus. *Scientific American* 258: 64–71.

Farmer, P. (1992). *AIDS and accusation. Haiti and the geography of blame.* Berkeley: University of California Press.

—— (1999). *Infections and Inequalities: the modern plagues.* Berkeley: University of California Press.

Fassin, D. (2000) Une crise épidémiologique dans les sociétés de post-apartheid: Le SIDA en Afrique de Sud et Namibie. *Afrique contemporaine* n° spécial "Situations nouvelles?": 105–115.

—— (1996). Ideology, pouvoir et maladie: eléments d'une anthropologie politique du sida en Afrique. In M. Cros (ed.) *Les maux de l'autre.* Paris: L'Harmattan, pp. 65–93.

—— (1999). L'anthropologie entre engagement et distanciation. Essai de sociologie des recherches en sciences sociales sur le sida en Afrique. In C. Becker, J.-P. Dozon, C. Obbo, and Moriba Touré (eds.) *Vivre et penser le sida en Afrique,* Dakar/Paris: CODESRIA/Karthala/IRD, pp. 41–66.

Feldman, D.A. (1986). Anthropology, AIDS and Africa. *Medical Anthropology Quarterly* 17(2): 38–40.

—— (1991). *Comments* on "Epidemiologists, social scientists, and the structure of medical research on AIDS in Africa." *Social Science & Medicine* 33(7): 783–784.

Freedman, D.G. (1979). *Human Sociobiology.* New York: Free Press.

Getchell, J.P., Hicks, D.R., Svinivasan, A., Heath, J.L., York, D.A., Malonga, M., Forthal, D.N., Mann, J.M. and McCormick, J.B. (1987). Human Immuno-deficiency Virus Isolated from a Serum Sample Collected in 1976 in Central Africa. *Journal of Infectious Diseases* 156(5): 833–837.

Gilman, S. (1985). *Difference and Pathology: Stereotypes of Sexuality, Race and Madness.* Ithaca: Cornell University Press.

Goody, J.R. (1976). *Production and reproduction: A Comparative Study of the Domestic Domain.* Cambridge: Cambridge University Press.

Gould, S.J. (1981a). *The Mismeasure of Man.* New York and London: W. W. Norton Company.

—— (1981b). *The Panda's Thumb: More Reflections in Natural History.* New York and London: W. W. Norton Company.

—— (1983). Of Crime, Cause and Correlation. *Discover* 4(12): 34–43.

Goze, T., and Séri, D. (1991). *Comportements sexuels et SIDA en Côte d'Ivoire.* Rapport d'étude présenté au GPA de l'OMS, Abidjan: Institut de sociologie et d'anthropologie.

Hacking, I. (1999). *The Social Construction of What?* Cambridge: Harvard University Press.

Héritier, F. (1984). Stérilité, aridité, sécheresse: quelques invariants de la pensée symbolique. In Marc Augé and Claudine Herzlich (editors) *Le sens du Mal.* Paris: Editions des Archives contemporaines, pp. 123–154.

Hooton, E.A. (1947). *Up from the Ape.* Revised Edition. New York: Macmillan.

Hrdy, D.B. (1987). Cultural practices contributing to the transmission of human immunodeficiency virus in Africa. *Review of Infectious Diseases* 9: 1109–1119.

Jacquemin, J.-P. (editor) (1991). *Le Noir du Blanc. Racisme. Continent obscur.* Bruxelles: Coopération par l'Education et la Culture.

Latour, B. (1999). *Pandora's Hope. Essays on the Reality of Science Studies.* Cambridge: Harvard University Press.

Le Blanc, M.-N., Meintel, D. and Piché, V. (1991). The African Sexual System: Comment on Caldwell et al. *Population and Development Review* 17(3): 497–505.

Leslie, C. (1990). Scientific Racism: Reflections on Peer Review, Science and Ideology. *Social Science & Medicine* 31(8): 891–912.

Lévi-Strauss, C. (1952). *Race et Histoire.* Paris: UNESCO.

Lock, M. (1993). The Concept of Race: An Ideological Construct. *Transcultural Psychiatric Research Review* 30(3): 203–228.

Lovejoy, C.O. (1981). The Origin of Man. *Science* 211: 341–350.

—— (1990). Comments on "Scientific Racism: Reflections on Peer Review, Science and Ideology." *Social Science & Medicine* 31(8): 909–910.

McEwan, P.J.M. (1990). Comments on Scientific Racism: Reflections on Peer Review. Science and Ideology. *Social Science & Medicine* 31(8): 911–912.

Miller, N. and Rockwell, R.C. (editors) (1988). *AIDS in Africa: the Social and Policy Impact.* Lewiston: Edwin Mellen Press.

Montagu, M.F.A. (1964). *The Concept of Race*. Toronto: Collier-MacMillan.

Mudimbe, V.Y. (1988). *The Invention of Africa. Gnosis, Philosophy and the Order of Knowledge*. Bloomington and Indianapolis: Indiana University Press.

Nau, J.-Y. (1987). "'L'épidémie sera à l'origine d'une mutation majeure de la société africaine,' nous déclare le professeur Clumeck." *Le Monde*, 28 November 1987.

Packard, R.M. (1989). *White Plague, Black Labour: Tuberculosis and the Political Economy of Health and Disease in South Africa*. Berkeley: University of California Press.

Packard, R.M. and Epstein, P. (1991). Epidemiologists, social scientists and the structure of medical research on AIDS in Africa. *Social Science & Medicine* 33(7): 771–783.

Pauw, C. (1774). *Recherches philosophiques sur les Américains*. Berlin.

Pellow, D. (1990). Sexuality in Africa. *Trends in History* 4(4): 71–96.

Peregrine, P.N., Carol, R. and Ember, M. (2000). Teaching Critical Evaluation of Rushton. *Anthropology News* (February) 41(2): 29–30.

Rigby, P. (1996). *African Images. Racism and the End of Anthropology*. Oxford, Washington, D.C.: Berg.

Rose, S. (1998). *Lifelines. Biology Beyond Determinism*. New York: Oxford University Press (see Chapter 10: The Poverty of Reductionism).

Rushton, J.P. (1990). *Comments* on "Scientific Racism: Reflections on Peer Review, Science and Ideology." *Social Science & Medicine* 31(8): 905–909.

—— (1999). *Race, Evolution & Behavior*. (Special Abridged Edition). Charles Darwin Research Institute.

Rushton, J.P. and Bogaert, A.F. (1989). Population Differences in Susceptibility to AIDS: An Evolutionary Analysis. *Social Science & Medicine* 28(12): 1211–1220.

Serwadda D., Mugerwa, R.D., Sewankambo, N.K., Lwegaba, A., Carswell, J.W., Kirya, G.B., Bayley, A.C., Downing, R.G., Tedder, R.S., Clayden, S.A., et al. (1985). Slim disease: a new disease in Uganda and its association with HTLV-III infection. *Lancet* 2(8460): 849–52.

UNAIDS (2000). Adults and children estimated to be living with HIV/AIDS at the end of 1999. Epidemic Update Report. http://www.unaids.org/epidemic_update/report/epi_core/index.htm

Van de Perre P., Clumeck, N., Carael, M., Nzabihimana, E., Robert-Guroff, M., De Mol, P., Freyens, P., Butzler, J.P., Gallo, R.C. and Kanyamupira, J.B. (1985). Female prostitutes: a risk group for infection with human T-cell lymphotropic virus type III. *Lancet* 2(8454): 524–527.

von Linné, K. (1735). *Systema Naturae*. Leyden: Haak.

Way, P.O. and Stanecki, K. (1991). *The Demographic Impact of AIDS in Sub-Sahara Africa*. Washington: Center for International Research, United States Bureau of the Census.

White, C. (1799). *An Account of the regular gradation in man and in different animals and vegetables*. London: C. Dilly.

WHO (1999). *The World Health Report: Making a Difference*. Geneva: World Health Organization.

Wilson, E.D. (1975). *Sociobiology: The New Synthesis.* Cambridge: Harvard University Press.

Wilson G.D. (1990). *Comments* on "Scientific Racism: Reflections on Peer Review, Science and Ideology." *Social Science & Medicine* 31(8): 910–911.

Chapter 7

"We five, our twenty-five"

Myths of population out of control in contemporary India

Patricia Jeffery and Roger Jeffery[1]

CHARAN SINGH:[2] I have three sons – the third came in the foolishness of looking for a girl. I will try to educate them all to MA level in the hopes they will get service. It doesn't matter if they all go away to work, I can always employ someone to do the farm work. Unless they get a good job, what benefit will there be from the education? Fortunately, my wife can supervise the children's study; I myself don't have the time.

ROGER: Why did you want a girl?

CHARAN SINGH: First to help her mother in the house, before she is married; secondly because if there is any work to be done (like getting a glass of water or some food) a girl will never refuse but a son will; also a daughter is needed for me to get the merit of giving a daughter in marriage.

ROGER: Why not have only one son, then he would get all the land?

CHARAN SINGH: Like I said, I need more than one in case that one son is bad.

ROGER: Then why not have many more sons?

CHARAN SINGH: Yes, that would be good for making the country strong; and would be important, for example in fighting, like against the Muslims, because their population is growing faster. But children are too expensive: the everyday costs are so high I couldn't afford any more.

Fertility in India has been declining since the early 1970s and numerous recent studies indicate that many people say that they can afford only a few children. In the same period, family planning has been ineluctably flavored by the communalization of politics at both national and grass-roots levels, with the widespread belief that Indian Muslims oppose family planning and do not adhere to the often-expressed ideal of "two boys and a girl." Thus, this interchange with a Hindu middle-to-rich peasant farmer from the locally dominant Jat caste in Bijnor district (Uttar Pradesh, north

India) encapsulates important themes in current understandings of India's fertility transition.

In this chapter we pick up one theme from the work of Charles Leslie: his willingness to confront issues over which he feels deeply. As he says, "Particularly in the social sciences we must examine what we are passionate about, and how our passions influence our work" (Leslie 1990b: 912). Charles made this comment in the context of a discussion of "scientific" racism: here, we confront arguments about Muslim Indians that are frighteningly similar to those Charles has helped to expose. Our paper has three sections. The first outlines "myths of population out of control," especially those about the scale and causes of fertility differentials between Hindus and Muslims that are associated with the so-called Hindu Right. These ideas have a common-sense quality, a pervasive but misplaced credibility, even for people with no active involvement in Hindu Right politics. The second section begins to challenge these views by examining how demographers have addressed Hindu-Muslim fertility through themes like regional differences, variations in socio-economic position, and occupation rather than religion as such. We are broadly sympathetic to their approach, yet demographers' elaborate statistical analyses on large-scale data sets are not readily sensitive to local-level variations. To conclude, we turn to our research in rural Bijnor to shed light both on Hindu Right political rhetoric and on the limitations of macro-level demographic analyses.

Communal politics and the numbers game

The Hindu Right comprises several organizations, including the Bharatiya Janata Party (BJP), Rashtriya Swayamsevak Sangh (RSS or National Volunteer Corps), Vishwa Hindu Parishad (VHP) and their associated women's and youth organizations.[3] These organizations epitomize an explicitly Hindu nationalist stance (as distinct from Nehru's "secular" nationalism). For instance, during the 1980s, they spearheaded a campaign to remove the Babari Masjid (a sixteenth-century mosque in Ayodhya), claiming that it was built over the birthplace of the Hindu god Ram. Their supporters demolished the mosque in 1992 and anti-Muslim riots flared around India.[4] The BJP (the Hindu Right's main political party) and allied parties have been elected in several Indian states at various times during the 1990s. In 1996, the BJP was the largest party in the central parliament in New Delhi, and its leader has been Prime Minister since 1998.

During the 1980s and 1990s, the Hindu Right echoed allegations repeatedly made in Hindu nationalist discourse since the early twentieth century that Muslims constitute a threat to the "Hindu community" (Datta 1993). A heightened pre-occupation with "community" numbers and population growth rates has been linked to colonial census operations and other aspects of British rule, especially from the latter part of the nineteenth century onwards (Appadurai 1993; Cohn 1987; Jones 1981; Pandey 1990). During the twentieth century, Hindu nationalist claims have focused *inter alia* on Muslim expansionism through invasions, forced conversions, and the abduction of Hindu women and have characterized Muslim men as militant, sexually predatory, and a danger to India's integrity (Bacchetta 1994, 1996; A. Basu 1993; Gupta 1998, 2002; Jaffrelot 1995; Pandey 1991). This discourse also portrays Indian Muslims as complicit with Pakistan, with their efforts to boost Muslim numbers supposedly entailing the conversion of poor Hindus (financed with Gulf state money) and schemes to infiltrate Muslims from Pakistan and Bangladesh into India (A. M. Basu 1996: 132–135; T. Basu et al. 1993: 74–75; Gupta and Sharma 1996; Jaffrelot 1996: 338ff.; Wright 1983).[5]

To argue on the Hindu Right's chosen ground of contrasting the demographic profiles of religious communities risks conceding that "the philosophical postulates of a particular religion ... constitute the exclusive, unchanging organisational principles for an entire people across all kinds of spaces, times and historical change" (T. Basu et al. 1993: 74). Differences in life-chances *within* the categories "Hindu" and "Muslim", however, are likely to be as significant as variations *between* the two categories. Essentializing Hindu and Muslim demographic behavior, though, is part of the Hindu Right's strategy to gain and retain political power, by creating an "Other" and reinforcing their own claim to represent all who regard themselves as Hindu. Given the Hindu Right's leading role in contemporary Indian politics, we would be evading our academic responsibilities if we refused to confront their myths of population out of control – even if, in doing so, we risk being mired in the numbers game (compare with A. M. Basu 1996: 154).

Islam and family planning

An enduring feature of the Hindu Right's anti-Muslim rhetoric is that Indian Muslims have a grand plan to render Hindus a minority in their "own country," a claim that relies heavily on asserting that Muslim fertility is significantly higher than that of Hindus. Since the early 1970s, Hindu Right propaganda has also vigorously insisted that Indian Muslims are antinational because of their supposed refusal to adopt "modern" contraception (for example, Hendre 1971 and Prakash 1979; A. M. Basu 1996, 1997; Wright 1983). Indeed, some Hindu religious leaders, with support from communal political parties (Jana Sangh [now BJP] and Shiv Sena), have advocated population growth for Hindus to avert the purported threat of being outnumbered (Mandelbaum 1974: 105).

The view that Islamic doctrine opposes family planning and that Muslims docilely respond to their religious leaders' propaganda draws on (and feeds into) a much wider pattern of portraying Muslims as dominated by Islam. Yet comparable assumptions are rarely made about adherents of other religions. Extrapolations are drawn from a few Islamic theologians, with little thought to their social locations, to disputes among different schools of Islamic thought, to changes through time, or to the complex relationships between theology and everyday social practices.[6]

Through the centuries, Islamic texts have lent themselves to diverse theological stances on family planning. Omran (1992), for instance, focuses on the lack of clarity in Islamic texts over the acceptability of different forms of contraception, noting that some sources condone *coitus interruptus* and suggesting (by extension) that all forms of non-terminal family planning are acceptable. Some theologians have regarded abortion as acceptable before "ensoulment," which occurs after the third month of pregnancy. Some authorities consider wanting to avoid poverty or to raise family living standards unacceptable motives for contraception, whereas wishing to avoid endangering the mother's health or transmitting a serious disease can be morally justified. Theological objections have been raised about sterilization – that the permanent prevention of conception signifies a lack of faith in God's capacity to provide – and it seems not to be actively endorsed by any school of Islamic jurisprudence (Khan 1979: 184–191).

In South Asia, Maulana Maudoodi argued in *Radiance* (the Jama'at-i Islami journal) that birth control produces sexual anarchy (Wright 1983).[7] In Pakistan, though, Maudoodi's position was not influential, and other Islamic leaders there have not denounced sterilization in particular, despite their generalized opposition to the government's family planning programs. In Bangladesh, the steep decline in the Total Fertility Rate and the rise in contraceptive prevalence rates since the early 1970s undermine the view that doctrinal opposition prevents South Asian Muslims from adopting family planning (Caldwell et al. 1999; Levin et al. 1999). In several other Muslim-majority countries, large numbers of men and women have undergone sterilization, including Iran where it was banned after the Revolution of 1979 but made available again after 1989 (Obermeyer 1994).

In India, some Muslim religious leaders have suggested that the political Emergency (1975–1977) was an era when family planning staff and other government workers disproportionately targeted Muslims for sterilization. Some Muslim clerics, indeed, have claimed that family planning (especially sterilization) is contrary to Islam, but their failure to endorse the Indian government's family planning program reflects the politics of minority status. Indian Muslims' fertility behavior cannot be attributed to a supposedly universal and timeless Islamic condemnation of contraception in general, or of sterilization in particular (A. M. Basu 1996: 139–141). In any case, if Muslim religious leaders in India condemn contraception, we must ask how far their audiences take this into consideration in their own fertility behavior (compare Cassen 1978: 56). This question is further complicated by the Indian family planning program's obsession with sterilization (see below).

The "backward" Muslim woman and polygamy

From the mid-nineteenth century, Christian missionaries and local reformers alike condemned the seclusion of women (*purdah*) for causing health problems, endangering women in childbirth, preventing girls from attending school, and ensuring that their "backwardness" would continue to undermine their role as mothers (Lal 1999; Minault 1998; Savage 1997). The most strictly secluded were women from the élite classes, whether Muslim or Hindu. In practice, then, *purdah* was not an Islamic institution, though it was often (erroneously) said to have been introduced into India by Muslim invaders.

A key strand in the Hindu Right's recent rhetorical demonization of Indian Muslims is how purportedly Islamic institutions, such as *purdah*, victimize Muslim women and perpetuate their "backwardness." This echoes (though with a communalist spin) contemporary demographers' preoccupations with the links between women's "autonomy," girls' schooling, and fertility (see below). Hindu Right claims about Muslim women's "backwardness", however, have generally been more indirectly linked to fertility through discourses on polygamy. Muslim men are stereotyped as more sexually active than Hindu men and as wanting more sexual partners and more children from them. Muslim women are cast as victims of Muslim men's (supposedly) excessive sexual appetites.[8]

Yet the proportion of Muslim men with more than one wife is small and about the same as or *less* than among Hindus (Krishnakumar 1991; National Committee on the Status of Women 1975: 21–23, 40–42). In rural Bijnor, polygamy is rare and it occurs about equally among Muslims and Hindus. Ethnographic accounts of Indian Muslims generally make only passing reference to polygamy. In practice, of course, there could be many polygamous marriages among Muslims only if Muslim men were marrying much younger women, or if (as the Hindu Right sometimes claims) women from other "communities" were converting and marrying Muslim men. There is, however, no credible evidence of conversions on a scale sufficient to create significant demographic shifts. In addition, the suggested link between polygamy and raised levels of fertility is problematic: what little evidence there is suggests that women in polygamous marriages usually have fewer not more children than comparable women in monogamous unions (A. M. Basu 1996: 138–139, 1997: 10–11).[9] In any case, polygamy has long been extremely contentious among Muslims. Conservatives generally say that Islam *permits* but does not actively encourage polygamy. Modernists argue that the Qur'anic verse that apparently permits polygamy sets such stringent conditions (that a man treat his wives equally) that it is effectively a prohibition, unless there are exceptional circumstances.[10]

Hindu Right rhetoric, then, rests on two crucial but false assumptions: that polygamy is common among Muslims but unknown among Hindus and that it is associated with high levels of fertility. Nevertheless, in 1968, the *Organiser* (the RSS journal) asserted that Muslims were using polygamy to activate the population bomb as a war tactic against Hindus (Bacchetta 1994: 198). During the Babri Masjid campaign, Sadhvi Saraswati claimed that polygamy "turns Muslim women into sexual objects and breeders", that for every five Hindu children born, Muslims have fifty and that Hindus would become a minority in India within twenty-five years (quoted in A. Basu 1998: 173; see also A. M. Basu 1996: 137), and Sadhvi Ritambara asserted that "The Muslims got their Pakistan. Even in a mutilated India, they have special rights. They have no use for family planning. They have their own religious schools. What do we have? An India with its arms cut off. ... The state tells us Hindus to have only two or three children. After a while they will say "do not have even one." But what about those who have six wives, 30–35 children, and breed like mosquitoes and flies?" (quoted in Kakar 1996: 225–226). The Indian government's family planning slogan advocating a small family norm for everyone – *"ham do, hamre do"* ("we two, our two") with its logo of a couple with their two children – has a public presence across India, from the walls of government buildings to postage stamps and railway tickets. The Hindu Right's distorted appropriation of this slogan neatly encapsulates their fallacies about Muslims and polygamy. A VHP pamphlet published during the Ayodhya campaign contained the riposte: while Hindus (supposedly) obey the government's slogan, Muslim men allegedly have four wives and say, *"ham pānch, hamāre pachīs"* ("we five, our twenty-five;" see Gupta 2002 and Sarkar 1993: 165).

This slogan and the assumptions that Islam is set against contraception and that Muslim men marry polygamously have attained a taken-for-granted quality. Paola Bacchetta and Pradip Datta (personal communications) both suggest that such claims do not figure as centrally in official publications of Hindu Right organizations (such as the RSS) as in verbal discourse, whether interviews or speeches made at rallies and other gatherings. Moreover, what Datta (1999: 23) has termed "a trope of extinction" has become part of the "common truth, a product of social 'good sense'" (Datta 1993: 1305) beyond Hindu Right activists (see also Wright 1983). Certainly, we often heard views such as these in Bijnor in 1990–1991, whether from urban middle-class people whom we met, or from villagers such as Charan Singh. Few were paid-up or active members of any Hindu Right organization (neither was Charan Singh).[11] Yet comments were often larded with the "we five, our twenty-five" slogan, which was also blasted out by the tannoy system at the BJP offices in Bijnor town during the general election campaign in Spring 1991. Even some Muslims we talked to believed that Muslims would outstrip Hindus in the foreseeable future.[12] Crucially, the Hindu Right's narrative rests on the belief that Indian Muslims' fertility behavior is part of a plan to outnumber Hindus, a claim that rests on several demonstrably false premises and that seriously misrepresents the complex social processes that influence fertility.

Demographers on fertility differentials

By contrast, demographers generally do not regard Islamic ideology as a key factor or, indeed, the categories "Hindu" and "Muslim" as sufficiently homogeneous for fertility differentials between them to be meaningfully analyzed.[13] Demographers systematically disaggregate the categories "Hindu" and "Muslim" along socioeconomic lines – region, place of residence (urban or rural), occupation, education (especially of the mother), class – rather than positing essential differences on the basis of religion *per se*. Thus they tend to undermine the very notion of "Muslim fertility". Further, while they might examine the impact of polygamy, along with age of marriage, length of breast-feeding, length of postpartum sexual abstinence, or sexual abstinence by couples whose children are married for instance, they treat these as proximate variables affecting fertility without making any assumptions about people's intentions. In recent years, demographers have also focused on gender politics, but in a decidedly different fashion from the Hindu Right. The findings of academic demographers, then, provide compelling critiques of the Hindu Right's simplistic claims about Hindu-Muslim differences in fertility behavior.

Region, class, and fertility

At the macro-level, Indian demographic statistics indicate that Muslim fertility rates are somewhat higher than those among Hindus, and that Muslims make up a (slowly) growing share of the Indian population (up from 10.5 per cent in 1951 to 12.5 per cent in 1991). Apart from some small-scale surveys and local case studies, demographers have mainly relied on special national surveys (Registrar General India 1982; International Institute of Population Sciences 1995) and the 1981 and 1991 national censuses for their analyses of interreligious fertility differentials in India. Selecting only one indicator (total fertility rate, TFR), the Infant and Child Mortality Survey produced all-India estimates for 1978 for rural Muslim TFRs about 12 per cent above those of Hindus (5.01 compared to 4.48) and somewhat more than 12 per cent for urban residents (3.98 compared to 2.97).

Disaggregated figures, however, provide a more complex picture. The regional distribution of Muslims is uneven: in 1981, 36 per cent of them lived in Bihar and Uttar Pradesh, which accounted for only 27 per cent of India's total population. These northern states have higher fertility and mortality rates than the rest of the country: the 1978 estimated rural TFR for Muslims was 6.39 and for Hindus was 5.82 in Uttar Pradesh (UP), and in Tamil Nadu the TFRs were 3.64 and 3.43 respectively; the urban rates were 3.88 and 3.21 in UP and 3.24 and 2.67 in Tamil Nadu. That is, Hindu fertility rates in north India are often higher than Muslim rates in central, eastern, and south India.[14] The national surveys also show sizable statistical effects for the literacy level of the mother, age at marriage, and total household expenditure, all of which are greater than the interreligious differentials.

Within north India, Muslims are more urbanized than Hindus (in UP and Bihar 29 per cent of Muslims live in towns, whereas only 15 per cent of Hindus do), but urban Muslims disproportionately occupy poorer housing areas with lower levels of public health infrastructure and have lower-paid jobs than their Hindu neighbors. More than half the urban Muslims are reported to have incomes below the poverty line, compared to 35 per cent of urban Hindus. In 1978, 79 per cent of rural Muslim households owned less than one hectare, compared to 68 per cent of rural Hindu households (Krishnakumar 1991; Shariff 1995; Sridhar 1991). In brief, Muslims are poorer and less educated than Hindus, as well as being distributed differently across the country (Registrar General, India 1982).

The independent effect of religion, however, seems not to have been analyzed using either of the large national surveys. Published analyses of the 1992–1993 data provide all-India comparisons of TFR (4.41 for Muslims and 3.30 for Hindus) but urban and rural rates by state have apparently not yet been systematically produced (Moulasha and Rama Rao 1999). Regional differences in fertility levels are still clear-cut (Mari Bhat and Zavier 1999). Multivariate analysis of the independent role of religion has been done only for contraceptive use – and then only controlling for education and region separately, and not for socioeconomic status (Ramesh and Retherford 1996). Large-scale survey data, then, indicate that there are interreligious fertility differentials, but not whether they would remain or how large they would be after controlling for other important variables.[15] The 1981 and 1991 census data, however, do present correlations between district-level characteristics and fertility, mortality, and female disadvantage (for example, Drèze and Murthi 1999; Kishor 1993; Mari Bhat and Zavier 1999; Mari Bhat 1996; Murthi et al. 1996). Sometimes religion is not mentioned at all (for example, Murthi et al. 1996) or only in passing (Kishor 1993). Mari Bhat (1996) and Drèze and Murthi (1999), though, find that the Muslim proportion of a district's population correlates positively with fertility indicators, even after controlling for other indicators.[16] In these and other studies, urban–rural residence, women's labor force participation, and mother's schooling have been the key indicators analyzed. Though the details are complex, demographers' analyses of large-scale data sets controlling for a range of social and economic variables significantly (but not wholly) reduce the Hindu–Muslim fertility differentials much trumpeted by the Hindu Right.

Women's "autonomy" and fertility

Since the early 1980s, "women's autonomy", or their capacity to make important decisions about their own lives, has been a preoccupation in demography. Most recent discussions focus on domestic politics – marriage arrangement, women's control over domestic resources, controls over women's mobility – as in Dyson and Moore's (1983) classic contribution. During the 1980s, labor force participation was considered crucial in enhancing women's domestic position and was central to discussions of regional differences in women's autonomy and discrimination against girls (Bardhan 1974; Miller 1981). But the unreliability of indicators of labor force participation derived from the Census proved a major limitation. Recently, only Kishor (1993) has treated it seriously as an explanatory variable, although Moulasha and Rama Rao (1999: 3048), using the National Family Health Survey, note that "only 15% of the Muslim women participated in work [economic activity] whereas for Hindu women the figure was 34%."

One of the most robust statistical relationships, however, is between girls' schooling and fertility decline. During the 1990s, extending girls' access to schooling became central in policy initiatives aimed at enhancing young women's autonomy, particularly with respect to fertility decision making. For India as a whole, survey and census data alike show that Muslims have less schooling than Hindus, reflecting and contributing to Muslims' generally weaker economic positions. Age for age, in rural and urban areas alike, a smaller proportion of Muslim than Hindu children is currently attending schools of any kind (Krishnakumar 1991; Shariff 1995). Up to age nine, approximately equal percentages of Hindu and Muslim boys (urban and rural) attend school; for girls, the situation is comparable, although the percentages of girls at school are lower. For older rural children, however, the gap between Muslim and Hindu enrollment levels widens markedly, especially for girls. In part, this reflects the relative concentration of Muslims in north India, where overall school enrollment rates are lower than elsewhere. Within north India, however, Muslim schooling rates are below those of Hindus in the same class position, especially for schooling beyond primary level.

Some demographic literature on the Middle East claims that features of gender politics that supposedly reduce Muslim women's autonomy (particularly seclusion) are key to understanding continuing high levels of fertility in the region.[17] Generally, though, analyses of women's autonomy have not regarded religious allegiance as a key issue. Krishnakumar (1991) and A. M. Basu (1996) are unusual in the emphasis they place on lower levels of literacy among Muslim women in India as a cause of higher fertility. Dyson and Moore (1983: 53), however, conclude that religious identification has relatively little influence on female autonomy, their main explanatory variable for demographic differences between north and south India.

Population increase, of course, is also a matter of mortality and migration. There is little information on mortality rates by religion in India. Infant death rates are higher in the north than in the south, yet, for the country as a whole, Muslim infant mortality rates were about 109 per 1,000 live births in 1978, compared with about 121 per 1,000 live births for Hindus, a difference of 10 to12 per cent (Registrar General of India 1981). Moulasha and Rama Rao (1999: 3049) quote figures suggesting a child survival rate of children born to Muslim mothers 20 per cent above that of children born to Hindu mothers. Unfortunately, there are few good multivariate analyses that combine factors like region, rural–urban residence, schooling of parents, and economic position to determine the net relationships between religion and mortality. Considering the large contribution of infant and child mortality to total mortality, though, Muslim total mortality might also be around 10 per cent below that of Hindus. If so, this could be almost as significant (in terms of differentials in population totals) as fertility differences but, unlike fertility, mortality has not been politicized by the Hindu Right. For most of India, migration rates are too small to be demographically significant (Moulasha and Rama Rao 1999: 3047), but migration has become politically contentious, with widespread anxiety about the infiltration of people from Bangladesh. In western UP, though, local migration patterns have not been an issue in communal politics.

In sum, demographic analyses indicate that Muslim and Hindu fertility levels alike are higher in rural areas, in north India, and among the poor and the poorly educated, than in urban areas, in south India, or among wealthier and educated couples, especially when the wife has more than eight years of schooling. After taking account of differences in the proportions who marry and in the age distributions of the two categories, demographic differences between religious communities can be largely (though not wholly) understood with reference to social and economic factors. Moreover, all these fertility rates are well below "natural" fertility and fertility was declining for all groups at about the same rate in the 1980s and 1990s, albeit from different starting points. Even if Muslim fertility rates fall more slowly and Muslim mortality rates remain lower than Hindu rates, the Muslim proportion of India's population is unlikely to reach 15 per cent by 2021.[18] This contrasts markedly with Hindu Right rhetoric that reifies the categories "Hindu" and "Muslim", assumes a homogeneity and potency to Islamic ideology, and claims that Muslims will soon outnumber Hindus.

Muslim and Hindu in rural Bijnor

We largely concur with demographers who argue that fertility differentials in India can largely be accounted for by analyzing social and economic variables and that the role of religion *per se* is relatively limited. Yet something still needs to be explained, for fertility differentials remain – albeit much smaller than those implied by Hindu Right rhetoric – even after regional and socioeconomic variables have been taken into account.

In analyzing our Bijnor data, however, we have become increasingly dissatisfied with conventional macrodemographic analysis. First, most demographers rely on special surveys or district-level data from the Census, but problems arise from working with units of analysis as large as a district (with perhaps several million people). When there is diversity below this level, excessive aggregation of data may mask variations between and within localities. Explanations of differences in fertility behavior, then, cannot be meaningfully carried out at the level of nation or even region. Second, demographers conduct elaborate statistical techniques to try to separate out the main elements in a causal model of demographic change, as in the recent emphasis on the widespread, statistically significant correlation between girls' education and low fertility. But our fieldwork suggests that this correlation is not necessarily straightforwardly causal (see below).[19] In general, detailed microstudies using local-level data and dealing with meaningful social groupings provide a better window into the fine-grain and locally specific processes that are likely to elude large-scale surveys. Differences exposed by large-scale statistical analyses, then, may suggest possible hypotheses, but not final answers.

Some social demographers, indeed, advocate amplifying data on measurable features of individuals (age at marriage, desired family size, and so on) derived from large-scale surveys with small-scale studies of the social relationships that link individuals' decisions (or nondecisions) to the collectivities to which they belong. Our experiences in rural Bijnor endorse Greenhalgh's view that we must "situate fertility, that is, to show how it makes sense given the sociocultural and political economic context in which it is embedded" (Greenhalgh 1995: 17). By locating people's approaches to fertility in the context of rural Bijnor, our "situated" account challenges both Hindu Right rhetoric and conventional demographers' accounts. We focus here on local perceptions of the family planning program, examine aspects of gender politics and women's autonomy at the domestic level, and, finally, outline local understandings of social and economic exclusion.

We conducted village surveys and interviewed people from many different caste and class backgrounds in rural Bijnor District. The material here, though, mainly concerns two roughly comparable caste groups, Sheikhs (Muslim) and Jats (Caste Hindu).[20] Muslims in Bijnor District, especially in urban areas, were particularly associated with artisanal and laboring activity. Rural Sheikhs, however, were the prime Muslim landowners, as were the Jats among Caste Hindus. Among Sheikhs and Jats alike there were class differences (assessed largely in terms of land ownership). Even when class was held constant, though, Sheikh fertility was slightly higher than Jat fertility. Hence, we must ask if there were features of the local situation that affected the Sheikhs *as Muslims* and contributed to higher fertility.

Muslims and family planning in rural Bijnor

The image of Muslims rejecting family planning because of Islamic doctrine and an ambition to outnumber Hindus is central to the Hindu Right perspective. Our data suggest that Sheikhs (indeed Muslims in general in rural Bijnor) did resist the government family planning program, but mainly for reasons of quality of service and the contraceptive technologies being offered.

We frequently observed the supercilious and disdainful manner of medical and paramedical staff (who were usually Hindus from relatively high caste urban backgrounds), especially with respect to Muslim and poor Hindu villagers. Semipublic consultations compromised patient privacy and confidentiality, and women were often chided for their childcare practices or their repeated pregnancies. Local sensibilities about family planning were particularly acute, because government health staff have had "targets" (the number of "cases" they should motivate for family planning) throughout much of the period since the mid 1970s. Consultations would routinely be diverted onto family planning (for example, Najma's visit to an ophthalmologist: Jeffery and Jeffery 1996a: 53–68). Many Muslims to whom we talked thought they were singled out by family planning workers, as they believed they had been during the 1975–1977 Emergency, when health workers and other government staff were put under greatest pressure to meet family planning targets. Health staff and many Muslims had diametrically opposed understandings: the former often commented adversely on Muslim views about family planning, the latter described the family planning program as a government initiative to eradicate Muslims. At the same time, health services in Muslim-dominated villages were of poorer quality than in Hindu-dominated villages. Many Muslims complained that they were ignored in public health campaigns, such as immunizations, although some regarded such services as mere sweeteners to persuade people to accept family planning.

Mistrust of government health and family planning services was undoubtedly exacerbated by a bias toward sterilization (overwhelmingly female sterilization since the late 1970s), despite supposedly offering a "cafeteria" service where people would select the family planning method that best suited their needs. Family planning workers not only had sterilization targets but received incentive payments for every case they motivated (with lower payments for IUCD, i.e. intra-uterine contraceptive devices); family planning acceptors also received small sums after sterilization or IUCD insertion. Pressure on staff was such that they sometimes exaggerated their achievements in the health center records (see P. Jeffery et al. 1989; Narayana and Kantner 1992 provide the national picture). Until the late 1980s, people in rural Bijnor generally thought that family planning and sterilization were synonymous and that family planning staff could or would offer only sterilization. Certainly, some women had IUCDs inserted and the contraceptive pill was available from pharmacies in Bijnor town, but a few women who wished their IUCD to be replaced or who wanted prenatal tetanus injections reported being pressured to become a sterilization "case." Many people, especially poor Hindus and Muslims, feared being coerced into adopting terminal methods such as sterilization. Although most women would have preferred spacing methods, mainly because of their fear of child mortality, it was widely considered futile to try to obtain them from family planning staff.

This led to popular resistance, as witness the requests we received during our research for alternative contraceptive methods, from Muslim and Hindu women alike. Certainly, rather than wanting numerous children, many of the Muslim women we talked to wished to limit their fertility, often pointing to the health costs to themselves and their children of repeated childbearing. Crucially, too, our data indicate significantly *higher* rates of infant and child mortality among rural Muslims in Bijnor than among comparable Hindus, in contrast to all-India statistics.

For Muslims in rural Bijnor, part of the story, but only a part, was certainly their belief that Islam prohibits sterilization and that they should not use the family planning method most readily available through the government health services (P. Jeffery and R. Jeffery 1996b; R. Jeffery and P. Jeffery 1997). But our field notes indicate that their reactions to the family planning program cannot be largely (leave aside wholly) attributed to their understandings of Islamic doctrine. The Muslims we talked to in rural Bijnor approached fertility limitation in a similar fashion to that of most of the other groups in the locality, with no generalized resistance to *spacing* methods of fertility limitation, but with an aversion to terminal methods and a mistrust of the government's family planning program. In other words, our research indicates that many women's needs for acceptable contraception were far from being met.

The Jats presented a striking contrast to this picture. Far more of them were actively limiting their families than were Muslims as a whole (including Sheikhs) and Hindus from the smaller, poorer, and lower castes. Of the Jat women we interviewed in 1991, 59 per cent of those aged 35 to 45 and 42 per cent of those aged 25 to 35 were using some form of modern contraception. They accessed health care and contraceptive services, including pills, IUCDs, and female sterilization via government family planning services as well as local private doctors. Does this mean, then, that instead of trying to account for the fertility differentials between Sheikhs and Jats in rural Bijnor in terms of Islamic doctrine, we should focus on women's capacity to implement their family planning preferences?

Women's autonomy, education, and fertility in rural Bijnor

Deconstructing the household can show that household members (such as husbands and wives) may have conflicting as well as common interests.[21] Gender politics at the household level, then, are likely to be crucial in many matters, including family planning decisions: as Greenhalgh (1995: 14) argues, reproduction is a "deeply gendered process." In recent demographic discussions of women's autonomy and fertility decline, girls' education has been a central concern.

In line with the national picture outlined above, girls from different castes and communities in rural Bijnor tend to have had different schooling experiences. Most Jat women had attended school. Sizable numbers, disproportionately from the wealthiest households, had obtained postschool qualifications such as BA or MA. By contrast, not even Sheikh women from rich peasant households were likely to have been educated outside the home. Those few who did attend school usually went to a *madrasā* (mosque school) rather than a secular school. Might the fertility differentials between rural Sheikhs and Jats that remained after controlling for class be attributed to different schooling experiences and different levels of autonomy among adult women?

Unfortunately, demographers have tended to treat both "education" (usually glossed as "years of schooling") and "autonomy" as black boxes that are simple variables consistently and causally linked to one another and to fertility. Thus Drèze and Murthi (1999: 3), for example, find that "women's education emerges as the most important factor explaining fertility differences across the country and over time". A local-level perspective, however, indicates that "autonomy" and "education" and their interrelationships are far more complex than this.

In rural Bijnor, it is doubtful that schooling experiences in themselves provided women with the capacity to act autonomously. School curricula, styles of classroom interaction, and the body language inculcated in girls at school seemed more likely to sustain conventional gender hierarchies than to enhance girls' autonomy, in the sense of capacity to think and act independently. At a *madrasā*, girls had to cover their heads and behave demurely while learning to recite the *Qu'rān Sharīf*; the wider curriculum did not always include Hindi and other subjects that might give access to knowledge beyond *Islāmiyāt* (Islamic ideas and history); and *madrasā* schooling was terminated once girls reached puberty. Secular schools also provided little scope for ensuring that pupils graduated with enhanced autonomy. In addition, many rural women who studied to BA and MA levels had done so as "private" rather than "regular" students, that is by correspondence courses at home – hardly an effective way of honing the skills and confidence to deal with the world beyond the home that are so often considered an important consequence of school attendance. Moreover, it was abundantly clear that parents did not send daughters to school in order to create autonomous women. Obtaining qualifications for paid employment was almost never considered (although some people said qualifications might enable a woman to stand on her "own legs" after a calamity such as widowhood or divorce). Rather, parents saw their daughters' schooling as a newly important (and quite costly) asset in the marriage market.

Measuring "education" in terms of "years of schooling," then, simply cannot grasp the local meanings attached to girls' schooling or the contrasts between different types of schools or different locations in which girls study. In any case, even if schooling could enable girls to *think* more independently, educated Jat women had no more control over the choice of their marriage partner or the timing of their marriage than women with little or no schooling. In rural Bijnor, young married women of all castes and communities, for whom decisions about fertility were particularly salient, operated within broadly comparable forms of domestic gender politics.

It is generally assumed that *purdah* disempowers women, for it restricts their mobility outside the home and may imply their lack of involvement in paid employment that could provide independent income. For the Hindu Right, *purdah* is a marker of Muslim women's "backwardness," but many ethnographic studies report on seclusion and veiling practices among Hindus, albeit often pointing to subtle differences between Hindu and Muslim *purdah* (see Jacobson and Wadley 1995; Mandelbaum 1986, 1988; Papanek 1982). Certainly, our data do not support an argument that Sheikh women (or indeed Muslim women as a whole) were more restricted by seclusion practices than Jat women (or Hindu women in general). Rather, seclusion practices reflected local ideas about family honor that were common to Hindus and Muslims.

Adult women's mobility beyond the domestic domain reflected differing work demands (relating primarily to the household's class position) and household composition and a woman's position in it (for example, as sole adult woman, or as mother-in-law or daughter-in-law), not religious allegiance. In the wealthiest rural households, women worked inside the house but rarely outside. In poorer households, women often had to work outside, whether as family labor or as employees of wealthier households in the locality, but such mobility was limited to the task at hand and did not imply enhanced autonomy or freedoms. One feature of gender politics remained constant, however: land, the major economic resource, was owned (albeit very inequitably) by men and not by women. Few women had any independent income; employed women worked out of necessity but usually earned very little as they had no marketable skills aside from domestic or farming work. Sheikh and Jat women as a whole, then, were not systematically differentiated in terms of mobility beyond the home, access to land and independent income: such contrasts as were present reflected class rather than community differences.

Our data highlights an additional problem with assuming that "education" straightforwardly enhances young married women's autonomy in their marital homes. The most educated Jat women were married into the richest households and were expected to be home-based. They were also more likely to be married to an only son and thus required to share a household with their mother-in-law. Yet women of all castes and communities thought sharing a household with the mother-in-law was more constricting than running their own household. Thus, girls' education neither correlates convincingly with differences in women's "autonomy" nor provides us with much insight into the fertility differentials between Jats and Sheikhs in rural Bijnor.

Further, low state school attendance by Sheikh and other Muslim girls cannot readily be explained by *purdah* restrictions (or Muslim "backwardness"). For many Muslim families, poverty was an important restraint on sending children to school. For more wealthy Muslims, though, low state school attendance by girls reflected (among other things) the tendency for state schools not to be located in Muslim villages or Muslim areas of mixed villages. Additionally, Muslim parents believed that Muslim girls were sexually and communally harassed at school and that the *madrasā* provided a more appropriate curriculum in a more protected environment.

None of these observations means that gender politics within the household are unimportant in decisions about girls' education (or fertility) in rural Bijnor. They do require, though, that we locate individual behavior and household dynamics within social and economic processes and relations of difference and inequality *beyond* the household (McNicoll 1994).

Perceptions of exclusion in rural Bijnor

For Greenhalgh (1995: 21), fertility transitions are the "products of changes in class-specific opportunity structures in response to transformations of global and regional political economies". Here, then, we want to account for the fertility differentials between Sheikhs and Jats in rural Bijnor in terms of their contrasting locations in local social and economic structures. We focus on the social and political implications of labeling oneself and being labeled by others as "Muslim" in rural Bijnor, not on Muslims as adherents of stereotyped Islamic spiritual beliefs and doctrinal commands.

Dyson (1991) considers that high fertility among poor rural populations does not need much explanation, largely because few people are making active decisions about family sizes. Fertility levels may be lower than "natural" fertility, but they may reflect unintentional factors such as age at marriage, length of breast-feeding, or sexual abstinence, rather than purposeful contraceptive use. By contrast, low or declining fertility in some sectors of the population does need explanation.

Were some Hindus in rural Bijnor, notably the Jats, experiencing social processes that led them to favor small families, whereas Muslims were not? As elsewhere in India, Muslims in rural Bijnor tended to be poorer and less educated. But school attendance by Muslim boys was lower than for Hindu boys even when class was held constant. Sheikh and Jat parents alike saw boys' schooling primarily as a resource in the job market and secondarily as an element in marriage arrangements. Charan Singh's comment quoted above is typical: "Unless they get a good job, what benefit will there be from the education?" Jats were generally optimistic that schooling enhances (though does not guarantee) the chances of obtaining white collar employment. Crucially, however, Sheikhs in Bijnor did not believe that their sons would get good jobs, no matter how much schooling they received. Sheikhs generally did not spend as much money on their children's schooling or put as much pressure on their children to attend school as did the Jats. Although Sheikh parents' views about schooling might adversely affect their sons' job prospects, several pointers suggest that the reverse is more plausible – that Sheikhs' experiences of exclusion from the job market led them to put a lower value on schooling than comparable Hindus.

First, Muslims are not covered by job quotas in government services, unlike members of the Scheduled Castes and Tribes (as defined in the Indian Constitution) and members of the Other Backward Castes (as defined in the government sponsored Mandal Commission Report of 1980). Nowadays, the practical significance of such exclusion is questionable, since there are very few "reserved" posts available. Nevertheless, many Muslims in Bijnor felt that their exclusion reflected other aspects of the Indian government's attitude toward Muslims. Second, our Muslim and Hindu informants generally claimed that job applicants in the public and private sectors alike needed either influence (*safarish*) through caste, kinship, or religious community networks or cash for a bribe (*rishwat*) or both to have much chance of being appointed. Firm evidence for these claims is hard to find. Yet the *belief* in such processes was crucial in parents' calculations about the value of investing in their sons' schooling. The absence (perceived or real) of Muslims from key positions damaged Muslims' access to future appointments, directly (because Muslim applicants have few people over whom they can exert "influence") and indirectly (by disheartening students and their parents at crucial stages of their progress through schooling). This also applied, of course, to poor Hindus who lacked the necessary networks and cash.

In addition, schooling is not standardized. Wealthier families, rural as well as urban, would pay for private schooling and for "tuition" after school hours for their sons, and expect women of the family to supervise children's homework. Poor rural families, however, could access only poor quality schooling and their low levels of social and cultural capital also restricted what their sons could gain from schooling. Muslims were differentially disadvantaged by poverty, yet, unlike children from the Scheduled Castes and Tribes, they were not entitled to scholarships and fee waivers. *Madrasā* schooling may have been more financially accessible, but it fed only into theological training and employment as an *imām* for a few able boys. Further, many Muslims believed that the ambience of mainstream schools was hostile to Islam and that Muslim children were subjected to harassment from other pupils and teachers alike. The uphill struggle to school their sons often hardly felt worthwhile, especially since the rewards, in terms of secure employment, seemed so elusive.

Girls' schooling certainly enters people's calculations about fertility and schooling, but not in the direct way posited by the demographic orthodoxy. Girls' schooling was valued for its contribution to marriageability, not employability. All girls' schooling was conditioned by the need to educate them to a level just below that of the kind of boy to whom their parents hoped to arrange their marriages. For many Jat girls, this could entail lengthy schooling and even college education. By contrast, Muslim girls' problems of harassment and of access to schools were compounded by the low levels of school attendance by Muslim boys, even among the relatively wealthy.

The crucial factor differentiating the fertility regimes of the Jats and the Sheikhs, however, was the Jats' relative success in the off-farm employment market. Most Jat men were limiting their families in pursuit of household goals: to educate their sons and place them in good employment, and to educate their daughters and arrange their marriages to educated young men with off-farm employment who would command increasingly larger dowries. Jat parents, then, obeyed the dictates of their pockets rather than the government's family planning slogan. As Charan

Singh put it, "But children are too expensive: the everyday costs are so high I couldn't afford any more." By contrast, the Sheikhs lacked access to influential people and processes of exclusion from sought-after employment effectively reduced the costs of child-rearing (school fees, bribes, dowry, for instance). Sheikh men were not unthinking followers of *molwis* who (allegedly) told them to have large families. Rather, they remained locked into the agrarian economy. Investing in schooling made little sense and they had little incentive to limit their fertility – calculations that also applied to smaller and poorer Hindu and Muslim groups in rural Bijnor. In these respects, then, there was nothing essentially "Muslim" about the Sheikhs' fertility regime.

Many Sheikh and other Muslim women articulated views on fertility akin to those of their husbands, emphasizing Muslims' difficult social and economic position. In addition, because of low school attendance, Muslim girls were available for marriage at younger ages than comparable Hindu girls. Many Muslim women were dismayed by the damage to their own health and the heavy workloads caused by lengthy childbearing careers. Muslim women wanting contraception often had no option but subterfuge. By contrast, Jat couples generally made family planning decisions jointly. Jat women's wishes usually coincided with their husbands' plans, although a few Jat women could not have as *many* children as they themselves wanted because their in-laws wished to prevent land fragmentation and limit the costs of child-rearing. In brief, Sheikh men did not especially oppress their womenfolk nor did Jat women have greater "autonomy". Rather, men's fertility rationales tended to prevail among Jats and Sheikhs alike.

Concluding thoughts

The communalization of politics in contemporary India has been buttressed by images of vulnerable Hindus (supposedly) doomed to be outnumbered. Assertions about Muslim fertility and about Muslim men's right to marry polygamously have been key to the Hindu Right's propaganda. Such communalist population myths are "short on facts, short on a proper understanding of the demographic situation – and short on honesty" (Krishnakumar 1991: 94) and dangerous propaganda in the victimization of minority groups that contributes to creating the very differences that are used to justify demonizing Muslims.

During our first fieldwork in Bijnor in 1982–1983, local Muslim commentaries on the family planning program and on boys' employment prospects already exposed Muslims' sense of marginalization and vulnerability. Political developments during the 1980s confirmed for them the government's ill intent toward Muslims and reinforced their distrust of the government machine. Muslims' insecurity was also exacerbated by sloganeering from the Hindu Right, by the communal disturbances in many parts of India during late 1990 (including in Bijnor: see A. Basu 1995; R. Jeffery and P. Jeffery 1994) and after the Babari Masjid was demolished in 1992, and by the BJP's subsequent electoral successes.

These physical and symbolic relations of dominance and subordination generated a sense of insecurity that structured the lives of Sheikhs in rural Bijnor simply because they were Muslims. The expense of schooling children and accessing employment was linked to fertility behavior just as much among Sheikhs as among Jat farmers, though with different outcomes. Far from higher fertility being an Islamic strategy for power or a plan to outbreed Hindus, it grew out of the Sheikhs' lack of power when compared with the locally dominant Jats.

Macrolevel data, on which demographers typically rely, mask the fine-grain and complex processes that result in fertility differentials within a locality. The move away from the construction of metanarratives of fertility behavior and toward "situated" accounts, however, offers the promise of greater explanatory potential that could be used to good effect throughout South Asia (though with the details certainly differing from our account here). The move would be important for this reason alone. Given the politicization of population issues in contemporary India, however, it has additional significance. "Situated" accounts allow us to undermine the Hindu Right's views on Indian demography. But we are contending with "a rhetoric that picks and chooses evidence, that ignores alternative hypotheses, that elides issues" (Leslie 1990a: 896) and we find so much wrong with their arguments that we despair of ever persuading them that their science is spurious (1990a: 894). Yet it is imperative and politically urgent to do so. Their views have achieved widespread acceptance and lie behind many acts of everyday routinized violence and discrimination against Muslims in India. We cannot leave the Hindu Right's myths of Indian Muslims' population out of control unchallenged.

Notes

1 This paper is based on fieldwork funded by the Economic and Social Research Council (1982–1983, 1985), by the Moray Fund of the University of Edinburgh (1985–1986), and by the Overseas Development Administration (1990–1991). We are grateful to them for their support; none of these organizations is responsible for the opinions expressed here. Our thanks also go to all the people in Bijnor who were so generous with their time and to our research assistants (Swaleha Begum, Radha Rani Sharma, Savita Pandey, Chhaya Pandey, Zarin Ahmed and Swatantra Tyagi). Earlier versions of this paper were presented at meetings in Edinburgh (1995), Heidelberg (1996) and Cambridge (2000) and we thank colleagues there and elsewhere for their comments, especially Michael Anderson, Paola Bacchetta, Alaka Basu, Pradip Datta, Christophe Jaffrelot, Donald MacKenzie, Mark Nichter, and Pravin Visaria.

2 Charan Singh is a pseudonym. This is our translation from the Hindi.
3 The Hindu Right is also known as the Sangh Parivar or "Family of the Sangh" (that is the Rashtriya Swayamsevak Sangh). Space precludes detailed analysis of differences in emphasis among these organizations.
4 On the Ayodhya affair and the communalization of politics in contemporary India, see A. Basu and Kohli (1998), T. Basu et al. (1993), Chakravarti et al (1992), Engineer (1991), Gopal (1991), M. Hasan (1997), Jaffrelot (1996), Ludden (1996), van der Veer (1994), Vanaik (1997). The Ayodhya affair was linked to the Shah Bano case, which revolved around the rights of divorced Muslim women. Space precludes detailed discussion of this case. It raised many issues, including (for Muslims) state intrusion into the "private" sphere of religious minorities (that is echoed in Muslims' responses to the family planning program) and (for the Hindu Right) the trope of the Muslim woman as victim (that also comes up in relation to polygamy; see below). The following provide useful accounts of the case: Chhachhi (1991), Engineer (1987), Z. Hasan (1989, 1993, 1994, 1998), Kishwar (1986), Kumar (1993), Mody (1987), Palriwala and Agnihotri (1996), Pathak and Rajan (1989). See also P. Jeffery (Forthcoming).
5 These allegations echo both the "Islamophobia" currently widespread in the West and classically Orientalist arguments (Obermeyer 1992; Said 1978). Sikhs and Christians have sometimes been accused of undermining Hinduism through religious conversions and faster population growth rates, but Muslims have been the target of most such claims in the 1990s (Krishnakumar 1991; van der Veer 1994; Wright 1983).
6 Writing about the Middle East, Fargues (1993) provides a recent example of the links drawn between Islamic fundamentalism, dreams of world conquest, and high fertility rates. By contrast, Obermeyer (1994: 60) highlights the tensions in Islamic doctrines between egalitarian and inegalitarian views and the "tremendous complexity and diversity that is found in the Muslim world"; see also Ahmed (1982).
7 Similarly, reversing Hindu communalist messages, G. M. Shah argued that every Kashmiri Muslim should have a dozen children because they were dying out (Pai Panandikar and Umashankar 1994). Shah's demography was as incompetent as that of his Hindu Right opponents: the Muslim proportion in Jammu and Kashmir was 57 per cent in 1947 and 64 per cent in 1981.
8 Widow remarriage was also central to early twentieth-century Hindu nationalist rhetoric. Muslim widows could remarry whereas Hindu widows prevented from remarrying within their own community were allegedly lured into marriages with Muslim men. Either way, it was claimed, Muslim numbers would grow at the expense of Hindus. With declining levels of widowhood and rising levels of widow remarriage among Hindus, however, widow remarriage is no longer as contentious as it once was (Gupta 2002; see also Datta 1993, Davis 1951: 79–82, Mandelbaum 1974: 35).
9 A first wife's failure to bear children (particularly a son) is a common reason for polygamy. Since male infertility may be the problem, second or later wives may also have difficulty in having children. Further, men marrying polygamously are generally older than those marrying for the first time and women in polygamous marriages are more likely to be widowed before menopause.
10 See Ahmad (1967: 63, 73, 95) for a discussion of nineteenth-century modernist views and Engineer (1992: 22, 98ff., 154ff.) for a contemporary argument against polygamy.
11 Several young Jat men from his village, however, became involved in the Ayodhya campaign in late 1990, courting arrest in Bijnor town and attending political rallies.

12 Such claims make no sense nationally but local situations may seem less clear-cut. In Bijnor, for instance, "caste Hindus" have gone from 46 per cent of the total District population in 1921 to about 37 per cent in 1991, and the Muslim share has risen from 36 per cent in 1921 to 40 per cent in 1991, despite some migration of Muslims to Pakistan in the late 1940s.

13 Goldscheider (1971) distinguishes three hypotheses linking fertility and religion. The first "particularized theology", attributes the effects of a religion to its doctrines about birth control and family size. The second, "characteristics", explains religious differences in fertility through the social, economic, and demographic characteristics that the members of a particular religion happen to have. The third, "minority group status", explains lower fertility among minority religious groups as a result of their insecurities. A fourth model, introduced by Chamie (1981) describes "interactions" that may change the relationships between fertility and religion through time. As Knodel et al. (1999: 163) point out, none of these is very satisfactory, either separately or together. We agree with their preference for a truly interactive model, one that acknowledges that "cultural, political, socio-economic, and historical factors interact with the relationship [between religion and fertility]" and that the "national and local context conditions the extent and perhaps nature of Islam's influence."

14 In these calculations, "Hindu" includes "Scheduled Castes" and "Scheduled Tribes."

15 In a small-scale study of rural Koil tahsil (Aligarh District, UP) the fertility differentials of caste Hindus, Scheduled Castes, and Muslims could be almost entirely understood in terms of the impacts of income, education, child mortality, and age at marriage (Khan 1991: 110–115).

16 It is likely that Hindus in these districts have higher fertility than Hindus in other districts, and that Muslim fertility in these districts is at least as high, and probably higher, but it is not clear why this might be.

17 Until the 1980s, Islamic countries in the Middle East were poor health achievers (relative to their wealth) and also, despite relatively high levels of female literacy, continued to have high levels of fertility. Caldwell (1986: 175) considered that "the central aspect of the relationship between Islam and mortality levels is undoubtedly the separate and distinctive position of women, operating partly through their access to education but also in many other ways." He has now shifted position somewhat, because fertility levels in the region have dropped dramatically without apparently being accompanied by major social and economic changes, especially in relation to women's autonomy (Caldwell et al. 1999).

18 Drèze and Murthi (1999) conclude that Muslims and Hindus differ neither in their preferences for sons nor in differentials in mortality rates by gender (see also Murthi et al. 1996). Sex ratios for Muslims in north India have historically been less "masculine" than those for Hindus, probably because of differences in mortality rates overall and the relationship of regional and socioeconomic factors to fertility (Agnihotri 1997).

19 See R. Jeffery and A. M. Basu (1996) and P. Jeffery and R. Jeffery (1998b) for critiques of this new orthodoxy and Drèze and Murthi (1999) for a response. We can note that neither Drèze and Murthi nor Mari Bhat (1996) elaborate on the correlation between high fertility and a high proportion of Muslims in a district, yet it is as strong as the links between girls' schooling and low fertility that are generally presumed to be causal.

20 This section draws on several of our publications on Bijnor, especially P. Jeffery (2001), P. Jeffery and R. Jeffery (1994, 1996a, 1996b), P. Jeffery, R. Jeffery,

and Lyon (1989), R. Jeffery and P. Jeffery (1993, 1997). As we indicated above, polygamy is extremely rare in Bijnor, so we do not discuss it further here.
21 See Agarwal (1997), Kandiyoti (1988, 1998), Sen (1990) for elaborations of these issues and also Kabeer (1999) on the problems of measuring women's empowerment and autonomy.

References

Agarwal, B. (1997). "Bargaining" and Gender Relations: Within and Beyond the Household. *Feminist Economics* 3(1): 1–51.

Agnihotri, S.B. (1997). Sex Ratio Imbalances in India: A Disaggregated Analysis. Doctoral dissertation, University of East Anglia.

Ahmad, A. (1967). *Islamic Modernism in India and Pakistan 1857–1964*. London: Oxford University Press (for Royal Institute of International Affairs).

Ahmed, L. (1982). Western Ethnocentrism and Perceptions of the Harem. *Feminist Studies* 8(Fall): 521–534.

Appadurai, A. (1993). Number in the Colonial Imagination. In *Orientalism and the Postcolonial Predicament: Perspectives on South Asia*, edited by C.A. Breckenridge and P. van der Veer, pp. 314–339. Philadelphia: University of Pennsylvania Press.

Bacchetta, P. (1994). Communal Property/Sexual Property: On Representations of Muslim Women in a Hindu Nationalist Discourse. In *Forging Identities: Gender, Communities and the State*, edited by Z. Hasan, pp. 188–225. New Delhi and Boulder: Kali for Women and Westview Press.

—— (1996). Hindu Nationalist Women as Ideologues: The Sangh, the Samiti and Differential Concepts of the Hindu Nation. In *Embodied Violence: Communalising Women's Sexuality in South Asia*, edited by K. Jayawardena and M. de Alwis, pp. 126–167. New Delhi and London: Kali for Women and Zed Books.

Bardhan, P.K. (1974). On Life and Death Questions. *Economic and Political Weekly* 9(32–34): 1293–1304.

Basu, A.M. (1996). The demographics of Hindu fundamentalism. In *Unravelling the nation: Sectarian conflict and India's secular identity*, edited by K. Basu and S. Subrahmanyam, pp. 129–156. New Delhi: Penguin.

—— (1997). The "politicization" of fertility to achieve non-demographic objectives. *Population Studies* 51: 5–18.

Basu, A. (editor). (1993). Women and Religious Nationalism in India. Volume 25 (4): *Bulletin of Concerned Asian Scholars*.

—— (1995). When Local Riots Are Not Simply Local: Collective Violence and the State in Bijnor, India 1988–93. *Theory and Society* 24: 35–78.

—— (1998). Hindu Women's Activism in India and the Questions it Raises. In *Appropriating Gender: Women's Activism and Politicized Religion in South Asia*, edited by P. Jeffery and A. Basu, pp. 167–184. New York: Routledge.

Basu, A. and Kohli, A. (editors). (1998). *Community Conflicts and the State in India*. Delhi: Oxford University Press.

Basu, T., Datta, P., Sarkar, S., Sarkar, T. and Sen, S. (1993). *Khaki Shorts, Saffron Flags*. Delhi: Orient Longman.

Caldwell, J. (1986). Routes to Low Mortality in Poor Countries. *Population and Development Review* 12(2): 171–200.

Caldwell, J.C., Khuda, B.E., Caldwell, B., Pieris, I. and Caldwell, P. (1999). The Bangladesh fertility decline: An interpretation. *Population and Development Review* 25(1): 67–85.

Cassen, R.H. (1978). *India: Population, Economy, Society*. London: Macmillan.

Chakravarti, U., Choudhury, P., Dutta, P., Hasan, Z., Sangari, K. and Sarkar, T. (1992). Khurja Riots, 1990–91: Understanding the Conjuncture. *Economic and Political Weekly* 27(18): 951–965.

Chamie, J. (1981). *Religion and Fertility: Arab Christian-Muslim Differentials*. Cambridge: Cambridge University Press.

Chhachhi, A. (1991). Forced Identities: the State, Communalism, Fundamentalism and Women in India. In *Women, Islam and the State*, edited by D. Kandiyoti, pp. 144–175. London: Macmillan.

Cohn, B.S. (1987). The Census, Social Structure and Objectification in South Asia. In *An Anthropologist among the Historians and Other Essays*, edited by B.S. Cohn, pp. 224–254. Delhi & London: Oxford University Press.

Datta, P. (1993). Dying Hindus: Production of Hindu Communal Common Sense in Early Twentieth Century Bengal. *Economic and Political Weekly* 28(25): 1305–1319.

—— (1999). *Carving Blocs: Communal ideology in early twentieth-century Bengal*. New Delhi and New York: Oxford University Press.

Davis, K. (1951). *The Population of India and Pakistan*. Princeton: Princeton University Press.

Drèze, J. and Murthi, M. (1999). Fertility, Education and Development: Further Evidence from India. London: STICERD, London School of Economics.

Dyson, T. (1991). Child Labour and Fertility: An Overview, an Assessment and an Alternative Framework. In *Child Labour in the Indian Sub-continent: Dimensions and Applications*, edited by R. Kanbargi, pp. 81–100. New Delhi: Sage.

Dyson, T. and Moore, M. (1983). On Kinship Structure, Female Autonomy and Demographic Behavior in India. *Population and Development Review* 9(1): 35–60.

Engineer, A.A. (editor). (1987). *The Shah Bano Controversy*. Bombay: Orient Longman.

—— (1991). The Bloody Trail: Ramjanmabhoomi and Communal Violence in UP. *Economic and Political Weekly* 26(4): 155–159.

—— (1992). *The Rights of Women in Islam*. Delhi: Sterling Publishers.

Fargues, P. (1993). Demography and Politics in the Arab World. *Population: an English Selection* 5: 1–20.

Goldscheider, C. (1971). *Population, Modernization and Social Structure*. Boston: Little, Brown.

Gopal, S. (editor). (1991). *Anatomy of a Confrontation: The Babri Masjid-Ramjanambhoomi Issue*. Delhi: Orient Longman.

Greenhalgh, S. (1995). Anthropology Theorises Reproduction. In *Situating Fertility: Anthropology and Demographic Enquiry*, edited by S. Greenhalgh, pp. 3–28. Cambridge: Cambridge University Press.

Gupta, C. (1998). Articulating Hindu Masculinity and Femininity: *Shuddhi* and *Sangathan* Movements in United Provinces in the 1920s. *Economic and Political Weekly* 33(13): 727–735.

—— (2002). *Sexuality, Obscenity, Community: Women, Muslims and the Hindu Public in Colonial India*. New Delhi: Permanent Black.

Gupta, C. and Sharma, M. (1996). Communal constructions: media reality vs. real reality. *Race and Class* 38(1): 1–20.

Hasan, M. (1997). *Legacy of a Divided Nation: India's Muslims since Independence*. Delhi: Oxford University Press.

Hasan, Z. (1989). Minority Identity, Muslim Women Bill Campaign and the Political Process. *Economic and Political Weekly* 24(1): 44–50.

—— (1993). Communalism, State Policy and the Question of Women's Rights in Contemporary India. *Bulletin of Concerned Asian Scholars* 25(4): 5–15.

—— (editor) (1994). *Forging Identities: Gender, Communities and the State*. New Delhi and Boulder: Kali for Women and Westview Press.

—— (1999). Gender Politics, Legal Reform, and the Muslim Community in India. In *Resisting the Sacred and the Secular: Women and Politicized Religion in South Asia*, edited by P. Jeffery and A. Basu, pp. 71–88. New Delhi: Kali for Women.

Hendre, S. (1971). *Hindus and Family Planning*. Bombay: Supraja Prakashan.

International Institute of Population Sciences (1995). *National Family Health Survey: India 1992–93*. Bombay: International Institute for Population Sciences.

Jacobson, D. and Wadley, S.S. (1995). *Women in India: Two Perspectives*. Delhi: Manohar.

Jaffrelot, C. (1995). The ideas of the Hindu race in the writings of Hindu nationalist ideologues in the 1920s and 1930s: A concept between two cultures. In *The Concept of Race in South Asia*, edited by P. Robb, pp. 327–354. Delhi: Oxford University Press.

—— (1996). *The Hindu Nationalist Movement and Indian Politics 1925 to the 1990s*. London: Hurst.

Jeffery, P. (2000). Identifying Differences: Gender Politics and Community in rural Uttar Pradesh. In *Invented Identities: The Interplay of Gender, Religion and Politics in India*, edited by J. Leslie and M. McGee, pp. 286–309. SOAS Studies in South Asia: Understandings and Perspectives. Delhi: Oxford University Press.

—— (2001). A Uniform Customary Code? Marital Breakdown and Women's Economic Entitlements in Rural Bijnor. *Contributions to Indian Sociology* 35(1): 1–33.

Jeffery, P. and Jeffery, R. (1994a). Killing My Heart's Desire: Education and Female Autonomy in Rural North India. In *Woman as Subject: South Asian Histories*, edited by N. Kumar, pp. 125–171. Calcutta & Charlottesville: Bhatkal and Sen & Virginia University Press.

—— (1996a). *Don't Marry me to a Plowman! Women's Everyday Lives in Rural North India*. New Delhi, Boulder: Sage/Vistaar, Westview Press.

—— (1996b). What's the Benefit of being Educated? Girls' Schooling, Women's Autonomy and Fertility Outcomes in Bijnor. In *Girls' Schooling, Women's Autonomy and Fertility Change in South Asia*, edited by R. Jeffery and A. Basu, pp. 150–183. New Delhi: Sage.

—— (1998a). Gender, Community and the Local State in Bijnor, India. In *Appropriating Gender: Women's Activism and Politicized Religion in South Asia*, edited by P. Jeffery and A. Basu, pp. 123–141. New York: Routledge.

—— (1998b). Silver Bullet or Passing Fancy? Girls' Schooling and Population Policy. In *Feminist Visions of Development: Gender Analysis and Policy*, edited by C. Jackson and R. Pearson, pp. 239–258. London and New York: Routledge.

Jeffery, P., Jeffery, R. and Lyon, A. (1989). *Labour Pains and Labour Power: Women and Childbearing in India*. Delhi and London: Manohar and Zed Books.

Jeffery, R. and Basu, A. (editors). (1996). *Girls' Schooling, Women's Autonomy and Fertility Change in South Asia*. New Delhi: Sage.

Jeffery, R. and Jeffery, P. (1993). A Woman Belongs to Her Husband: Female Autonomy, Women's Work and Childbearing in Bijnor. In *Gender and Political Economy: Explorations of South Asian Systems*, edited by A. Clark, pp. 66–114. Delhi: Oxford University Press.

—— (1994b). The Bijnor Riots, October 1990: Collapse of a Mythical Special Relationship? *Economic and Political Weekly* 29(10): 551–558.

—— (1997). *Population, Gender and Politics: Demographic Change in Rural North India*. Cambridge: Cambridge University Press.

Jones, K.W. (1981). Religious Identity and the Indian Census. In *The Census in British India: New Perspectives*, edited by N.G. Barrier, pp. 73–101. Delhi: Manohar.

Kabeer, N. (1999). Resources, Agency, Achievements: Reflection on the Measurement of Women's Empowerment. *Development and Change* 30: 435–464.

Kakar, S. (1996). The construction of a new Hindu identity. In *Unravelling the nation: Sectarian conflict and India's secular identity*, edited by K. Basu and S. Subrahmanyam, pp. 204–235. New Delhi: Penguin.

Kandiyoti, D. (1988). Bargaining with Patriarchy. *Gender and Society* 2(3): 274–290.

—— (1998). Gender, Power and Contestation: "Rethinking bargaining with Patriarchy". In *Feminist Visions of Development: Gender Analysis and Policy*, edited by C. Jackson and R. Pearson, pp. 135–151. London: Routledge.

Khan, M.E. (1979). *Family Planning Among Muslims in India: A Study of the Reproductive Behavior of Muslims in an Urban Setting*. Delhi: Manohar.

Khan, M.F. (1991). *Human Fertility in Northern India*. Delhi: Manak Publications.

Kishor, S. (1993). "May God Give Sons to All": Gender and Child Mortality in India. *American Sociological Review* 58(2): 247–265.

Kishwar, M. (1986). Pro Women or Anti Muslim? *Manushi* 6(2): 4–13.

Knodel, J., et al. (1999). Religion and reproduction: Muslims in Buddhist Thailand. *Population Studies* 53(2): 149–164.

Krishnakumar, A. (1991). Canards on Muslims: Calling the Bluff on Communal Propaganda. *Frontline* 8(21): 93–98.

Kumar, R. (1993). *The History of Doing: an Illustrated Account of Movements for Women's Rights and Feminism in India, 1800–1990*. New Delhi: Kali for Women.

Lal, M. (1999). Purdah as Pathology: Medical Research and Reproductive Health in twentieth-century India: School of Oriental and African Studies (Conference on "Population, Birth Control and Reproductive Health in late Colonial India" 18–19 November 1999).

Leslie, C. (1990a). Scientific racism: reflections on peer review, science and ideology. *Social Science and Medicine* 31(8): 891–905.

—— (1990b). Rejoinder. *Social Science and Medicine* 31(8): 912.

Levin, A., Caldwell, B. and Khuda, B.E. (1999). The Effect of Price and Access on Contraceptive Use. *Social Science and Medicine* 49(1): 1–15.

Ludden, D. (editor) (1996). *Contesting the Nation: Religion, Community, and the Politics of Democracy in India*. Philadelphia: University of Pennsylvania Press (also published as "Making India Hindu" by Oxford University Press).

Mandelbaum, D.G. (1974). *Human Fertility in India: Social Components and Policy Perspectives*. Berkeley: University of California Press.

—— (1986). Sex Roles and Gender Relations in North India. *Economic and Political Weekly* 21(46): 1999–2004.

—— (1988). *Women's Seclusion and Men's Honor*. Tucson: University of Arizona Press.

Mari Bhat, N. and Zavier, F. (1999). Findings of National Family Health Survey: Regional Analysis. *Economic & Political Weekly* 34(42–43): 3008–3032.

Mari Bhat, P.N. (1996). Contours of Fertility Decline in India: A District Level Study based on the 1991 Census. In *Population Policy and Reproductive Health*, edited by K.N. Srinivasan, pp. 96–177. Delhi: Hindustan.

McNicoll, G. (1994). Institutional analysis of fertility. New York: The Population Council.

Miller, B.D. (1981). *The Endangered Sex: Neglect of Female Children in Rural North India*. Ithaca: Cornell University Press.

Minault, G. (1998). *Secluded Scholars: Women's Education and Muslim Social Reform in Colonial India*. Delhi: Oxford University Press.

Mody, N.B. (1987). The Press in India: The Shah Bano Judgment and Its Aftermath. *Asian Survey* 27(8): 935–953.

Moulasha, K. and Rao, G.R. (1999). Religion-Specific Differentials in Fertility and Family Planning. *Economic and Political Weekly* 34(42): 3047–3051.

Murthi, M., Guio, A. and Drèze, J. (1996). Mortality, Fertility and Gender Bias in India. In *Indian Development: Selected Regional Perspectives*, edited by J. Drèze and A. Sen, pp. 357–406. Delhi: Oxford University Press.

Narayana, G. and Kantner, J.F. (1992). *Doing the Needful: The Dilemma of India's Population Policy* Boulder: Westview Press.

National Committee on the Status of Women (1975). *Status of Women in India: A Synopsis of the Report of the National Committee (1971–74)*. New Delhi: The Indian Council of Social Science Research/Allied Publishers.

Obermeyer, C.M. (1992). Islam, Women and Politics: The Demography of the Arab Countries. *Population and Development Review* 18(1): 33–60.

—— (1994). Religious Doctrine, State Ideology and Reproductive Options in Islam. In *Power and Decision: the Social Control of Reproduction*, edited by G. Sen and R.C. Snow, pp. 59–75. Boston: Harvard School of Public Health.

Omran, A.R. (1992). *Family Planning in the Legacy of Islam*. London and New York: Routledge.

Pai Panandikar, V.A. and Umashankar, P.K. (1994). Fertility Control and Politics in India. In *The New Politics of Reproduction (Supplement to Population and Development Review, volume 20)*, edited by J. L. Finkle and A. A. McIntosh, pp. 89–104. New York: Oxford University Press.

Palriwala, R. and Agnihotri, I. (1996). Tradition, the Family, and the State: Politics of the Contemporary Women's Movement. In *Region, Religion, Caste, Gender and Culture in Contemporary India*, edited by T. V. Sathyamurthy, pp. 503–532. Delhi: Oxford University Press.

Pandey, G. (1990). *The Construction of Communalism in Colonial North India.* Delhi: Oxford University Press.

—— (1991). Hindus and Others: the Militant Hindu Construction. *Economic and Political Weekly* 26(52): 2997–3009.

Papanek, H. (1982). Purdah: Separate Worlds and Symbolic Shelter. In *Separate Worlds: Studies of Purdah in South Asia*, edited by H. Papanek and G. Minault, pp. 3–53. Delhi: Chanakya Publications.

Pathak, Z. and Rajeshwari, S.R. (1989) "Shahbano". *Signs* 14(3): 558–582.

Prakash, I. (1979). *They Count Their Gains – We Calculate Our Losses.* New Delhi: Akhil Bharat Hindu Mahasabha.

Ramesh, B.M. and Retherford, J. (1996) *Contraceptive Use in India 1992–93.* Volume 2. Mumbai: International Institute for Population Studies.

Registrar General India (1982). *Levels, Trends and Differentials in Fertility 1979.* New Delhi: Vital Statistics Division, Office of the Registrar General India, Ministry of Home Affairs.

Registrar General of India (1981). *Survey of Infant and Child Mortality, 1979.* New Delhi: Ministry of Home Affairs, Government of India.

Said, E.W. (1978). *Orientalism: Western Conceptions of the Orient.* New York: Pantheon.

Sarkar, S. (1993). The Fascism of the Sangh Parivar. *Economic and Political Weekly* 28(5): 163–167.

Savage, D.W. (1997). Missionaries and the Development of a Colonial Ideology of Female Education in India. *Gender and History* 9(2): 201–221.

Sen, A. (1990). Gender and Co-operative Conflicts. In *Persistent Inequalities: Women and World Development*, edited by I. Tinker, pp. 123–149. New York: Oxford University Press.

Shariff, A. (1995). Socio-Economic and Demographic Differentials between Hindus and Muslims in India. *Economic and Political Weekly* 30(46): 2947–2953.

Sridhar, V. (1991). Fiction and fact: the real plight of the minorities. *Frontline* 8(21): 99–101.

van der Veer, P. (1994). *Religious Nationalism: Hindus and Muslims in India.* Berkeley: University of California Press.

Vanaik, A. (1997). *The Furies of Indian Communalism: Religion, Modernity and Secularization.* London: Verso.

Wright, T.P. Jr (1983). The Ethnic Numbers Game in India: Hindu-Muslim Conflicts over Conversion, Family Planning, Migration and the Census. In *Culture, Ethnicity and Identity*, edited by W.C. McCready, pp. 405–427. New York: Academic Press.

Chapter 8

Establishing proof

Translating "science" and the state in Tibetan medicine[1]

Vincanne Adams

> The structures of meaning in diagnoses of illnesses are not limited to the technical meanings of medical concepts, but are situated in and draw significance from other cultural domains.
>
> (Leslie 1992: 179)

In his numerous contributions to the field of medical anthropology, Charles Leslie demonstrated that a medical system ought to be understood not just as a system of knowledge, belief, and practices, but as a set of social, historical, political, and economic forces that are set in motion through medical personalities. Through portraits of individuals who in some cases were explicitly concerned with such things as nationalism, resisting colonial hegemony, alternative scientific truth, and marketplace advantage, he showed how practical engagements with medicine reveal these larger forces and concerns (Leslie 1976, 1980, 1986, 1992). In doing so, Leslie foreshadowed contemporary science studies insights that empirical medical truths are contingent on much larger political, economic and social negotiations. In this essay, I follow Leslie's example by exploring the larger forces at work in contemporary practices of Tibetan medicine in modern-day Tibet. In particular, I focus on one physician's efforts to establish "proof" of the effectiveness of Tibetan medicine by using empirical evidence. I suggest that claims to empirical truth found in this case should be understood as both products of competing political, nationalist, religious, economic, and culturally historical influences in China's Tibet, on the one hand, and on the other, products of the particular medical methods of those individuals who live through these influences.[2]

In China's Tibet, debates about medical legitimacy are articulated in debates about the meanings of medical "science" and the limits of empirical validity. At the outset, one should understand these debates as a product, in part, of conditions of ongoing Chinese rule in the Tibetan Autonomous Region, and what some would call conditions of "colonialism."[3] Tibetan doctors increasingly use a language that politically legitimizes their presence and their practices in the eyes of those who represent larger forces of social change in Tibet. In other words, this colonial language is not just Mandarin. In the halls of Tibetan medicine, the colonial language of Chinese sovereignty and international market capitalism are articulated as a language of "science." Thus, the commonly heard refrain in the Tibetan medical hospital (Mentsikhang) that "Tibetan medicine is a science" remains surprisingly unchallenged, despite the fact that the meaning of "science" in Tibet is hotly debated and despite Tibetan medicine's ongoing reliance on the religious precepts which underlie the theory of both physiology and disease. What exactly, then, are the meanings of science as they can be seen in the practices of individual practitioners in contemporary Tibet?

The study

This is the story of a "scientific" study recounted to me during fieldwork in Lhasa in 1998 by a physician in the women's ward at Mentsikhang, whom I will call Dr Dawa. She told me that in 1997 Tibetan physicians in the women's ward undertook a retrospective scientific study of the outcomes of female patients diagnosed with a condition called "bile-related womb disorder" (*mngal nad mkhri gyu*). The reason for the study was that during the past ten years physicians had noticed remarkable recovery rates for women with this condition. The study, she explained, was carried out to "prove" the effectiveness of Tibetan medicine. She then told me the following.

In all there were 60 records of patients who had bile-related womb disorders. In addition to being diagnosed with similar disorders, all of the patients also had in common that they were treated with the medicine *yu kyong ka tsar* (a compounded medicine) in the afternoon during the course of their treatments at the inpatient ward. The outcomes for all the patients were determined by evidence of the elimination of symptoms of pain, and on pulse, urine and tongue diagnoses. The outcomes were very good, she said. All of the women who had bile-related womb disorder were either entirely or nearly entirely cured of their disorders. The results showed 100 per cent effectiveness in the Tibetan treatment.

She then went on to offer what, for me, was more confusing evidence. The findings of the study also included information from ultrasound diagnostic techniques. Since the hospital had been given several ultrasound machines, doctors were increasingly asked to include ultrasound diagnostic information in their reports. Most women who came to the clinic also had ultrasound reports, either taken at the local biomedical hospital or at the Mentsikhang itself. Thus, the study had to account for this information as well.

When ultrasound information was included, the results of the study looked different. Instead of all having bile-related womb disorders, the patient diagnoses were broken down into more specific maladies and their outcomes looked, to me, slightly less glorious than those recorded when the broader category of bile-related womb disorder alone was considered. Of the 60 women in the study, ultrasound showed that 30 of the women had inflammation in the fallopian tubes (*gyushap gyi nyentse*), among whom 28 (were cured and 2 showed partial improvement only. Fifteen women had "water behind the uterus" (fluid in the cul-de-sac) (*mngal la chu gyaba*); only 10 of these were cured and 5 showed no improvement. Ten women had growths in the ovaries (*min skran*), of whom only 5 were cured, 4 showed partial improvement, and 1 showed no improvement. Finally, one woman had a "flesh" growth in the uterus (fibroids) (*sha skran phembo*) and were totally cured. The remaining 4 patients were unaccounted for in the study.[4]

The results seemed confusing, I told Dr Dawa. How could they record that they had 100 per cent cures when they called it *mngal nad khri gyu*, but then indicate by ultrasound that the disorders persisted? To answer, she referred to the conclusions of the study. The doctors undertaking the study concluded that since they were working in a Tibetan medical hospital and were committed to the advancement of Tibetan medical science, they ought to rely solely on the Tibetan medical methods of diagnosis and outcomes and these showed total effectiveness.

Instead of answering my inquiry, this response simply raised more questions. How was the doctor able to say that the ultrasound showed that in some cases the disorders persisted and simultaneously claim that, by the Tibetan methods, these patients were fully recovered from their disorders? At one point, she suggested that the diagnoses made with the use of ultrasound were, in fact, diagnoses of biomedically named disorders. How was this possible, I asked. The disorders identified through ultrasound looked to me as if they were well established in Tibetan medicine, *nyentse* being the Tibetan term for infection caused by agitation of the bile humor. "Water behind the uterus" is not necessarily identified as pathology in biomedicine (particularly not the small amounts seen in these reports). Although "growths" of a wide variety were known in biomedical diagnoses, they were also discussed in the Tibetan system (being of two sorts: blood and flesh). When I asked her again, she explained that the ultrasound diagnoses were not showing diagnoses different from those identified as *mngal nad mkhris rgyu*. In what seemed like a contradiction with her previous statement, she said that the ultrasound merely showed refinements of the *same* diagnosis; the diagnosis of *mngal nad mkhris rgyu* encompassed and included these disorders rendered visible in more detail through ultrasound. Her reference to their being "biomedical" diagnoses meant that they were also known to "outside" medicine.

Dr Dawa clearly was not just dismissing the diagnostic evidence that the ultrasound made visible. On many other occasions Dr Dawa had explained to me that ultrasound was useful in *confirming* Tibetan diagnoses. She told me that it was important for the doctors at Mentsikhang to use these Western technologies, not just because they were modern and scientific but because they could "prove" the effectiveness of Tibetan medicine. However, she had also reminded me on numerous occasions that ultrasound reports were not the most reliable source of information for Tibetan doctors. They could be "wrong," in the sense that they were misleading and, more importantly, they did not necessarily tell physicians the most relevant information about patients' disorders.

In her reading of the results of this study, however, it was not that she saw the evidence in them as wrong. The evidence in them was, for her, correct. At the same time, the fact that the report indicated that some patients showed "no improvement" was not for her a basis for undermining her claim that all of the patients were successfully treated. Something about the way she was reading the information in them enabled her to suggest that these ultrasound data were not, of their own evidentiary power, able to unseat her claim that Tibetan medicine was 100 per cent effective. What, then, was she to make of these data in the ultrasound tests that showed persistence of the symptoms that were being identified as indicators of disorder?

I was also curious about the study's method: the idea that a single medicine should end up being the focus for research was not entirely consistent with traditional Tibetan medical methods. The medicine *yu kyung ka tsar* was a relatively new medicine compounded with more than 33 ingredients; highlighting it as the key to successful remedies ran counter to all I had learned about Tibetan medicine, in which one medicine was given in conjunction with a variety of other medicines and external treatments in patterns that were idiosyncratically tailored to the particular humoral pathologies of each individual patient. Rarely were all the treatment protocols exactly the same for any two patients with the same named disease. What, then, was the significance of and impetus for this study's focus on a single drug?

Although I could not see it at that time in my conversations with Dr Dawa, I came to realize later the epistemological richness of her study. Her report was a good indicator of the complicated cultural negotiations undertaken by traditional Tibetan medical practitioners in order to awkwardly both accommodate and distinguish their medicine from its "modern medical" counterpart (*phyi-lu* or "outside" medicine, as it is referred to in Tibet). "Outside" medicine, by its official support and prolific visibility throughout China's urban Tibet, consisted of various practices of Sinicized biomedicine. It had achieved political hegemony in the domain of medical "science," a process that was put in motion swiftly during the

Cultural Revolution and is sustained today under conditions of post socialist market liberalization and "development" modernization. The task of figuring out where Tibetan medicine stood in relation to the dominating claims of "outside" medicine was made doubly hard for doctors like Dr Dawa by the arrival of biomedical technologies that seemed to hold the promise of superior, but more importantly "swift," benefits to health and health care for a medically needy public.

Dr Dawa's study, I realized, offered a compelling instance of this hegemony in that it suggested an opposition to "outside" medicine while also obtusely incorporating its linguistic and cultural practices to establish legitimacy for itself therein (Lock 1990). I could only understand her conclusions, I realized, if I read them as a product of the historical forces and cultural negotiations that prevailed under a new medical hegemony in Tibet (Janes 1995). In other words, there are other ways to explain Dr Dawa's conclusions, but explaining them in terms of historical and cultural contingencies is more fruitful and instructive than would be a simple reading of what Leslie (above) identified as the "technical meanings of medical concepts."

For example, one way to read Dr Dawa's conclusions might be to turn to the particular theoretical foundations of anatomy, physiology, and pathology within Tibetan medicine, as Kuriyama (1994) has shown for Chinese medicine. Surely, Tibetan theories can explain how ultrasound evidence might be "read" differently by Tibetan doctors than "outside" medical doctors because Tibetan doctors read data humorally. From the perspective of humoral approaches to healing, the signs of having successfully eliminated a disorder are found in those diagnostic techniques that indicate humoral function (pulse, urine, and so on). Once these signs point to a healthy state, the residual traces of disorders are not necessarily immediately destroyed; this takes time. Evidence of a previous imbalance may remain indefinitely, even leaving scars, and it appears as remaining growths, inflammation, and the like in ultrasound photos.

Dr Dawa's conclusions might be understood from the perspective that Kuriyama (1994) takes regarding Chinese approaches to anatomy, a particular way of "seeing" evidence in relation to establishing the existence, or lack of existence, of anatomical facts.[5] But such an approach would necessitate that Dr Dawa herself advocate a theoretical appreciation for the different modes of knowing that could be applied to ultrasound evidence. I found, however, that these theoretical foundations were seldom at the forefront of Dr Dawa's approach. In fact, the more I asked her about theory, the more murky her explanations became. Although surely her theoretically unreflective training led her to read evidence "humorally," it could not explain her approach sufficiently. Rather, her conclusions about the ultrasound evidence were best explained by looking at the historical, political, and economic forces that gave rise to her particular engagement with, and her vision of, Tibetan medicine. Dr Dawa's way of "seeing" and then making sense of "evidence," surely had as much to do with the historical contingencies of this medicine at the time as it did with the implicit epistemologies of humoral medicine that might be embedded in her practices.[6] I turn, then, to these historical contingencies as a way of exploring how she, and other Tibetan doctors, establish "proof" of the efficacy of Tibetan medicine in very particular ways.

Particular contexts and histories as the basis for explaining evidence

The context of the disclosure of this Tibetan physician's study is revealing. I learned about it while talking with Dr Dawa about the methods Tibetan doctors used for making drugs. The study came up almost coincidentally. I had noted that despite the fact that we daily emptied the cold remainder of our hot water and tea into the flowers that decorated the center of our large conference table, where we met each day to talk about patients and their treatments, the plants appeared to be dying. "It isn't the lack of water," she finally told me. "They are dying because Dr Trinley (her colleague) used the room last year to make his new medicine for *marutse* (a venereal disease) and the vapors from the medicines were too strong for the plants." For this reason, the plants were all dying now.

Her point was well-taken in that she had, for weeks, been trying to impress upon me the potency of Tibetan medicines and the "modern" approach that they, in the women's ward, took to them as shown by their experimentalism. Many of the new medicines, she reminded me, were invented by individual doctors who noticed the effectiveness of some ingredients or some combinations of ingredients for certain intractable or new disorders for which old medicines no longer seemed to work. On this basis, she said, they sometimes compounded new medicines that were very potent and, with permission from the head of the hospital division, the director of the hospital, and the research division in the hospital, they tested them in practice.

Dr Dawa's emphasis on the empirical and experimental approach in Tibetan medicine was not missed. Nor could it have been, since this was her primary and sole emphasis. In our months of research, she and I had spent a good deal of time struggling over my questions. Dr Dawa was a strict empiricist (in at least one sense) in the traditional Greek sense of the word (Hankinson 1994). She cared little for explanations of the theoretical bases for Tibetan medical efficacy. I, on the other hand, was primarily interested in questions of theory in practices that evidently worked. I would ask how exactly had diet produced humoral imbalances? What theory linked them? What was the relationship between physical symptoms and humoral excesses? I wanted to know how Tibetan doctors explained the biological outcomes of their treatments; what was the logic of their interventions? Her answers were always elusive. For her, it was surely that I was asking the wrong questions; for me, it was as if she was simply not understanding my questions. Often, to answer my questions, she would reach below her desk and pull out her copy of the medical chapters of the *rGyu bShi* (Four Tantras, the main medical treatises) that were directed to the disorders in question. Then, she would begin to read, from these pages, the menu like lists of disorders as they were categorized under humoral classifications. The problem with the book, I would say, is that it does not explain the theory underlying Tibetan medicine. How did ideas about causation fit with ideas about physiological imbalance and, in turn, the development of symptoms, humoral function, and the appropriate cures? She would just smile and nod, then, and remind me that Tibetan medicine was very complex, not simple or easy to understand.

I did find other doctors who were able to clarify the theories for me. Both younger doctors and older doctors who knew medical theory, explained that the principles of the relationships between the five elements (earth, wind, fire, water, space) also underlay all of the relationships between humors, diet, symptoms, and outcomes. These relationships were explained in the *Kalachakra Tantra* as part of a larger set of cosmological insights about the nature of the universe (including astrology). Others reported that the theory of the poisons (the faults of anger, ignorance, desire) underlay the whole medical approach. Both of these theories, I was told, explained such basic things as the humoral constitution of the individual, his or her susceptibility to disease, the pathways of disease in the body, the manifestation of symptoms through time, and even the likelihood of a successful outcome of treatments based on the particular constitution of the patient. Simply, if one understood how the humors themselves emerged embryologically from the presence of the three poisons (faults) in the transmigrating soul (consciousness) of the person, one could understand their relationship to these defective emotions in the adult body. Moreover, if one understood how the humors were made up of the same elements as the other body constituents (phlegm of earth and water, bile of fire, wind of wind) in the same way that everything our bodies come into contact with (from food to climate) are also made up of these elements, then one could understand how diet, behavior, climate, and mood all affect one's bodily function by augmenting or decreasing the humoral potencies. In the more esoteric explanations, even such things as tantric blessings and exorcisms were believed to produce effects on the elements, and so also on patients' bodies in an amerliorative manner.

Armed with these insights, I realized that Dr Dawa's approach was not exemplary of Tibetan medicine, but neither was it unusual. Dr Dawa's approach was typical of a certain generation of scholars. Her reluctance to explain theory was not surprising. She had come of age in medicine during the Cultural Revolution, when it was forbidden to learn medical theory or speak it. The particular conditions of her medical training, and the history of a whole generation of scholars like her, could, I realized, account in part for her "reading" of the ultrasound. In other words, her conclusions could be understood as a product of a particular history as much as they were a product of a peculiar theoretical approach in Tibetan medicine. This, too, needs an explanation.

Particular histories: the rise of modern science

Dr Dawa had seen it all. In the early days of the socialist regime, Tibetan medicine was legitimized by its cultural appeal to the masses as an instrument of winning over the hearts and minds of Tibetans to communism. It won hers. A medical historian told me that in those days Tibetan medicine was supposed to appeal to the masses by its practical interventions not by its training in esoteric theory. And so, the halls of the Tibetan medical college had been closed at first and then reopened to only a few students, those who performed well in school and those from old elite families who had demonstrated "progressive" political attitudes.[7] These students were charged with modernizing Tibet from the "outside" in, that is from the countryside first, and according to the principles of materialist and progressive advancement.

By the mid 1960s, traditional Tibetan medicine was, some Tibetans say, nearly totally destroyed by its submission to the particular version of Marxist empiricism and materialism (Janes 1995). Many of the doctors from her generation, however, felt they had learned a usefully streamlined and pared down version of Tibetan medicine that fit into the model of the barefoot doctor and was empirical to a fault, socialist to perfection, and sufficient for training medical cadres for the masses. Practices were reduced to simple lists of diseases and standardized treatments, and references to religious or esoteric theories underlying the medicine (and even to the less complicated theories of elements, humors as poisons, and so on), such as those found in its primary esoteric referent, the *Kalachakra Tantra*, were both outlawed and deemed extraneous to medical practice. Many of the country's most skilled religious medical figures were either sent to the most remote regions and barred from teaching or, in some cases, imprisoned.

It was this period of time that actually marked the second offering of a rhetoric of "modern science" to Tibetan doctors. Some forty years earlier, in 1916, during the reign of the 13th Dalai Lama, efforts were made to modernize Tibetan medicine as part of a more general campaign to modernize Tibet. These efforts were instigated by the influence of British imperialism and other forms of political diplomacy that attempted to impress upon Lhasa officials the benefits of modern political secularism. This resulted in the opening of the Mentsikhang, College of Medicine and Astrology, Tibet's first non-monastic institution for higher education. Although the selection of students for this college was not based on monastic achievement (children of aristocracy and military families were allowed entrance), the subjects taught at the college were essentially the same as those taught in Lhasa' premier monastic medical college, Chags po ri. In other words, this modernization amounted to a form of "new bottles for old wine." Students at Mentsikhang studied the five major and five minor sciences (including medicine) as did monastically trained physicians, with the exception that the Mentsikhang had no tantric colleges.[8] Without actual exposure to the practices and technologies of "outside" medicine in Tibet, there was little impact of these forms of modern science on Tibetan medicine. By the time of Chinese rule and the Cultural Revolution, however, this all changed.

Before and during the Cultural Revolution in Tibet, "scientific" principles were substituted for religious belief. But even scientific principles were only adhered to if they were politically correct: not too expert or esoteric. If they made reference to religious or superstitious ideas that were shown to justify the old "feudal order" of society, they were eliminated on grounds that they represented elite knowledge that served only the aristocracy. Similarly, scholars with too much expertise, or who stressed the need for greater training requiring deeper levels of both pedagogy and intellectual practice of the Buddhist tantras, for example, were likewise deemed unsuitable for socialism.

Dr Dawa was one of those students invited to receive training in the practical techniques of Tibetan medicine, in service to the revolution. She, of all people, understood this form of the "modern scientific" in Tibetan medicine. Stressing medical outcomes over theory was a way for her to not simply practice Tibetan medicine but to meet the terms and conditions for its survival that had been put in place by the state.[9] Ever committed to the socialist vision herself, Dr Dawa also promoted a form of Tibetan medicine that was driven primarily by its practical and political, not theoretical, possibilities. In this effort, she placed greater stress on dietary and behavioral pathogens while totally eliminating spiritual or karmic pathogens. She placed greater emphasis on drug treatments than on combination therapies that included ritual cures, incense, cupping, massages. Dr Dawa's approach was to match standardized symptoms to politically "acceptable" diseases and, in turn, to known politically "acceptable" treatments. This formed the backbone of good medical practice. As a result, Dr Dawa could tell me which named diseases corresponded to which pulses, urine symptoms, and dietary excesses, but she could not tell me how these disorders came about physiologically in relation to larger theories of humors, their basis in the afflictive emotions of greed, anger, and ignorance, nor their correspondence to more esoteric principles used in Tibetan medicine, such as the five elements, the consciousness, or the astrological considerations. These, for her, were not necessary aspects of medical practice.

In Dr Dawa's world, evidence consisted of visible signs and symptoms, such as frothiness of stirred urine; pulse strength and rapidity; confessions on the part of patients that they drank a lot of beer, ate too much spicy food, had too many abortions, lived too long in a damp and cold environment, and the like. Just how such factors affected the strength of a patient's inner winds, how moral infractions (related to desires or anger, for example) might arise from these winds, or how the elements were mapped out in humoral capacities, was never something she could tell me about. For other doctors, the move to theory was essential: how else could one know the true nature of the disorder, its cause, and likely cure? Unless one recognized the links between, for example, bile-fire-anger-fevers or phlegm-earth-water-ignorance, one could not truly know how to help a patient. For Dr Dawa, however, it was not important how theory pulled all the practices together and made them part of a coherent and logical system, not least because this theory was so haunted by religious ideas that were part of the "old" feudal society. What mattered was that patients could be diagnosed by considering the signs and symptoms presented and that certain treatments worked to cure them and others did not.

With Dr Dawa's emphasis on the empirical, however, we might once again question her reading of the ultrasound results in her study. How is it that she was able to see the evidence of, for example, ongoing growths in the ovaries, and yet not consider this information valid enough to change her opinion of the efficacy of the Tibetan treatments for all of the patients in the study? What was it about the ultrasound evidence that looked different from other kinds of evidence she found useful in determining outcomes? Also still unexplained was why her study emphasized a single drug. To answer these questions, we have to spend even more time on history and the powerful social forces that conditioned her "vision" of medical practice.

Legitimizing practices: debating science

By the time I got to know Dr Dawa, Tibetan medicine had undergone something of a sea change from the days of her training. From 1979 onward, Tibetan medicine was reinvested with government support, including the construction of new medical hospitals, the opening of new medical schools, and even efforts to recuperate lost religious elements of the practices. By the 1990s, the government's efforts to rebuild Tibetan institutions had become a way of mediating political tensions in this minority region. Many of the great religious scholar lamas of medicine were brought back from their rural posts or, in some cases, from prison, and put back in the medical institutions. There was even an effort to recover and revitalize those aspects of Tibetan medicine that were now deemed "religious" by modernizing forces Tibet.

But the government that wanted to remake its history in Tibet has also had to do so under conditions not of its own choosing, a cruel irony in the case of the early Marxist regime. By 1993, the government's fear of religion was rekindled, in part by recognition of the extraordinary levels of devotion still held by Tibetans for their exiled ruler, His Holiness the Dalai Lama, China's declared enemy of state for supporting the campaign for Tibetan independence. Thus, by the mid-1990s, even though the government was investing time and money in the revitalization of Tibetan medicine, this effort was constrained because of Tibetan medicine's theoretical foundations in religion, and the fact that religion continued to be a political problem. The extraordinary suspicion that the government continued to have toward religion, because it was always potentially read by the government as a sign of political dissent, meant that medico-religious figures supported by the government were (and are) carefully watched for signs of political separatism.

One effect on medical doctors of the politicizing of religion has been linguistic. Because socialist development so skillfully deployed the Marxist rhetoric of distinctions between material forces and metaphysical and cultural outcomes, the idea that science could be viewed as oppositional to religion became widely accepted.[10] Thus, Tibetan doctors today call their medicine a "science." This is sometimes in opposition to calling it a "religiously-based" tradition in order to avoid arousing political suspicion (an ironic depoliticization at the same time that it politicizes; Janes 1995). Sometimes this claim is made in reference to something else. Some medical intellectuals claim that there is no linguistic shift at all; Tibetan medicine has always been a "science," they say. Reference is often made, for example, to the fact that medicine (*gso wa rig*), one of the five major "sciences," was always distinguished from "religion" (*nang rig*). Herein the term *rig* is translated as "science" although it might just as easily be read as "field of knowledge." In this sense, it seems perfectly reasonable to call all of Tibetan medicine's theories "scientific." At the same time, one would then also have to call Tibetan "religion" a "science" since it, too, is a *rig*. Hence, this effort often takes doctors in the direction of having to dance that delicate and complex dance that will establish what Tibetan medical sciences are (considering that they are based on religious ideas) in relation to "modern medical science."

Dr Dawa never had conversations about the "scientific" status of Tibetan medicine with me. She was not very religious, herself. And, she made a point of reminding me that doctors in her ward were not allowed to take time off from work for religious activities (such as circumambulations around holy cites of the city, pilgrimages to distant holy places, or even visits to monasteries on traditional holy days). One of her doctors who persisted in keeping a photograph of His Holiness the Dalai Lama in his home shrine had become a serious problem for her, and she made this clear by restricting his activities in the wards. She was devoted to implementing official policy for government work units like the Mentsikhang, even when this meant undertaking denunciations like those carried out during the Cultural Revolution.

It was also clear that Dr Dawa was not well informed, or willingly able, to talk with me about religiously significant episodes that occasionally came up, uninvited, with her patients. When patients mentioned to me that they had visited lamas for treatments of their disorders (including medical drugs), they noted that the doctors in the Mentsikhang neither asked nor seemed to care about these actions. When I mentioned references in the medical texts to spirit causes of disorders, karma, or even to the religious foundations of the humoral theories, Dr Dawa would plead ignorance of these things, remind me that they were not very important these days to Tibetan medicine and, after persistent questioning on my part, refer me to an older practitioner in her ward who had a better sense of them than she did. This doctors could only tell me that these "superstitious" ideas were no longer considered valid in Tibetan medicine. "Spirits" he said, "was the name for things like epilepsy and parasites before we knew the real causes of these diseases."

When she suggested that I talk with one of Tibet's great medical historians, however, I learned that Dr Dawa's approach might be more complex than a simple abandoning of traditional religious ideas for the sake of Western science. When I asked him about the religious underpinnings of Tibetan medicine amidst claims that it was a "science" today, he offered particularly useful insights about how the effort to establish that Tibetan medicine is a science requires showing how Tibetan sciences are like, while still being different from, the modern science of "outside medicine" (western medicine, *phyilu sman*). He told me:

Tibet is the highest country in the world. People have existed in this country for thousands of years. If there was no science in the Tibetan medical system, then no doubt all the Tibetans would have died many years ago. Long before Western medicine came into being, Tibetan medicine was already doing prevention work and giving medical cures in society. Even Western doctors have commented on the immense scientific knowledge in Tibetan medicine, especially when it comes to human medicine. Doctors who are very advanced in science, using proofs, etc. are still very impressed with what Tibetan medicine has been able to do in its own scientific ways.

In the effort to distinguish a Tibetan medical science from its "outside" medical counterpart, one also detects in this doctor's comments a desire to draw upon "modern science" (or its representatives who arrive in Lhasa) as a basis for legitimizing Tibetan medicine. The effort to establish Tibetan medicine as a unique science of its own also reveals how deeply entangled in the reference of "modern science" it already is. This is partially born from political necessity today. It is expressed as a new self-consciousness about what it means to be deemed "scientific" by those who carry authority within modern sciences. Historically, the idea that there were religious foundations of the basic fields of scientific knowledge was not something that Tibet's educated writers or thinkers were self-conscious about. Today, this has all changed. Today, there is a need to establish that Tibetan medicine is a science, in reference to what Westerners and political officials in China think modern science is – the kind that is visible in practices of "outside medicine."

In addition to his explanation of the "scientific" qualities of Tibetan medicine, this doctor also alluded to the internal politics of religion that, in the contemporary moment, compel Tibetan doctors to locate the epistemological basis for their practices in "science" rather than religion. When I initially brought up the subject of religious foundations in Tibetan medicine, he told me that he would be frank with me. He had lived through the Cultural Revolution and had suffered the humiliation of being made to wear the cap and placard for public trials targeting his own "crimes" against the state. He was not ashamed now to explain that it is important to recognize that historically there were religious elements of Tibetan medicine, and that this is true for most medical sciences. But, today, he noted, Tibetan medicine has progressed in a scientific manner that is based on observation of effective remedies. We should recognize, he said, that Tibetan medical sciences differ from modern medicine in the manner of treating the whole body and relating each symptom to the entire humoral functioning of the body, which he said was different from "modern medicine." He concluded by telling me that

> The five elements, the humors, the consciousness (*rnam shes*), all of this may seem very different to a Western scientific person, but greed, anger, and ignorance, these three, we consider these part of a scientific explanation. There are many people who have high prestige but they may completely ignore the fact that scientific explanations can be different in Tibetan medicine because they are so pro-Western medicine. All of these must be recognized as scientific ideas.

Although Dr Dawa herself seldom talked about Tibetan medical theory in this way, the words of her colleague revealed a commitment that Dr Dawa also held to the idea that Tibetan medical science offered cures that could be proven in Tibetan medical ways. This approach, I think, offers the first insight into Dr Dawa's conclusions in the case of the retrospective study of bile-related womb disorders. What, finally, might be said about Dr Dawa's reading of the ultrasound tests was that beyond her reluctance to theorize at all, Dr Dawa was "seeing" the data in the photos in ways that were conditioned by this internal political history that had required Tibetan medicine to be "scientific" in its "own" way, that is, in a way that both made use of and yet distinguished itself from modern medicine. Her repeated admonition that I should not use Western medical ideas to understand Tibetan medicine made sense, in this light, as did her explanation that the ultrasound reports were not necessarily the definitive factor in determining outcome.

In this sense, it was neither that the ultrasounds showed contrary evidence, nor that Dr Dawa simply dismissed the ultrasound information as being from "outside" and therefore only useful in relation to modern medical standards. It was rather that what she "saw" in the ultrasounds had to enable her to both acknowledge the presence of contrary evidence and at the same time confirm Tibetan medical methods. The presence of growths revealed in the ultrasound did not mean there was still a disease, from a Tibetan perspective. It was not that the ultrasound did not show the growths or the infections, but simply that these visual cues could be read from the perspective of Tibetan medicine in a way that did not suggest evidence of failure of Tibetan medicine.

Dr Dawa's reading of the ultrasound evidence could be explained on the basis of humoral theories. She could see both that there was ultrasound evidence of "no improvement" and that, from evidence from other visual and observational cues of Tibetan medicine, there *was* improvement, and cure, in all cases. As Kuriyama has shown for how we might approach Chinese medicine, the fact that symptoms remained visible in the ultrasounds did not necessarily mean that the patients were still sick, from a humoral perspective. Again, humoral perspectives would suggest that cures that begin by addressing and rectifying the root source of disorders – that is humoral imbalance – can be cured from the root first. The last signs of cure in such a case would be visible in things like ultrasound photos. But this interpretation would have required Dr Dawa to adopt and then be able to explain the humoral basis – the theory – upon which such claims could be made.

But Dr Dawa did not deploy a theoretical approach to reading the ultrasound reports. She could never explain the outcome in this way, for her ability to define the links between symptoms and humoral function, let alone between the theory of humoral medicine and the diagnostic signs within Tibetan medicine, was never shown. If anything, she indicated the opposite insight: that from the perspective of the ultrasound reports, some patients had shown "no improvement." In other words, Dr Dawa knew that she had to validate Tibetan medicine by the use of foreign technologies that carried with them their own epistemological demands regarding evidence. This epistemology asked Dr. Dawa to recognize the persistence of some disorders and different rates of success than the Tibetan methods suggested. Thus, the data from the ultrasound diagnoses were left in the report. The fact that ultrasound photos suggested ongoing disorders had to be acknowledged *and* rendered irrelevant at the same time. What Dr Dawa "saw" in the ultrasound evidence was in this sense viewed through the politics and historical forces of this act. Her vision was a product of the political and historical forces that made it important for her to both include the ultrasound readings and the outcomes from a Tibetan medical perspective in order to be scientific but also absorb the evidence in them into a framework that, for political, historical, and cultural reasons, proved that Tibetan medicine was efficacious in its own unique and uniquely empirical ways. For Dr Dawa this vision did not amount to a contradiction of evidence. It was an avowal that evidence can mean different things in different political and cultural contexts, even when it appears, from some viewpoints, to contravene "shared" standards of empiricism. It was this recognition that allowed her to treat the ultrasound evidence as subordinate, in terms of relevance, to the evidence gathered by Tibetan "scientific" techniques, and it was this approach that explained her commitment to the "advancement" of Tibetan medicine in its own terms.

Selective studies of efficacy: the impact of the market

If particular historical contingencies partially explained Dr Dawa's reading of the "evidence" of Tibetan efficacy, might they also answer the second question I posed about Dr Dawa's study, the question of why it focused on a single medicine? I suggest that they do. However, the answer to this question takes us to other political and, this time, economic forces acting on her and her colleagues. The validation of Tibetan medicine as a "science" is not just a product of the Socialist project mixed with exposure to Western forms of biomedicine and its own particular history in China's Tibet. This validation is tightly interwoven with the new economic liberalization throughout China. In the state's drive to privatize and liberalize to a market economy, the project of identifying aspects of Tibetan medicine that are marketable in an international arena has compelled Tibetan doctors to affirm single drug therapies rather than medical models that emphasize the multiplicity of treatments, flexibility, and variation in therapies even for those with the same named disorders. But the way this has come about is neither simple nor straightforward.

International health development organizations from Western countries are now invested in the development of Tibet. More often than not these organizations are committed to handing down to Tibetans the terms of medical legitimacy that valorize only one medical model. Typically this effort relegates all other medical knowledge to a space wherein validity can only occur in the reductionistic terms set forth by biomedicine. But in the case of China's Tibet, this effort is mediated by China's own commitment to an already Sinicized biomedical development and a strong state interest in promoting its indigenous medical systems, such as Zhongyi (Traditional Chinese Medicine, TCM) and Tibetan Medicine (*rGyu bShi*), as equally capable of effective interventions as biomedicine. Tibetan medicine, however, is rendered distinct from Zhongyi because it is from a minority (*minzu*) group and the government has invested great time and money in promoting the cultural traditions of the minorities as part of its effort to arouse state nationalism among all the potentially separatist minorities.[11]

With this in mind, one might note that the conditions that produced Dr Dawa's retrospective study might also include the situation these doctors find themselves in as minorities in China. Their interest in meeting the state's claims that their medicine is "scientific" needs to be understood, in addition to the forces already described, in relation to the fact that they are told their medicine holds the same position among the Tibetan minorities as Zhongyi TCM holds for the Han majorities. That is, the effort is to affirm that Tibetan Medicine represents one of the indigenous Chinese treasures, that it affirms traditions of science preceding Western or "modern" medicine, and that it should be made available not just to non-Tibetans within the motherland, but to patients in the international arena, much as the state has supported efforts to internationalize TCM.

This appeal to internal Chinese nationalism is one that gives the appearance of great tolerance for the minorities. But it is coupled with market reforms that undermine this state support. Privatization efforts on the part of the government increasingly tell the minorities they need to achieve greater financial independence, particularly because most of the minorities are in rural areas that are viewed as a "drain" on state resources in contrast to coastal areas of Eastern China that have seen great economic and industrial development and greater economic self-sufficiency. As the state shifts over to privatized market economic models, the minority institutions of traditional medicine have been asked to take on more responsibility for their financial survival than those of Sinicized biomedicine. For Tibet's Mentsikhang, this has meant converting their streetside property to commercial rental space, deploying fee-for-service policies in the hospitals, and positioning themselves as a resource in the international medical market.

In this way, state pressures from within China to make Mentsikhang achieve financial independence have indirectly pressured doctors to focus on those strategies already validated in the international market, including the single drug approach, regardless of whether or not single drugs were emphasized in traditional Tibetan treatments. This approach, along with changes in the pharmaceutical packaging of Tibetan drugs has, in fact, enabled Mentsikhang to advertise and sell its medicines in an international market, already putting three new drugs into United States markets as "food supplements."

The more dramatic evidence that economic pressures played a role in Dr Dawa's retrospective study was that it was financial pressures of the new market economy that had made the doctors interested in doing the study in the first place. Of late, it had become more difficult to get one of the most important ingredients (out of 33) used in this medicine. The ingredient was the seed of a plant grown on rural mountainsides in the southern part of Tibet, typically harvested by villagers and sold to physicians at the women's ward where doctors, for ten years, had made the medicines themselves in the hospital.

In order to convince the administration of the need to subsidize this medicine by turning over its production to the main Tibetan medical factory, thereby hoping to increase the price paid for the ingredient and to stimulate its harvesting by villagers, they undertook this scientific study. The same pressures doctors felt to privatize and subsidize their medical system in ways that were internationally recognized through their pharmaceutical projects were the same pressures that were placed on villagers who were no longer willing to harvest the seed ingredient needed for the drug because they were too busy trying to earn a living in more profitable, privatized ways. This situation, too, should be considered in an attempt to explain why Dr Dawa read the results of her study the way she did.

Despite the fact that these patients were given all sorts of other treatments besides *yu kyung katsar* in their stays at Mentsikhang, and in most cases they were given a variety of different treatments, it made sense that Dr Dawa would "see" the results primarily in terms of the single medicine. Although it in some way runs counter to Tibetan medical epistemology, a study like this could prove Tibetan medicine's usefulness not only in view of competing market trends in Lhasa but also in the larger international community, as it was envisioned by Mentsikhang researchers. The goal was to legitimize Tibetan medicine in the global market at the same time that it was legitimized as a minority tradition worthy of increased state support within China. Convincing the pharmaceutical factory to pick up payment for production, and thus raising the price that could be paid to villagers who might then be more inclined to harvest the plant, was an immediate goal, but the survival of Tibetan medicine under new economically privatized conditions was the ultimate goal.

Conclusion

I began this essay with the comment that the language of colonialism that is spoken in Tibetan medicine in contemporary Tibet is that of science, but that the question of who stands behind this colonizing force and what its outcomes are in terms of the way evidence is read and used to establish proof of efficacy are complex questions. What I have attempted to show here is that answers ought best be sought not simply in terms of political domination by China, nor solely in terms of theoretical explanations and reference to alternative epistemologies found in traditional Tibetan "scientific" practices. Rather, we might also seek answers by looking at the multiple forces of history, internal and international politics, transnational medical culture, and modern economics that have and continue to actively produce the need for claims about a "science" of Tibetan medicine in the first place.

In the case of studies like that undertaken in the women's ward, it is possible to see all sorts of competing and contradictory impulses produced from these forces, some that see "science" as a rigid empiricism focused on outcomes and single drugs, and some that see science as a form of theoretical engagement that is broad enough to encompass religious ideas by renaming them as "scientific." Other outcomes are unique ways of "seeing" evidence produced by biomedical technologies – in particular, one finds efforts to both deflect and make use of epistemological demands that some technologies, like ultrasound, bring with them. One result is that what might seem like a contradiction of evidence to some looks noncontradictory to others, and in fact it is that noncontradictory quality of such aberrant data that forms a basis for "proof" of the efficacy of Tibetan medicine for doctors like Dr Dawa.

In this sense, I would say that it is not in the statistical outcomes that we find the basis for establishing "proof" in Tibetan medicine. "Proof" is rather found in the particular demands that have been placed on Tibetan doctors and on this medical system in the form of historical, political, and economic trends, all of which have skillfully articulated the state's needs in and through the medical resources of Tibetan medical professionals and all of which have enabled them to "read" evidence in particular ways. Proof, in this sense, becomes not just a question of epistemology (however important that remains) but rather a question of the way epistemology is made to speak for politics, history, and free markets in a changing world.

Notes

1 I would like to thank Dechen Tsering and Yangdron Kelsang, as well as the physicians and nurses and director of the Mentsikhang in Lhasa, TAR. Thanks also to Mark Nichter and Kim Gutschow for suggestions that improved this

essay. Thanks are also extended to the Wenner Gren Foundation, the National Science Foundation, and UCSF for their generous support of the research upon which this article is based.

2 Others who have made this point include Lock (1980, 1990), Nichter (1992).

3 With this in mind, I turn also to the work of Ashis Nandy, who argued in relation to his postcolonial Indian identity that it should not be held against the once colonized that he must speak in the language of the colonizer (Nandy 1983). Across the Himalayas in China's Tibet, doctors in the wards of Tibet's traditional medical hospital might also be given this consideration.

4 The results of this study were read to me from a preliminary report in 1998. In 2000, on a return visit, I obtained the published version of this study, and it had removed much of the qualitative data on outcomes or changed the data, leaving only summaries of how, generally, the outcomes were very promising.

5 Kuriyama argues that the way historical Chinese doctors "saw" the body was based on not seeing anatomies as consisting of objects, *per se*, but as processes that linked together functioning systems in the body. Obeyesekere (1976) makes arguments like this for Ayurveda also.

6 Langford (1995, forthcoming) makes this argument about Ayurveda, noting that Ayurveda is not a formal, theorized, or objectified system that has a scholarly basis in shared practices among its many varied practitioners. Rather, it is a collection of varied and disparate practices that are deployed differentially by various practitioners, and understanding these varied practices is best done through exploration of the historical forces of modernity, colonialism, and romantic nativism that bear upon them, particularly and idiosyncratically.

7 See Janes (1995) for a history of this period of time.

8 These fields are translated differently in different sources. One translation includes: grammar, logic, technology, medicine, and religion as the major fields, and rhetoric, epistemology, drama, poetry, and astrology as the minor fields.

9 Farquhar (1987, 1992, 1994a, 1994b) shows how this has worked in Chinese medicine. She notes that Chinese doctors found ways to incorporate Marxist dialectical materialism into their theories of yin and yang, and how the history of efforts to modernize Chinese medicine has meant transforming disparate and idiosyncratic, lineage based sets of practices into formal, standardized objectified theories of the body and its processes has only been partially complete. Farquhar argues that Traditional Chinese Medicine did not historically deploy "theory" in the sense that biomedicine refers to theory. I am suggesting that Tibetan medicine actually did have "theory" historically, and that that "theory" was rendered less visible during certain socialist times by the fact that it was associated with religion. Official efforts focused on replacing religious theory with socialist political rhetoric.

10 Of course, this distinction is not unique to communist polities. Latour's (1993) exegesis on Durkheimian social science, in which the idea that "nature" was separate from "society" came to form the basis of Western epistemology, offers a good critique of this history and the culturally constituted "distinction" between domains it brought about. One must also include Marxist-Leninist political rhetoric in this history, in that it, too, deploys the same distinctions and rationalizes it in a method for social change.

11 See Schein (2000), for the case of other minorities. An example of this in Tibet is the Chinese Medical Association of the Minorities that was formed by the government to promote medical systems like Tibetan medicine and that hosted its first International Conference on Tibetan medicine in the year 2000 in Lhasa, Tibet. This followed closely on the heels of the First International

Congress on Tibetan Medicine, sponsored by a United States group and held in Washington DC, November 1999. There were only two representatives from China at this US conference.

References

Farquhar, J. (1987). Problems of Knowledge in Contemporary Chinese Medical Discourse. *Social Science and Medicine* 24(12): 1013–1021.

—— (1992). Time and Text: Approaching Chinese Medical Practice through Analysis of a Published Case. In *Paths to Asian Medical Knowledge*, edited by Charles Leslie and Allan Young, pp. 62–73. Berkeley: University of California Press.

—— (1994a). Multiplicity, Point of View, and Responsibility in Traditional Chinese Healing. In *Body, Subject and Power in China* edited by A. Zito and T. Barlow. Chicago: Chicago University Press pp. 78–102.

—— (1994b). *Knowing Practice: The Clinical Encounter of Chinese Medicine*. Boulder: Westview Press.

Hankinson, (1994). The Growth of Medical Empiricism. In *Knowledge and the Scholarly Medical Traditions* edited by D. Bates. Cambridge: Cambridge University Press pp. 60–83.

Janes, C. (1995). The Transformations of Tibetan Medicine. *Medical Anthropology Quarterly* 9(1): 6–39.

Kuriyama, S. (1994). The Imagination of Winds and the Development of the Chinese Conception of the Body. In *Body, Subject and Power in China* edited by A. Zito and T. Barlow. Chicago: Chicago University Press pp. 23–41.

—— (1995). Visual Knowledge in Classical Chinese Medicine. In *Knowledge and the Scholarly Medical Traditions* edited by D. Bates. Cambridge: Cambridge University Press pp. 205–234.

Langford, J. (1995). Ayurvedic Interiors: Person, Space, and Episteme in Three Medical Practices. *Cultural Anthropology* 10(3): 330–360.

Latour, B. (1993). *We Have Never Been Modern*. Cambridge: Harvard University Press.

Leslie, C. (editor) (1976). *Asian Medical Systems*. Berkeley: University of California Press.

Leslie, C. (1980). Medical Pluralism in World Perspective. *Social Science & Medicine* 14B(4): 191–196.

—— (1986). Indigenous Pharmaceuticals, the Capitalist World System and Civilization. *Preceedings of the Kroeber Anthropological Society Meetings*. University of California, Berkeley, 8 March 1986.

—— (1992). Interpretations of Illness: Syncretism in Modern Ayurveda. In Charles *Paths to Asian Medical Knowledge* edited by Leslie and Allan Young. Berkeley: University of California Press pp. 177–208.

Lock, M. (1980). *East Asian Medicine in Urban Japan*. Berkeley: University of California Press.

—— (1990). Rationalization of Japanese Herbal Medication: The Hegemony of Orchestrated Pluralism. *Human Organization* 49: 41–47.

Nandy, A. (1983). *The Intimate Enemy: Loss and Recovery of Self Under Colonialism*. Delhi: Oxford University Press.

Nichter, M. (editor) (1992). *Anthropological Approaches to the Study of Ethnomedicine*. Gordon & Breach, Science Publishers.

Obeyesekere, G. (1976). The Impact of Ayurvedic Ideas on the Culture and the Individual in Sri Lanka. In *Asian Medical Systems* edited by Charles Leslie. Berkeley: University of California Press pp. 201–226.

Schein, L. (2000). *Minority Rules: The Miao and the Feminine in China's Cultural Politics*. Durham: Duke University Press.

Chapter 9

Notes on the evolution of evolutionary psychiatry

Allan Young

> Srinivasa Murti had written, "We should not torture Ayurvedic texts
> to read into them modern Allopathic teachings through forced compar-
> isons and fanciful interpretations." Dwarkanath was convinced that his
> ... interpretations avoided this error. But self-deception is not the most
> interesting issue for us in considering his work.
>
> (Leslie 1987: 27)

In 1984, Charles Leslie participated in an international symposium on the
comparative history of medicine, held in Japan. His paper was an account
of the people, philosophies, and controversies that have shaped modern
ayurveda. One of the individuals mentioned in the paper was Chandragiri
Dwarkanath, who served as Advisor on Indian Systems of Medicine in
the Ministry of Health (India) from 1959 to 1967. His *magnum opus* was
a three volume monograph titled *Fundamental Principles of Ayurveda
(1954)*. In it, Dr. Dwarkanath compared the epistemologies of ayurveda
and Western science. Western science, he observed, had devised procedures that allowed researchers to incrementally eliminate the errors and
misconceptions of their predecessors. In contrast, the traditional system
of Hindu philosophy, the *Darsana*, lacked equivalent procedures. Yet this
was a sign of strength and not weakness, for the knowledge of the *Darsana*
was the telos toward which Western science was moving. As science
progressed, its findings confirmed "the unchanging, complete, and perfect
truths of Hindu theory." Evidence in support of this conclusion could be
found in correspondences, notably between ayurvedic humoral functions
and Western physiological science. The ayurvedic concept of *vata* [wind]
corresponded to the "processes of the central, vegetative, and autonomous
nervous system." *Pitta* [bile] matched the functions of the nutritional
system, including the "activities of glandular structures, especially enzymes
and hormones, whose functions [are] tissue building and metabolism."
Kapha [phlegm] referred to the skeletal and anabolic systems as they are
described by Western physiologists (Leslie 1987: 22).

According to Leslie, the "motive force of Dwarkanath's career was an effort to translate between ayurveda and cosmopolitan [Western] medicine, to prove thereby that Hindu theories were more inclusive and valid than the limited and changeable truth of modern science" (1987: 25). Yet the correspondences on which Dwarkanath based his claim were problematic. It was not Western science that had moved in the direction of ancient Hindu truths, but rather ayurveda that had shifted in the direction of the West. Ayurvedic medicine had been "revived" during the nineteenth and twentieth centuries. The goal of the revivalists was to purge ayurveda of corrupt interpretations and alien accretions and to facilitate its development as a system of practice. Revival meant both restoration and transformation, continuity and change. The ancient Hindu conceptions represented in ayurveda were "unchanging, complete, and perfect truths." At the same time, this perfect wisdom anticipated modern science's most formidable discoveries. In this way, the revivalist rhetoric

> provided the ideological platform for an indigenous movement that ... transformed traditional medical learning in modern South Asia. The leaders of this movement adopted technology, ideas, and institutional forms from the evolving cosmopolitan [Western] system to found pharmaceutical companies, colleges, and professional associations, and to reinterpret traditional knowledge.
>
> (Leslie 1987: 9)

This is the background to Dwarkanath's comparison between ayurvedic and Western concepts of the body and physiology. The correspondences that he discovered were conceivable precisely because *vata*, *pitta*, and *kapha* had acquired a new context, shaped by the events, collective desires, and politics of the last two centuries. Dwarkanath did not recognize this historical transformation. His second error was in believing that Western science had a telos, that it was moving inevitably toward unchanging perfect truths. Yet there is nothing particularly Indian about Dwarkanath's style of reasoning and, more particularly, the pursuit of correspondences in support of eternal truths. There is no shortage of this kind of thinking in Western medicine. This chapter describes a recent example: the re-emergence of *evolutionary psychiatry*.

The principles of evolutionary psychiatry

The term "evolutionary psychiatry" is used by psychiatrists and psychologists to label an assortment of theories and proofs that explain the origins and significance of mental disorders. Monographs and articles published in mainstream psychiatric and psychological journals during the past fifteen years have provided evolutionary accounts of schizophrenia (Crow 1991,

1993, 1995), major depressive disorder (Nesse 2000), post-traumatic stress disorder (Silove 1998), bipolar affective disorder (Gardner 1982), panic disorder (Marks and Nesse 1994), antisocial personality disorder (Mealey 1995), and substance use disorders (Nesse and Burridge 1997).

Many of these contributors believe that it is possible to discover an evolutionary origin or context for most of the disorders in *The Diagnostic and Statistical Manual of Mental Disorders* (DSM-IV 1994), the official nosology of the American Psychiatric Association. This system, which originates with the 1980 edition of the nosology (DSM-III), is modeled after the classification of infectious diseases, in that each named mental disorder is identified with a unique set of diagnostic features and is assumed to have a distinctive etiology. This is a radical departure from the previous nosologies, in which disorders were represented in dimensional rather than categorical terms – that is, as expressions of intersecting biological, psychological, and social vectors. The tendency in psychiatry today is to regard biological factors as causal and to treat psychological and social factors as affecting "risk" or vulnerability. Because these evolutionary accounts generally correspond to individual disorders, they have two effects. They explain the origins and pathogenesis of the disorders and, at the same time, they vindicate the correctness of the categorical perspective.

Interest in the evolutionary origins of mental disorders and related conditions dates to the second half of the nineteenth century. One theory, promoted by Cesare Lombroso, was that there are individuals who fail to evolve through all of the stages of human biological evolution. They are atavists and behave in ways that, although once adapted to our species' life conditions, are now abnormal and often dangerous to the fully evolved members of society. Herbert Spencer and the great neurologist John Hughlings Jackson believed that stages of evolutionary adaptation are "sedimented" neurologically and thus part of our biological makeup. In normal individuals, primitive neurological structures are controlled and inhibited by other structures, in the neocortex, acquired at a later stage in the evolution of the species. Under conditions of great duress and in certain cases of biological impairment, even previously normal individuals would regress to earlier stages and more primitive structures, and they could be expected to think and behave in irrational and pathological ways. Sigmund Freud and W. H. R. Rivers, among other twentieth-century doctors, adopted versions of this principle. A British army doctor in World War I, Rivers promoted the idea that the paralyses, contractures, anaesthesias, mutism, and other motor symptoms characterizing traumatic hysteria among soldiers are products of a transient neurological regression and represent an archaic response to danger, viz. the freeze aspect of the fight-flight-freeze response (Rivers 1922). Freud's concept of primary process thinking that he associated with the unconscious reflects a similar perspective. In common with both Lamarck and Spencer, Freud imagined that evolutionary sediments could also take the form of phylogenetic memories. This process is described in *Totem and Taboo, Group Psychology and the Analysis of the Ego*, and *Moses and Monotheism*, where Freud tells and retells the Oedipal origins of psychoneurosis (Young 1999).

These evolutionary ideas died with their authors. By World War II, Rivers' psychiatric writings were largely forgotten. Freud's Lamarckianism proved to be an embarrassment to his followers, who either rejected or ignored his phylogenetic thesis. In the 1960s, when interest in the evolutionary origins of mental disorders revived, the stimulus came from ethological research on primate societies rather than the speculations of Rivers and Freud.

As the term is used now, "evolutionary psychiatry" labels a variety of neo-Darwinian perspectives, rather than a unitary theory. One finds a range of unconnected starting points and theoretical positions based on archetypes (Carl Jung), attachment theory (John Bowlby), the triune brain (Paul Maclean), modular processing (Jerry Fodor), and so on. Nevertheless, the studies that are published and cited in the leading psychiatric journals tend to share a distinctive set of premises – a common theoretical framework, if not a full-blown theory:

1   Most (all?) mental disorders can be traced to specific evolutionary adaptations. A feature is "adaptive" if it provides an individual with a reproductive advantage over individuals, within the same species, that lack this feature.

2   These adaptations are equivalent to problem-solving mechanisms. They are hard-wired and possess a heritable identity. They are known by various names, including "modules," "design features," "inference engines," "mental organs," "neurological circuits," and "neural programs." They increase reproductive success by satisfying significant "environmental demands" and "functional requirements," and their operations are characteristically domain-specific, rapid, and hierarchical. These operations contrast with the much slower and more flexible processes characteristic of the individual's general purpose intelligence.

3   These domain-specific mechanisms correspond to ways of thinking about objects and events – more especially thinking about physical causality, the features and properties of objects and events of the biological world, the manufacture and employment of artifacts, sources of danger, and ways of responding to danger. In this context, "thinking" means simply cognition and does not imply "consciousness," which is itself an adaptation that emerged long after many of these other ways of thinking.

4   Some domain specific mechanisms are adaptations to the *social environment*. There is a looping effect (mutual enhancement) between these mechanisms and the increasing complexity of the social envi-

ronment throughout the course of human evolution. The most frequently mentioned of these mechanisms is "Machiavellian intelligence." It represents the modular capacity to decode the perceptions and motivations of other individuals. This is the basis for complex forms of cooperation and competition; for instance, via the ability to detect cheating.

5   Most of these adaptive mechanisms evolved during the foraging or paleolithic stage of human and proto-human development, a period lasting about five million years. This represented a relatively stable period and would have provided sufficient time for the mechanisms to emerge and become part of the human genome. The subsequent history of humanity was brief and accompanied by rapid and continual change, especially during postneolithic times. The entire period lasted only 10,000 years in southwest Asia, about as long in China, and was appreciably shorter in other parts of the world. The time-span was too brief and the challenges too unstable for new hard-wired mechanisms to emerge.

Mental disorders are puzzling phenomena from an evolutionary point of view, since they are clearly maladaptive. Schizophrenia is an obvious example. Impairment is severe and chronic, age of onset (in males) coincides with the beginning of the period of normal reproductive activity (Crow 1993: 594–595). Nonpsychotic disorders, such as depression, are likewise associated with significantly reduced fertility. Why were these disorders not eliminated in the course of human evolution, assuming that each one has a genetic basis other than recurrent spontaneous mutations (cf. achondroplastic dwarfism)? The solution consists of three elements: a mental disorder, a scenario explaining the evolutionary origins of a heritable adaptation, and a mechanism that connects the disorder with the adaptation. For the moment, I want to concentrate on the connections that are most often mentioned in this literature.

One of these is the notion of *genome lag*. The idea is that our paleolithic bodies are seriously mismatched to the "demand characteristics" of postindustrial society. Take the example of this diagnostic classification, "agoraphobia without history of panic disorder." The essential feature of this disorder is the fear of finding oneself in a place or situation from which escape might be difficult, or where help might be unavailable if one were incapacitated. Because of this fear, patients avoid crowds, refuse to travel by bus, train, car, or airplane, and require a companion whenever they leave home. Typically the disorder persists for years and impairment is usually severe. Yet the same tendency would be highly serviceable under paleolithic conditions, where individuals would have been at risk for a wide variety of environmental hazards and entirely dependent on the support and attention of close kin.

Adaptions and disorders are also connected through evolutionary trade-offs. The idea here is that adaptations have costs as well as benefits. It is the ratio between these two that will determine whether or not a feature provides a reproductive advantage. For instance, there was a point in the past when the ability to experience fear (a characteristic we share with most vertebrates) was extended to include anxiety. Primal fear is oriented to the present, to concrete threats and dangers. Anxiety is a later development and is oriented to the future. It imagines possibilities, it considers associations, and it lacks closure. (Fear ceases with the elimination or evasion of the source of danger.) The advantage of anxiety under paleolithic conditions should be obvious. An individual would remain vigilant, sensitive to environmental cues. The feature would be especially advantageous whenever he entered a novel environment. The evolutionary trade-off is that anxiety produces frequent false alarms, during which the individual is unnecessarily aroused. The arousal state is also intrinsically unpleasant, but this quality is part of the adaptation and helps to explain the effectiveness of anxiety. The distress is an advantage from an evolutionary point of view, because it is difficult to ignore. From a subjective point of view, it would be a cost but probably irrelevant to reproductive success. Fast forward to modern times, where the anxiety feature becomes a psychiatric problem. Leave aside the fact that its adaptive value may have diminished as a consequence of our enhanced ability to control our natural and social environments. The more important point is that the anxiety mechanism expresses itself differentially. In most individuals, its evolutionary by-product (distress, false positives) falls within nondebilitating limits. In a minority of people however, the mechanism is either hypertrophied (reflecting normal variation within a population) or defective, producing clinically significant chronic anxiety and episodes of recurrent or acute anxiety.

Another way in which psychiatrists and psychologists speak about the evolutionary origins of mental disorders is in terms of "harmful dysfunctions" (HD), a term coined by Jerome Wakefield (1999). A harmful dysfunction represents the failure of a psychobiological mechanism to perform its natural function. Every mental illness described in the official nosology corresponds to a distinctive harmful dysfunction. Because the epistemology of the HD concept is based on the "natural functions" of failed mechanisms, it is antithetical to the ideas that mental disorders and classifications are historical products. The problem, of course, is to justify the use of "natural functions," to show that the term does not simply mask or "naturalize" the way in which the HD advocate selects the individual "functions." Wakefield is attentive to this requirement. He defines a natural function as a product of adaptation, which, in turn, can be judged against objective standards of fitness and reproductive advantage. Here again, the standard is not being based on the current utility of the feature or its subjective quality, but its evolutionary history.

One might argue that most psychobiological mechanisms are not products of adaptation, but rather might be by-products of adaptations – evolutionary "spandrels" as described by Stephen Gould and Richard Lewontin. In such a case, the evolutionary history of a feature would be irrelevant to explaining or justifying the diagnostic classification to which it corresponds (Lewontin 1998). We would have to look for other ways – perhaps to socially determined ideas about disability and abnormality – to explain why psychiatrists would classify a given constellation of mental states as a distinctive disorder. This line of reasoning assumes that a feature can be stabilized within a phylogenetic line even if it is not favored by natural selection. Wakefield rejects this assumption. He argues that the ultimate origin of a feature is irrelevant: a feature that emerged as a by-product will be stabilized if it acquires a function and a selective advantage. Otherwise, it will degenerate into a vestigial form, as in the blindness of cave dwelling fish. In other words, the persistence of a feature is evidence of its selective advantage – at least until the close of the paleolithic period.

The evolutionary origins of depression

In *Instinct and the Unconscious* (1922), W. H. R. Rivers constructed an evolutionary theory that explained the origins of traumatic hysteria. Following the lead of Hughlings Jackson, he distinguished between "positive symptoms" and "negative symptoms." The onset of positive symptoms reflected the disinhibition of primitive neurological structures and archaic adaptations, negative symptoms were products of organic pathologies and lacked an evolutionary meaning. Rivers died in 1922, he left no intellectual heir, and his theory concerning the origins of mental disorders was soon forgotten. Walter Cannon constructed a similar theory in an article on Voodoo Death, published twenty years later (Cannon 1942). Cannon's article was frequently cited, but it inspired no sequel. Another dead end.

The revival of interest in evolutionary origins dates to 1967, with the publication of an article in *The Lancet*, entitled "Hypothesis: the dominance hierarchy and the evolution of mental illness." Its author is John Price, a British clinical psychiatrist interested in ethological research. Price's starting point in the article is an epidemiological puzzle. Mental disorders are associated with reduced fertility and, under ancestral conditions, even mild depression would confer a disadvantage. Yet the prevalence of clinically significant depression, anxiety and irritability is consistently high, affecting one person in seven in the general population. Since human beings are the products of a ruthless process of natural selection, how is this possible?

Price's article lists fifteen sources. Two of the studies are psychiatric and are cited for their epidemiological data. The other sources are animal studies (mainly primates) and recent accounts of the social life of early man. The accounts are interchangeable, for the prevailing wisdom at the time was that "early man lived in small social groups ... organised into dominance hierarchies, much as the groups of baboons and macaques are today" (Price 1967: 245). These societies, monkey and hominid, are composed of aggressive individuals. Within them, one finds a characteristic economy of emotions: "irritability towards inferiors, anxiety towards superiors, elation on going up the hierarchy and depression on going down." According to Price, this ability to experience depression satisfies a functional requirement for the survival of these societies, by providing stability and limiting intragroup violence. "[D]epression ... prevents the descending animal from fighting back; the fight goes out of him and it 'gives up the sponge', the sponge being essentially precedence and status, but such things as food, sexual outlets, and choice of sleeping quarters are likely to be lost as well." Factors undermining stability – the presence of evenly matched alpha males, environmental change leading to increased competition for essential resources, etc. – would increase the incidence of depression and anxiety. Factors that reduce this kind of competition would have the opposite effect.

Price's first step was to reconstruct the emotional economy of paleolithic society via ethological accounts of contemporary baboon social life. The second step is to connect the mental life of contemporary humans with the experiences of their reconstructed ancestors. This connection is genetic (the heritability of archaic predispositions) and also clinical, for Price believes that the scenario is mirrored in his own practice. Behavior patterns at the bottom of the baboon hierarchy (as in paleolithic society) resemble

> the sort of behaviour and symptoms that we observe in depressed patients. The ideas of inferiority and unworthiness, the withdrawal, the selective forgetting of memories conducive to self-esteem, the loss of appetite and libido: these might have been designed to prevent an individual from desiring and attempting to regain former status.
>
> (Price 1967: 244)

Thus among humans, we can expect less depression and anxiety in groups that have unquestioned leaders and that are aggressively involved with external enemies. Would one expect autocracy, patriarchy, militarism, and warfare to be associated with reduced levels depression and anxiety? But egalitarian societies are not without resources in this respect, since levels of depression and anxiety will be low where individuals have access to alcohol, other sedative drugs, and "the emotion of love, especially in its religious form."

> One might mention, at this point, the position of the doctor in the patient's hierarchy. Perhaps much of his ability to comfort the

disturbed patient lies in the fact that he is perceived as powerful, confident, assured, and yet strongly committed to the patient's interests. So do baboons in time of insecurity turn to their overlord for reassurance.

(Price 1967: 245)

An article published in the *Archives of General Psychiatry* in 1982 extended Price's social hierarchy thesis to manic-depressive illness (bipolar affective disorder). In it, Russell Gardner proposed a correspondence between mania and depression in humans and the psychological state of alpha males (dominant rank) and omega animals (lowest rank) in baboon troops. According to Gardner, alpha and omega states occur in humans, as normal, hereditary responses to social rank. In some individuals, however, the states are cyclical, abnormally easy to stimulate, and disconnected from social reality – a condition said to originate in "an unstable component in the susceptible person's neural organization" (Gardner 1982: 1439). While no equivalent of bipolar disorder has been observed among nonhumans, animal studies are nonetheless useful, permitting the dissection of bipolar illness into component parts (alpha and omega) and providing a "better understanding of the evolutionary context" of affective disorders (Gardner 1982: 1440–1441).

An article published a decade later in the *British Journal of Psychiatry* turned to the subjective component of depression. According to the authors (who included Price and Gardner), in human and monkey societies, each individual possesses an "animal self-concept" that reflects its place in the social hierarchy. In these same societies, individuals are engaged in competition with one another for limited resources. Social life is a zero sum game and this circumstance affects the ways individuals assess themselves. An individual's self-concept will be based on its knowledge of its fighting capacity, its strength and skill, its previous successes and failures in competition, the support that it might expect from allies and kin, and its access to weapons (or so it is assumed: this self-concept would seem more appropriate for males than females; I will return to this point.) Thus self-concepts (satisfying and unsatisfying) will vary according to the individual's capacity to acquire and retain resources, such as food and sexually active females. Fast forward to our own times, where the animal self-concept is transmogrified into that state of awareness known to mental health experts as "self-esteem."

Price had previously made the point that social hierarchies require a mechanism for closing violent episodes between competitors – something short of the physical elimination of the loser. (At this point, the authors replay the fascinating account of "symmetrical schizmogenesis" provided by Geoffrey Bateson in his monograph, *Naven* (1959).) The burden for this falls on the loser. He must have a means of communicating with the dominant animal (and with his own allies) and it must be sufficient to stop the aggression at this point. The evolutionary solution is a "yielding mechanism," which the authors identify with depression:

> Depression can be seen as a ritual form of losing behaviour producing a temporary psychological incapacity which signals submission to the winner but preserves the loser without physical damage. It performs the function which death performs in unritualised fighting, and which the referee performs in culturally ritualised competition.
>
> (Price et al. 1994: 310)

Ritualized depression (yielding) is hard-wired, reactive, stereotypic, functional, and transient. Clinical depression shares this circuitry and replicates the behavior. The disabling, vegetative symptoms that accompany depression are "a ritual (psychological) substitute for the physical damage which is suffered by the loser in an unritualised contest." The depressed person's perception of the external world is based on erroneous perceptions and reasoning (Beck 1967, 1987). However, it is his distorted self-concept and self-esteem that count and, to a degree, transform the external reality:

> [T]he world of the depressive is not a favourable arena for competing; and the pessimism of the depressive is in stark contrast to that optimism which seems required for successful competition. The depressive . . . [also] has a distorted view of the past in which former rank, ownership and success seem . . . like a sham . . . not to be regained.
>
> (Price et al. 1994: 312)

There are situations in which the onset of the omega state follows a real, socially patterned decline in status and self-efficacy. This explains the increased prevalence and severity of depression among the elderly (Price et al. 1994: 312). The ticklish part of the theory concerns women. The epidemiology of clinical depression is strongly gender-biased. Being female is a significant risk-factor for this illness. Why should this be true? In the primal society, females do not compete for alpha status. Their size consigns them to subordinate status, and they are one of the "resources" for which males compete and on which the males' animal self-concept is based. Can we conclude that women are the eternal victims of their evolutionary history? A reassuring *No*: "Our argument is that agonistic behaviour [aggression, competition] is more conspicuous but not more common in males, and, in any case, there is evidence that when women have equal opportunities, the female excess of depression disappears" (Price et al. 1994: 312).

The "yielding hypothesis" confirms the therapeutic wisdom of targeting interpersonal conflicts, cognitive distortions, and unrealistic self-appraisals.

Patients can be helped to "substitute voluntary yielding in the form of conscious submission for the involuntary and unconscious yielding of depression." This can take the form of penitence, atonement, and forgiveness. If negotiation and reconciliation are unlikely to yield results, the therapist can help to facilitate the patient's physical separation and mental detachment from the adversarial person. On the other hand, "insufficiently self-assertive" patients can be helped to win conflicts (Price et al. 1994: 313–314).

A recent article in *Archives of General Psychiatry* returns to the yielding hypothesis and the notion that depression encourages disengagement. Experiments with animals and humans confirm that when efforts to attain a goal are frustrated, the individual experiences a strong negative effect and its motivation to continue with the current effort declines. Depression generalizes this response. Pessimism is pervasive and associated with low self-esteem.

Depression is disabling, but it can also be an adaptive mechanism that helps individuals to cope with situations where continuing engagement is futile and dangerous, e.g., the case where an unrelenting weaker competitor invites his own destruction. Depression can also be adaptive when a person or proto-human must cope with the failure of a major life enterprise – e.g., the ecological exhaustion of a band's home territory, the end of marriage or a career in our own case. The individual must avoid rash situations. The start-up costs of new enterprises are high and, under the sway of positive effect, he may be inclined to ignore the possible dangers and exaggerate his chance of success. "In this situation, pessimism, lack of energy, and fearfulness can prevent calamity even when they perpetuate misery" (Nesse 2000: 17). At the same time, the "low mood system" is prone to getting stuck in positive feedback loops – pessimism depletes energy and drives low self-esteem, which, in turn, feeds pessimism. Nesse suggests that serious depression may have been less persistent and severe in the past, when circumstances more closely resembled the evolutionary *Ur*-situation: "Mood dysregulation may now be so prevalent because we are bereft of kin, beliefs, and rituals that routinely extracted our ancestors from such cycles" (Nesse 2000: 17).

Psychiatric just-so stories?

Evolutionary accounts are organized around three elements: a current diagnostic classification, an evolutionary scenario involving an adaptation (a trait), and a mechanism connecting the past (the trait) to the present (mental disorder). Concepts such as "genome lag" and evolutionary "trade-off" refer to the contexts within which these mechanisms might function.

Lewontin argues that these evolutionary accounts are equivalent to just-so stories, and that knowledge concerning the mental life of our archaic ancestors is necessarily a matter of conjecture, notwithstanding analogies based on empirical studies of nonhuman primate societies. Is he correct? To answer this question, we need a satisfactory understanding of these "traits," predispositions that are said to start out as adaptations and end up as mental disorders. For an evolutionary account to be credible, it must establish that the trait in question is *heritable as such* – that it is a distinctive neurological structure. On the other hand, if it can be shown that the trait is actually generated by a general purpose intelligence, then it is not heritable as such, regardless of whether it is a helpful behavior. If a trait is not heritable as such, it cannot be a mechanism that connects past with present in the manner described by evolutionary psychiatry. In which case, we can look no further than the faculty that generates the trait. And while our general purpose intelligence does have an evolutionary history that may illuminate clinical conditions, it cannot provide histories that are specific to multiple mental disorders.

A recent paper by Leda Cosmides and John Tooby helps to illustrate this point. The authors explore the evolutionary origins of obsessive-compulsive disorder (OCD). These patients are "identified as reasoning oddly ... [therefore] it is vital for neuropsychologists and therapists to be able to characterize exactly what pieces of functional machinery are impaired. To do this, one needs to correctly inventory and characterize the set of species-typical reasoning competences in normal humans" (Cosmides and Tooby 1999: 462). The phrases, 'pieces of functional machinery' and 'inventory of reasoning competences,' imply the existence of a dedicated neural mechanism, and this is exactly what is required for their evolutionary story. There is another possibility, that the authors ignore. OCD might be a breakdown in normal cognitive-affective functions; it could be a condition that Rivers or Hughlings Jackson would have associated with "negative symptoms." If so, the symptoms would be without an evolutionary subtext. In both of these versions, OCD is traced to a neurological structure. In the alternative version, the structure is responsible for a wide variety of cognitive-affective states and functions, of which the OCD symptoms are only one expression. If this is the case, there is no way (or cause) to link OCD to a paleolithic adaptation.

Even if one assumes, without argument, that certain symptoms are "positive" in the Jacksonian sense – that is, they express an archaic adaptation – problems remain, since it is possible to discover rival accounts likewise based on evolutionary premises. Recall the yielding thesis, said to explain the epidemiology of depression: men and women share a single evolutionary history; men have subordinated women (omega status) in the status hierarchy throughout this entire time-span; and these circumstances help to explain the higher prevalence of depression in women. A British psychologist, Anne Campbell (1999), has recently proposed an alternative evolutionary scenario. It is based on the idea that females give a higher value to protecting their lives than to competing for status. This preference would be adaptive because it favors reproductive success, that is, the survival of infants and *ipso facto* the survival of the genes of women who refrain from competition. According to Campbell, females behave this way today because of an "evolved mechanism" that is expressed in an inherited low threshold for fear in situations that threaten bodily injury. Disputes among females are usually restricted to indirect aggression and low-level fighting, and women (then and now) are characteristically concerned with acquiring and defending scarce resources, not status.

So here are two problems associated with evolutionary accounts: the problems of alternative origins (modularity versus domain general intelligence) and alternative modularity-based narratives. There are ways to address these problems, the most important being via clinical and experimental evidence. When Jerry Fodor first proposed the notion of modularity (1983), he listed nine features. They included domain-specificity, obligatory firing, rapid speed, inaccessibility to consciousness, and dedicated neural architecture. Two of the features are clinically significant: age of onset and "the characteristic pattern of breakdown." They are also the source of compelling evidence supporting the modularity position (see Baron-Cohen 1995 on autism and the concept of Machiavellian intelligence). This is important research, but I have no room to explore it here. It will be enough to say that there is likewise compelling clinical and experimental evidence that would lead one to the opposite position and would give modularity a much restricted meaning (see Karmiloff-Smith 2000 on Williams syndrome).

The road not taken

If one thinks of *Just-so* stories not as a category but rather as a spectrum, progressing from zero (Baron-Cohen) to ten (Dr Dwarkanath), then it is fair to say evolutionary accounts of mental disorders are *Just so* stories. They are characterized by varying degrees of conjecture, analogy, and tendentious reasoning. Something similar can be said about other fields of psychiatric research. So, evolutionary psychiatry is unexceptional in this respect. Perhaps we should not be asking whether evolutionary accounts are *Just so* stories, but whether they are useful. Do they provoke interesting research? Do they help clinicians, researchers, and readers to see patients and mental illness in fruitful and novel ways? Unfortunately, the answer to these questions is *no*. Generally speaking, the stories vindicate rather than challenge conventional wisdom.

Things did not have to turn out this way. The evolutionary perspective does not lead inevitably in this direction. As we have seen, the revival of interest in evolutionary psychiatry began in 1967 with John Price's article on the puzzling relationship between depression and natural selection. But it was only fifteen years later that evolutionary psychiatry took off as an identifiable discourse and presence in mainstream journals. In between, there was a revolution in American psychiatry. Its most visible moment was the publication, by the American Psychiatric Association, of a nosology based on categorical principles and modeled after the infectious disease model of classification (see above, my comments on DSM III). From this point forward, the DSM III editors wrote, diagnostic criteria would exclude any reference to causal mechanisms (such as psychoneurotic processes), except in the case of organic brain disorders and the one syndrome that is defined by its etiology, posttraumatic stress disorder.

One of the first DSM III era articles to adopt an evolutionary perspective was Russell Gardner's account of the origins of bipolar disorder (mentioned above). In introducing his topic, he writes:

> However, this idea, namely, that triumph may stimulate mania, and defeat, depression, remains of interest, even in an era when the major paradigm guiding research on affective disorders eschews reactivity to provocative stimuli as a significant variable (in contrast, eg, to the earlier Meyerian concepts embodied in DSM-I).
>
> (Gardner 1982: 1437)

The phrase "major paradigm" refers to DSM III's epistemology, and "Meyerian concepts" identifies the dimensional approach, in which disorders are represented as expressions of intersecting biological, psychological, and social vectors. (Adolph Meyer was the editor of the first two editions of the DSM). Gardner's caution is understandable, but it also proved unnecessary. Evolutionary theory offered an intellectually satisfying accommodation with the austere, postneurosis principles imposed by the new DSM. And the theory came in a form that did not interfere with the new diagnostic conventions. Indeed the theory, as represented in Gardner's paper and those of later writers, had no clinical implications at all, other than naturalizing the mandatory diagnostic classifications. It included a causal account, but likewise an account that did not interfere with the newly adopted diagnostic conventions.

Things could have been different. One can imagine an evolutionary perspective that would challenge and provoke what is merely taken for granted. I have room to mention one of several possibilities. Gordon Claridge's *Origins of Mental Illness* was published in Britain in 1985. Claridge wished to address a paradox that Walter Cannon had previously explored, namely "how illness can flow from health, normality become abnormality ... [and] mechanisms that have *utility* for the organism can nevertheless bring about a derangement of function." Claridge's thesis was that mental illness originates in a person's "pre-existing tendency to disorder." This tendency manifests itself as a variation in normal function and, in appearance, it corresponds to what we once called "temperament." But it is also a biological phenomenon, rooted in "potentially discoverable processes in the brain." Clinically, this tendency to disorder is expressed *across a spectrum of diagnostic categories* (Claridge 1985: 13, 15; Canguilhem 1991: Sec. 1, Ch. 4 and Sec. 2, Ch. 2). This is not to argue that diagnostic labels are not clinically useful, only that they do not correspond to infectious diseases.

This perspective would yield a repertoire of evolutionary stories quite different from the ones that we are currently reading. We would not get one story for depression, another for panic disorder, and a third for PTSD. The new stories would not provide matching modules. (However, there is nothing in Claridge's theory to suggest that the notion of modularity is without merit.)

Lessons from psychopharmacology

There are some indications that psychiatry may be moving back to a dimensional understanding of mental disorders. Let us go back to the origins of DSM III. The new system followed a classificatory model first applied to infectious disease. At first glance, the model seems singularly inappropriate, since each infectious disease category is associated with a distinctive etiology and pathogenesis, while DSM III postponed any mention of etiologies in the absence of compelling empirical evidence. Thus no etiologies are mentioned, except for a handful of disorders. Why then would one assume that the DSM categories are distinct and separate? The framers of DSM III had various grounds for making this assumption. For example, a syndrome (category) might be distinguished from other syndromes by its distinctive course over time (known as "predictive validity"). One starts with a valid clinical description of a syndrome and then proceeds to undertake research to discover its etiology. This approach had been advocated at the turn of the century by the pioneering German psychiatrist, Emil Kraepelin. The framers of DSM-III, happy to call attention to this precedent, identified themselves as "neo-Kraepelinians."

The correctness of the new system seemed to be confirmed by developments in psychopharmacology, beginning with the discovery of chlorprozamine. Here was a drug whose effects appeared to be specifically antipsychotic. In the decades leading up to DSM III, pharmacologists succeeded in producing a series of drugs whose effects were similarly specific – antidepressant, anti-anxiety, anti-bipolar disorder. Efficacy was interpreted as evidence of each disorder's distinctive (but yet to be discovered) etiology.

So much for appearances. In the years since publication of DSM III, it has become clear that the specificity of these agents has been greatly exaggerated. Here is a recent example. Pfizer pharmaceuticals initially marketed the drug Zoloft (sertaline) for major depressive disorder. Subsequent clinical trials permitted Pfizer to market Zoloft for panic disorder and obsessive-compulsive disorder. In 1999, Pfizer acquired the approval of the Food and Drug Administration to market Zoloft for an additional illness, post-traumatic stress disorder (e.g., see the monthly Pfizer advertisements in the *American Journal of Psychiatry*, beginning with the June 2000 issue). This is good news for Pfizer, since it greatly expands the market for its drug. Other pharmaceutical companies have taken the same path, crossing diagnostic boundaries that were once regarded as secure.

According to David Healy, an authority on the history of psychopharmacology, the "antidepressant" drugs are misbranded. Drugs like Zoloft are effective for a wide range of "neurotic" conditions. The terms "tonic" and "psychic energizer" would be more accurate, but they lack the suggestion of specificity and are politically incorrect (Healy 1997: 256). Neurotic conditions, tonics, and psychic energizers imply a dimensional approach to mental disorders and deprive current diagnostic classifications of their biological individuality. This conclusion is antithetical to the DSM epistemology, but also unwelcome in a health care system "in which the only act of a psychiatrist that is reimbursed is the act of prescribing. Lengthy amounts of time put into managing nonspecific aspects of care count for nothing" (Healy 1997: 262).

Conclusion

Evolutionary psychiatry, as we know it today, may have a dubious future. The revival of dimensional thinking in diagnosis would leave the current batch of *Just so* stories high and dry. For the present, however, evolutionary psychiatry still has possibilities. It has demonstrated its capacity for discovering dedicated neurobiological mechanisms tailored to current classifications. And it has a largely unexploited potential for reconstructing human nature – at least at the edges, where pathology shades into abnormality.

Take the example of Robert Spitzer, writing about homosexuality. Spitzer was the editor-in-chief of both DSM III (1980) and the revised edition, DSM IIIR (1987), and a leading neo-Kraepelinian. The DSM III editorial task force had a special interest in the psychiatric status of homosexuality. Previous to this edition, homosexuality was regarded as a disorder, a clinical "condition." Gay rights groups objected to this characterization. Their position was that homosexuality is neither a pathology nor an abnormality, but rather a sexual orientation that is comparable to heterosexuality. Spitzer agreed with this position and advocated the demedicalization of homosexuality in DSM III (Spitzer 1981). Thus the manual included only ego-dystonic homosexuality – the patient who believes that his homosexual desires and behavior are alien to his character and wants to remove his condition.

By 1999, Spitzer had changed his mind about homosexuality, with guidance provided by the harmful dysfunction (HD) branch of evolutionary psychiatry:

> Recently I presented the HD concept of mental disorder to a group of psychiatric residents ... I tried to show that ... one could argue that certain forms of homosexuality are disorders ... [T]he residents had no problem with the HD concept of disorder ... What they took strong exception to was my suggestion that evolution has produced built-in mechanisms to ensure heterosexual arousal and that failure to have that capacity could be a dysfunction in sexual development.
>
> (Spitzer 1999: 431)

The controversy over whether this dysfunction is "a harmful or negative condition" may ultimately be about values, he concludes. However, "the HD view nicely illuminates what the argument is about" (Spitzer 1999: 431). But what *is* the argument about? Spitzer treats it as something that we come to discover, rather than create. Evolutionary psychiatry, including the HD approach, does not illuminate the argument, rather it defines an argument.

Of course there is nothing intrinsically wrong with defining one out of many possible arguments or frames of reference. Spitzer's point is that the HD argument is privileged. Its terms mirror a condition of nature, that is, a place beyond values and discourse. Cosmides and Tooby take a similar position:

> [A] scientific account of the underlying psychological or biological situation ought to be kept separate from and undeformed by such questions of value ... [but] there will be an endemic and motivated temptation to confuse these issues in order to spuriously "win" moral disputes under the guise that they are factual disputes.
>
> (Cosmides and Tooby 1999: 457)

The consequence has been "the naturalization or medicalization of morals." And it is an antidote to these confusions that these writers now recommend evolutionary psychology and the HD approach.

This is not the first time that the psychiatric remedy is a symptom of the disorder that it proposes to cure.

References

Baron-Cohen, S. (1995). *Mindblindness: An essay on autism and theory of mind.* Cambridge MA: MIT Press.

Bateson, G. (1959). *Naven: A survey of the problems suggested by a composite picture of a New Guinea tribe from three points of view.* Stanford, California: Stanford University Press.

Beck, A. (1967). *Depression, clinical, experimental, and theoretical aspects.* New York: Hoeber.

—— (1987). Cognitive models of depression. *Journal of Cognitive Psychotherapy* 1: 5–37.

Campbell, A. (1999). Staying alive: Evolution, culture, and women's intrasexual aggression. *Behavioral and Brain Sciences* 22: 203–252.

Canguilhem, G. (1991). *The normal and the pathological.* Cambridge: MIT Press.

Cannon, W. (1942). Voodoo death. *American Anthropologist* 44: 169–181.

Claridge, G. (1985). *Origins of mental illness: Temperament, deviance and disorder.* Oxford: Blackwell.

Cosmides, L. and Tooby, J. (1999). Towards an evolutionary taxonomy of treatable conditions. *Journal of Abnormal Psychology* 108: 453–464.

Crow, T.J. (1991). The origin of psychosis and "The Descent of Man." *British Journal of Psychiatry* 159(supplement 14): 76–82.

—— (1993). Sexual selection, Machiavellian intelligence, and the origins of psychosis. *Lancet* 342: 594–598.

—— (1995). A Darwinian approach to the origins of psychosis. *British Journal of Psychiatry* 167: 12–25.

Dwarkanath, C. (1954). *The Fundamental principles of Ayurveda, Part III, Ayushkamiya and Dravyadi Vignana (including Rasabhediya) of Ashtanga Hrdaya.* Mysore: Hindusthan Press.

Fodor, J. (1983). *Modularity of mind: An essay on faculty psychology.* Cambridge MA: MIT Press.

Gardner Jr, R. (1982). Mechanisms in manic-depressive disorder: An evolutionary model. *Archives of General Psychiatry* 39: 1436–1441.

Healy, D. (1997). *The antidepressant era.* Cambridge: Harvard University Press.

Karmiloff-Smith, A. (2000). Why babies' brains are not Swiss Army knives. In *Alas poor Darwin: Arguments against evolutionary psychology* edited by H. Rose and S. Rose, pp. 173–187. New York: Harmony Books.

Leslie, C. (1987). Interpretations of illness: Syncretism in modern ayurveda. In *History of Diagnostics: Proceeding of the 9th International Symposium on the History of Medicine – East and West,* edited by Yosio Kawakita, pp. 7–42. Osaka, Japan: Taniguchi Foundation.

Lewontin, R. (1998). The evolution of cognition: Questions we will never answer. In *Methods, models, and conceptual issues,* edited by D. Scarborough and S. Stemberg, pp. 107–132. Cambridge: MIT Press.

Marks, I.M. and Nesse, R.M. (1994). Fear and fitness: An evolutionary analysis of anxiety disorders. *Ethology and Sociobiology* 15: 247–261.

Mealey, L. (1995). The sociobiology of sociopathy: An integrated evolutionary model. *Behavioral and Brain Sciences* 18: 523–541, 587–599.

Nesse, R.M. (2000). Is depression an adaptation? *Archives of General Psychiatry* 57: 14–20.

Nesse, R.M. and Burridge, K.C. (1997). Psychoactive drug use in evolutionary perspective. *Science* 278: 63–66.

Price, J. (1967). Hypothesis: The dominance hierarchy and the evolution of mental illness. *The Lancet* 2: 243–246.

—— (1969). The ritualization of agonistic behaviour as a determinant of variation along the neuroticism/stability dimension of personality. *Proceedings of the Royal Society Medicine* 62: 1107–1110.

Price, J., Sloman, L., Gardner Jr, R., Gilbert, P. and Rhode, P. (1994). The social competition hypothesis of depression. *British Journal of Psychiatry* 164: 309–315.

Rivers, W.H.R. (1922). *Instinct and the unconscious: A contribution to a biological theory of the psychoneuroses* (2nd ed.). Cambridge: Cambridge University Press.

Silove, D. (1998). Is posttraumatic stress disorder an overlearned survival response? An evolutionary-learning hypothesis. *Psychiatry* 61: 181–190.

Sloman, L. (1976). The role of neurosis in phylogenetic adaptation, with particular reference to early man. *American Journal of Psychiatry* 133: 543–547.

Spitzer, R.L. (1981). The diagnostic status of homosexuality in *DSM-III*: A reformulation of the issues. *American Journal of Psychiatry* 138: 210–215.

—— (1999). Harmful dysfunction and the *DSM* definition of mental disorder. *Journal of Abnormal Psychology* 108: 430–433.

Wakefield, J.C. (1999). Evolutionary versus prototype analyses of the concept of disorder. *Journal of Abnormal Psychology* 108: 374–399.

Young, A. (1999). W. H. R. Rivers and the war neuroses. *Journal of the History of the Behavioral Sciences* 35: 359–378.

Chapter 10

Utopias of health eugenics, and germline engineering

Margaret Lock

Over the course of the past decade billions of dollars have been invested in the "Holy Grail" of biology – the mapping of the human genome. The rough first maps are now complete and published; one created with public funding appeared in *Nature*, and the second map, carried out with private funding, in *Science*. Knowledgeable commentators suggest that these maps are equivalent to having a list of parts for a Boeing 747, but with no idea as to how they go together and no knowledge of the principles of aeronautics.

It is undeniable that we are able to manipulate nature as never before; biology is increasingly malleable in our hands, and for some advocates this newfound ability to tinker with the basic building blocks of life itself has kindled a vision for the transformation of both the human body and society for the better. However, the startling promise made when the mapping of the human genome was first embarked upon will not be kept: that the "full sequence of the human genome will teach us, finally, 'what it means to be human'" (Gilbert 1992: 96) and will enable us "to decipher the mysteries of our own existence" (Fox Keller 1992: 293). Of course many of us have been deeply skeptical of this claim all along and take exception to the utopian rhetoric associated with the endeavor.

One of the features of modernity is the tenacity of a widely shared belief that scientific progress, particularly in the form of new technologies, will lead to a global utopia of health: a condition where our control over nature will enable us to eradicate its capriciousness. Two decades ago Charles Leslie, with his abiding interest in medical pluralism, argued that one of the ideals of biomedical practice was to transform local medical systems everywhere so that they would become part of an internationally standardized medical system persuing the rational and laudable goals of biomedicine. Leslie (1980: 191) argued that this ideal is a powerful force in modern history "because it expresses the dream of a future good society in which modern science will be used benevolently and rationally to relieve human suffering and distress."

Utopias of health have a long history, of course, but the good and healthy society was never visualized as global until recently. On the contrary, more often than not, early utopian thinkers strongly supported the idea that in order to prosper and have health society would have to dispose of its "dregs" in some way, by symbolically sealing them off as outsiders or as slaves or else literally casting them adrift. Utopian visions of health became expansive only after the seventeenth century. When coupled later with the mid-nineteenth-century science of eugenics, it became possible to think about the betterment not only of individual health but the improvement of the health of future generations through the application of state control over the reproductive practices of the population at large. Instead of deporting the unwanted, their ability to reproduce was forcibly terminated. The history of modern genetics has been plagued by its close association with eugenics.

In this paper, focusing on the rhetoric associated with germline engineering, I argue that in spite of the utopian claims made about the Human Genome Project and the practices of the new genetics associated with it, the specter of eugenics hovers over this endeavor. Enhancement of the human genome, the explicit goal of several of the loudest proponents of the new genetics, means, by definition, that some individuals are judged inadequate to contribute to the "good society" or the "human race." This rhetoric is masked, however, because enhancement of the human genome is justified in the modern guise of progress associated with benevolence, human dignity, and the relief of individual suffering. Of course critical commentators, among them geneticists, counter this discourse, but much of the dissent focuses on the uncertainties and false claims made for the science itself or else on ethical issues raised by possible abuses of individual rights. A critique of germline manipulation in terms of its possible social consequences is less often expressed, as is the case with the new genetics as a whole.

Utopias of health

It was common in premodern utopias of health to associate "healthy" minds and correct behavior with the health not only of individual bodies but with the collective of society. One of the best known examples is that of Plato's *Republic*, where he argued that social justice would come about naturally if individuals conducted themselves correctly and virtue was lauded as salubrious. Thomas More coined the term "utopia" in 1516, for which the original Greek meaning of "No place" is usually conveniently forgotten. In More's book, *Utopia*, a calm and regular functioning of the body is considered one of the greatest pleasures in life, and pleasure, provided it does not impinge on others, is synonymous with virtue. In order for his ideal society to thrive, however, More argued for the necessity of practicing active euthanasia.

More's utopia, like so many similar premodern fantasies, was located on an island; a space removed from the "real" world. Samuel Butler's 1872 *Erewhon* (an anagram for nowhere) was perhaps the last example of this grand escapist tradition. Erewhon is set somewhere in New Zealand, among the exotic Other of the last century. It is a society with technological expertise, but use of machines has been deliberately discarded in order to advance to a post-technological Utopia, something for which the European narrator of the book is totally unprepared. He is filled with wonder, comes to understand that "man's moral nature" is not adequate to rule machines, and that society will unavoidably be made corrupt by the materialism of a technologically dominated society. Butler, writing at the same time as Herbert Spencer and later Charles Darwin, was accused by his contemporaries of inappropriately criticizing the insights of this duo, and of being actively opposed to the advances of science.

Earlier, in the first quarter of the seventeenth century, *New Atlantis,* the South Sea island utopia visualized by Francis Bacon, in contrast to Butler's *Erewhon*, had been hailed as a triumph of the imagination. *New Atlantis* went through eight editions shortly after its publication, was translated and distributed throughout Europe, and became a model of the "moral intent" for the new scientific academies founded in the seventeenth and eighteenth centuries (Manuel and Manuel 1979: 258). Bacon believed that prolongation of life on earth was not contrary to God's will, and the most powerful people who populate his utopia of Bensalem are 36 Elders living in a house of inventions known as Solomon's House. These Elders are scientist-priests whose charge is to conduct experiments that will securely establish a medical utopia dedicated to the curing of disease and the prolongation of life (Bacon 1942). Bacon was a sickly child and he and his brother were regularly dosed with all manner of compounds, so it is perhaps not surprising that medicine should be the liberating force in his utopia (Manuel and Manuel 1979: 256). Even though *New Atlantis* is not a utopia in which ordinary people may participate (the masses are lost forever in the embrace of their dark superstition and foreigners are excluded entirely), Bacon makes low cost medicines prepared in dispensaries available for everyone.

Dissection of animals and birds and the biological engineering of new forms of birds, animals, and humans are carried out by the Elders of Solomon's House, even though "in creating animals that Adam himself had not named Bacon approached a religious abyss" (Manuel and Manuel 1979: 257). Above all, Bacon is concerned with experimental sciences and their application, and he shows few sympathies for theoreticians who work with abstractions. The scientist has a religious duty to inquire into God's creation: "If God made the winds, Bacon reasoned, and man's science through an understanding of winds invented sails, then man was merely bringing to realization what had always been present, though hidden, in that initial creation" (Manuel and Manuel 1979: 260).

The Elders form a unified community of scientists, there are no *virtuosi,* and they travel widely, gathering information relevant to their research, ensuring that Bensalem will have superior science. The guiding principle is one of *caritas* (charity), but the Elders do not always reveal their findings to the State, for Statesmen are not held in high regard. Above all, the sacerdotal nature of the scientific enterprise must be preserved while the Elders seek out the knowledge of causes, the secret motion of things, and seek to enlarge the human Empire. This last endeavor, novel to utopian thinking, was one of the first moves toward globalization.

Tommaso Campanella, who lived at almost exactly the same time as Bacon, was enraged, as was Bacon, by the reverence given to Greek "pagan" thinking throughout Christian Europe. Campanella, son of a Calabrian shoemaker, became a monk, but was nevertheless accused at one stage in his career of having a familiar spirit. He wrote about a utopia that, although somewhat different from that of Bacon, had a lasting influence. Campanella's fantasy was decried as a heresy and blasphemous because he went so far in his early days as to deny the existence of God. He was tortured, tried, found guilty, and thrown into prison for life. It is possible that he escaped the death penalty because he was deemed mad. *The City of the Sun* was published in 1602. This utopia is located in Taprobane, the ancient name for Sumatra or possibly for what is now Sri Lanka. As is typical of early utopias, a wanderer, in this case a Genoese sea captain, returns to report about the fabled place (Campanella 1981). In Taprobane the supreme ruler, Metafiscio, is all-powerful and all loving. Scientific knowledge, pictorialized so as everyone, even children by the age of 10, can understand it, is used to administer the city efficiently.

Apart from the supreme ruler, life is conceptualized as communal and egalitarian, although the aged and city officials have privileges. Men and women are of equal status, there is no disease, cleanliness is valued, and the freedom of will of each individual is respected. Knowledge is pursued as a means to reduce drudgery and pain and to enhance the "pleasantness" of life. Nevertheless, Taprobane is a rigid enclave, where eugenics is practiced by controlling sexual behavior to bring about the improvement of the race. *City of the Sun* depicts violence and depravation raging all around Taprobane. Campanella's vision is inspired in part, it seems, by the urgency he experiences of the necessity to convert infidels – Jews, Mohammedans, and Protestants – to Catholicism, while at the same time transforming the Catholic faith into a rational, scientifically grounded religion (1981). Campanella recants on his early claim that there is no God, but nevertheless supports the philosophical study of nature through reasoned activity. For Campanella, as for Bacon, science and religion must strive to create a new synthesis that will bring about a spiritual renewal of mankind.

Closely associated with the spread of secular thought, commencing in the early nineteenth century and continuing into the latter part of the twentieth century, rationalist, utopias were envisioned whose provenance was the everyday world, and most serious thinkers abandoned the idea of an enclosed space of fantasy for their location. Utopian thought was transformed fully into a platform for political action, and the requirements of human freedom and even future happiness became intrinsic to it. In his three volume *Principles of Sociology* published between 1876 and 1896, Herbert Spencer is explicitly concerned with the achievement of individual freedom, but it was his ideas about social evolution and the superiority of certain peoples that proved influential in the shaping of what was to become a dominant style of utopian thought that long exceeded Spencer's lifetime.

Spencer, linking Darwin's theory of evolution with his own previously formulated theories, vigorously supported the idea that organic changes in human biology are intimately associated with social progress. As is well known, progress, and hence social evolution, manifests itself for Spencer as a hierarchy of increasing social complexity, with the European "race" as the most advanced. Prior to the nineteenth century it had been widely accepted that, as people migrated around the world from the original site of the Garden of Eden and moved into different environmental niches, a certain amount of "degeneration" from the primordial human form had taken place. This degeneration accounted for visible physical variation, but was not necessarily negatively valued.

Once Georges Buffon's concept of distinct human races was firmly established, the original meaning of degeneration became transformed in a subtle but insidious fashion. Georges Cuvier, for example, argued that certain races were "by nature" inevitably degenerate and could never be stimulated by their physical or social environment to achieve greatness, "to become, in essence, whitened, "physically, mentally, or morally" (cited in Leys Stepan 1986: 264). Degeneracy, understood as "process" gone into reverse, was used to assign people to their "correct" place in the new global order.

By the end of the nineteenth century the urban poor, prostitutes, criminals, and the insane were all thought of as "degenerate" types whose purported deformed skulls, protruding jaws, and low brain weights marked them as "races apart" from other more fortunate individuals in whom evolutionary progress was evident. Similar arguments were made by analogy about the intellects and physical bodies of women, who, although of the same race as their men folk, were nevertheless systematically ranked as lower and inferior to them (Leys Stepan 1982). This type of nineteenth-century thinking remains evident in the blatantly racist research of Philippe Rushton and others (1989) so cogently criticized by Charles Leslie (1990). I argue below that it is also detectable in more subtle form in some of the writings and declarations made by several of the leading geneticists and molecular biologists of today.

Technology and boundary transgressions

Following Spencer and like-minded thinkers of his time, the idea that, through the appropriate application of science and technology, we can improve on the health and well-being of individuals and society, has been an ideology that has gone largely unquestioned. The history of technology, for the most part, has been transmitted in Europe and North America as a narrative of progress and of the betterment of social life in general. Brian Pfaffenberger (1992) characterizes this history as the Standard View of technology; we create tools, devices, and artifacts that permit us to lead, we believe, increasingly rational, autonomous, and prosperous lives, liberated from the constraints imposed by individual biology, oppressive human enemies, and the environment.

It has been argued that embedded in the Standard View are two sets of tacit meanings that at first glance are contradictory. The first assumes that the relationship of humans to technology is too obvious to need examination. Organizations, industries, technicians, craftspeople and so on simply make things that are in themselves neither good nor bad. This is what Langdon Winner (1977) has labeled "technological somnambulism" – an unreflective acceptance of technological innovation. The second approach, one of technological determinism, conceives of technology as a powerful and *autonomous* agent, inherent to progress, and therefore by definition an unquestionable good, but one that inevitably dictates the form that human social life will take (see, for example, Robert Heilbroner 1967).

Autonomy in the Kantian tradition is, of course, associated with the concept of free will and with the idea that individuals can free themselves from domination by laws external to social life. But the very idea of an autonomous technology raises an "unsettling irony," for the assumed relationship of subject and object is reversed (Winner 1977: 16). We humans have apparently lost out to the monster, but nevertheless rush eagerly ahead creating new devices in the belief that we will achieve yet more control and autonomy.

The tacit assumption embedded in both the somnambulist and autonomous technology views is that material artifacts are things-in-themselves, and therefore ethically and morally neutral. However, philosophers of science, among them Michel Callon (1992) and Bruno Latour (1993), as well as the feminist theorist Donna Haraway (1991), together with a burgeoning number of sociologists and anthropologists of science, argue against this position. Many of the new biomedical technologies (and genetic engineering is among them), permit us to radically reconstruct the boundaries between culture and nature so that we are busy today creating new entities, hybrids of what was formerly thought of as distinctly in the domain or either nature or culture (see, for example, Franklin 1997; Lock 2000, 2001; Strathern 1992).

We are also for the first time creating new cross-species hybrids of nature with nature: the gene from the flounder that permits it to survive in frigid waters has been inserted into tomatoes and strawberries to enable them to cope with northern winters, and a rhesus monkey was recently born with a jellyfish gene inserted into its genome. Proponents of genetically modified organisms claim that we have been creating hybrids of plants and animals for centuries, that this is what agriculture and husbandry has always been about, and that nothing radically new has taken place. But we have not been able to hybridize *across* species before; this technology is radically new.

Debates surrounding this type of reconstruction of nature and culture and the disputes about possible consequences for individual and social well being are inevitably molded in part by the possibilities that specific technologies make imaginable. Of our own making, technologies enable our knowledge and practices to move in certain directions while other paths are closed off, temporarily at least. Styles of reasoning come to dominate in scientific discourse to which technologies themselves contribute, even though inevitably culture, economics, and politics put brakes on what is actually doable (Galison and Stump 1996; Lock 2002).

Of course utopian visions about the freedom that technologies will bring us have not been entirely hegemonic, but have all along been opposed by counter discourse about the dystopias we are bent on creating for ourselves, replete with warnings about the consequences for society of technology gone wild. From the Frankenstein story of Mary Wollstonecraft Shelley on to Charles Dickens's *Hard Times*, H. G. Wells's *Dr Moreau,* Aldous Huxley's *Brave New World*, George Orwell's *Nineteen Eighty-four* and Margaret Atwood's *The Handmaiden's Tale,* among many others, we read in novels and treatises of the havoc and misery that technologies can potentially create. These are societies where technology rules, where eugenics and thought reform have taken hold.

Among those who earlier this century perceived the effects of technological innovation principally as a form of dystopia was Lewis Mumford. In his extensive writings he was one of the first to sow the seeds of a more complex approach to our understanding of the relationship between technology, society, and culture and, with fascism very much in mind, he wrote critically about technology. Mumford referred to "our over-mechanized culture," a condition that he feared would lead to a "final totalitarian structure." He believed that the new international competitiveness associated with globalization would eventually produce a "dominant minority" who would manipulate the majority through the creation of depersonalized organizations constituting a "megamachine." This megamachine Mumford visualized as an inclusive but "invisible" entity, embracing not only technical and scientific expertise and artifacts, but also the bureaucratic structures designed to organize and control the whole enterprise. Mumford (1934) explicitly understood this massive apparatus as male dominated. Apparently some citizens fear that we have reached this condition, judging by the demonstrations outside the meeting of the World Trade Organization in 1999 and more recently in Washington and several European cities.

Writing in the late 1950s, the biologist René DuBos was less concerned about control, but nevertheless highly critical of nineteenth-century Utopian treatises. Neither God nor science can restore a mythological time of well being argued DuBos (1959), who was insistent that health is a "mirage," and that maintenance of human life as a harmonious equilibrium is an impossibility. He insisted that neither health nor happiness can be permanent conditions because biological fitness requires "never-ending efforts of adaptation to the total environment, which is ever changing." DuBos was concerned because, thanks to technology, many people survive to reproductive age today that prior to this century would have died as children. He ruminated, purely as a biologist and without moral judgment, as to what this would do over time to the gene pool. This concern is explicit in current discourse about genetic engineering, and extremists argue that we should work toward eliminating unsuitable genes from the gene pool of future generations. Maynard Smith (1988: 75) is quick to point out that one difficulty with such a policy is that virtually every human being has genes that could be designated as unsuitable for transmission to the next generation. It is frightful to contemplate who should be delegated to make decisions as to how to go about a neoeugenics of the genepool.

In summing up prevailing attitudes Pfaffenberger (1992: 495) suggests that technology, like Shiva in Hindu iconography, as seen through a Modernist lens, is both creator and destroyer, an agent of future promise and at the same time of culture's destruction. The fundamental tension continues to be about whether we are slowly destroying that which makes us human, and in doing so denying freedom to many people, or if we are indeed liberating ourselves from oppressive forces formerly beyond our control, including the forces of nature.

Enhancement of human populations

Before turning to genetic engineering, one more facet of recent biological history must be considered, namely the train of activity set in motion by Charles Darwin's younger first cousin, Francis Galton. In writing an introduction to the 1972 edition of Galton's book *Hereditary Genius,* originally published in 1869, Darlington (1972: 9) captures Galton's excitement:

> If, Galton thought, we can observe men as we observe animals, if we
> can measure their abilities, their faculties of mind and body, if we can

follow them as individuals through life and in families from generation to generation, then we shall be able to understand man in an
altogether new way. We may even be able to use our knowledge for
the benefit of society. The prospect was splendid. The task was waiting
for him.

The task Galton set for himself was to investigate the origins of "natural
ability," and he gave the name "eugenics," meaning "good in birth," or
"noble in hereditary," to the program he devised, the ultimate objective
of which was human improvement. Galton was the first investigator to
apply mathematics to biological problems when he made use of the newly
formulated Gaussian concept of "normal distribution" to human populations. This method of estimating variation around a mean is today known
more familiarly as the Bell curve. Galton set up an anthropometric laboratory in London and was joined by Arthur Pearson, described by one of
his colleagues as "a lump of ice," who worked to transform the vague
language of the biology of the day into something resembling a hard
science. As a result of his research, which included setting out for the first
time a theory of correlation, Pearson declared: "We are forced, I think
literally forced, to the general conclusion that the physical and psychical
characters in man are inherited within broad lines in the same manner,
and with the same intensity" (cited in Kevles 1984a: 83). In giving the
1903 Huxley lecture to the Anthropological Institute in London, Pearson
argued that: "No training or education can *create* [intelligence], you must
breed it" (Kevles 1984a: 85).

It was in the United States that eugenics was firmly consolidated. As
Kevles (1984b: 92) notes, "Eugenics was British by invention and American
by legislative enactment." Charles Davenport, a biologist well versed in
the science of his day, devoted his time to the creation and collection of
family pedigrees. Among other things, he observed that "pauperism,"
"criminality," and especially "feeble-mindedness" were, in his estimation,
heritable. On the basis of these observations Davenport argued that individuals with such traits should be prohibited from reproducing so that
defective protoplasm might be eliminated from the gene pool. Davenport's
work was well publicized, and thousands of Americans gave financial
support to the activities of the Eugenics Record Office in Cold Spring
Harbor, of which he was the director. Eugenics was transformed rapidly
in the early part of the twentieth century from a rather obscure science
set out by Galton and his colleagues into a major political movement.

It was primarily white middle and upper-middle-class citizens, notably
scientists and other professionals, who actively supported the eugenics
movement; similar programs developed at the same time in Japan and
China were also spearheaded by intellectuals (Otsubo and Bartholomew
1998). What is perhaps not well recognized today is that many of the early

eugenicists were progressive-minded socialists, among whom Emma Goldman, George Bernard Shaw, H. G. Wells, and Margaret Sanger were prominent. Eugenics for these writers and activists would become the foundation for social reform. H. G. Wells claimed, for example, that "the children people bring into the world can be no more their private concern entirely, than the disease germs they disseminate, or the noises a man makes in a thin-floored flat." For Wells eugenics is a facet of public health (Kevles 1995: 92).

Margaret Sanger (1922: 98) wrote that "Those least fit to carry on the race are increasing most rapidly. . . . Funds that should be used to raise the standard of our civilization are diverted to maintenance of those who should never have been born." The early birth control movement strongly supported Sanger's position, and a 1940 joint meeting of the Birth Control Federation of America and the Citizens Committee for Planned Parenthood was entitled "Race Building in a Democracy." The eugenics movement grew stronger during the depression and was generally supported by geneticists (Paul and Spencer 1995). In Japan, where abortion is legal, to this day it is carried out under the Eugenic Protection Law passed in 1948, something about which Japanese feminists vehemently protest (Hara 1996).

Throughout the early part of this century, eugenically minded scientists were concerned with rooting out the causes of social degeneration and highlighting its cost to the public purse. Research into diabetes, epilepsy, syphilis, feeble mindedness, and other diseases was motivated not merely by an interest in the mechanism of the diseases, but by a concern about their financial burden to society. It has been documented that as recently as the 1960s the practice of "negative eugenics" (forced sterilization of individuals designated as biologically inferior, thus "eliminating" the birth of impaired individuals) was widespread, and a 1999 newspaper report comments on a "sterilization drive" currently under way in Peru (*Guardian Weekly* 1999). In America it is estimated that something like 50,000 individuals were forcibly sterilized during the first half of the twentieth century. This practice was replicated in Canada, South Africa, and northern Europe, including the socialist countries of Scandinavia and, in the most systematic and ruthless fashion, Germany. Lawsuits in connection with these practices continue to the present day.

Continuities between the rhetoric employed in early twentieth century eugenics and some of that associated with the Human Genome Project are not hard to see. By 1988 the European Commission, the executive arm of the European Community, had set out in writing a platform for what was termed "Predictive Medicine: Human Genome Analysis." This document notes that the major diseases of our time – diabetes, cancer, stroke, coronary heart disease, and so on – are the products of interactions between genes and the environment. However, the rationale for

Predictive Medicine rests on the assumption that we cannot hope to control the environment, and hence we should "seek to protect individuals from the kinds of illnesses to which they are the most vulnerable and, where appropriate, to prevent the transmission of genetic susceptibilities to the next generation." (Kevles 1992: 71). This neo-eugenics, designed to eliminate unsuitable embryos and fetuses through the implementation of genetic screening programs followed by abortion, was fostered in the conservative 1980s and early 1990s with the blessing of Margaret Thatcher and like-minded politicians specifically in order to allay future health care expenditure (Kevles 1992: 72). In contrast to the 1930s, the proposal for Predictive Medicine met with considerable opposition in which the German Greens, activist Catholics, and some British conservatives formed an unlikely alliance. In the end, when the European Community's human genome program was funded, the program for Predictive Medicine was removed from it, and prohibitions on genetic manipulation of human embryos and germ cell research were put in place.

Laissez-faire eugenics

The historian of science, Edward Yoxen, points out that we are currently witnessing a conceptual shift that was not present in the language of geneticists prior to the advent of molecular genetics. While the contribution of genetics to the incidence of disease has been recognized throughout this century, it has only been in the past two decades [that is, from the 1960s] that the notion of "genetic disease" has come to dominate discourse such that other contributory factors are obscured from view (Yoxen 1984). Fox Keller (1992) argues that it was this shift in discourse that made the Human Genome Project both reasonable and desirable in the minds of many involved researchers. In mapping the Human Genome, the objective is to create a baseline norm, but it is one that will correspond to the genome of no living individual so that we will all, in effect, become deviants from this norm (Lewontin 1992). Moreover, with this map in hand, the belief is that we will rapidly move into an era in which we will be able to "guarantee all human beings an individual and natural right, the right to health" (Fox Keller 1992: 295). Fox Keller cites a report put out by the Office of Technology Assessment in the United States in which it is argued that genetic information will be used "to ensure that ... each individual has at least a modicum of normal genes" – this is defined as a "eugenics of normalcy" and is based on the idea that "individuals have a paramount right to be born with a normal, adequate hereditary endowment" (Office of Technology Assessment 1988).

Although improvement of the quality of the gene pool is being aired in documents such as these, as Fox Keller (1992: 295) and others have pointed out, the language used is no longer one that focuses on social policy, the good of the species, or even the collective gene pool. We are now in an era dominated by the idea of individual choice in connection with decision making relating to health and illness. Genetic information will furnish the indispensable knowledge that individuals need in order to realize their inalienable right to health. A *laisser-faire* eugenics – a "utopian eugenics" (Kitcher 1996) – is already in place, one that depends upon decisions that individuals and families must make, usually about abortion, on the basis of the results of genetic testing and screening programs. The iron grip of Foucault's microphysics of power (1980) is at work.

It is now agreed by virtually everyone that the eugenics of the first part of the twentieth century was grounded in invalid science, and its practices are roundly criticized. However the cost to health care systems of treating and caring for "defective" children is still made explicit when justifying the implementation of screening programs. The State of California introduced maternal serum α-fetoprotein screening for all pregnant women more than a decade ago in the hope of reducing the number of infants born with neural tube defects and thereby saving costs (Caplan 1993). The 1990 guidelines of the International Huntington Association make it clear that it is acceptable to refuse to test women who do not give a complete assurance that they will terminate a pregnancy if the Huntington gene is found. As Paul and Spencer (1995) point out, "Those who made this recommendation certainly did not think they were promoting eugenics. Assuming that eugenics is dead is one way to dispose of deep social, political and ethical questions. But it may not be the best one."

Genetic screening and germline engineering

Human eugenics is a fact of life because of consumer demand, a 1989 editorial proclaimed in *Trends in Biotechnology*. We are encouraged to believe that the public is pushing the scientists. This may be the case where certain middle-class families with high expectations about the promise of technology are concerned, but research has shown that only between 15 and 20 per cent of individuals designated at risk for genetic disease have made use of testing (Quaid and Morris 1993; Beeson and Doksum 2001) and others, when tested, have ignored the results (Hill 1994; Rapp 1999).

In any case, as pointed out by Daniel Kevles (1984c), who has written extensively on eugenics, the ability of scientists to meet the desires and hopes of consumers is still a long way off, despite the rapid progress being made with locating genes, or markers for them, on chromosomes. As more knowledge is accrued and we become increasingly aware of the complexities of gene-gene and gene-environment interactions, it is undeniable how little we know. Even the mechanisms of the "straightforward" genetic diseases that follow well-defined Mendelian inheritance patterns are proving to be only sketchily understood. For one thing, we are often unable to predict disease severity that may range from mild to devastating. Until recently it was assumed that if someone has the gene for Huntington's disease it would inevitably be expressed, but now it is known that this is not the case.

Beyond these technological limitations, the social consequences of genetic testing and screening can easily backfire. The sickle cell screening programs set in place in the 1970s in the United States, often with active support from the African-American community, reveal in retrospect how programs designed to reduce suffering through genetic interventions can go badly wrong when this type of information gets into the hands of employers and school boards and is used to reinforce exclusion and racism (Duster 1990). Questions about who should have access to the results of genetic testing remain unanswered and firm policy recommendations have not been made, and yet today screening for sickle cell disease is mandatory in 33 of the United States.

Another troublesome example is that of the screening program set up by the Colorado school board to detect Fragile X syndrome (Nelkin 1996). The incidence of this disease, associated with mental impairment among other things, is estimated to be about one per 1,500 males and one per 2,500 females. In common with a good number of other similar diseases, the involved genes exhibit "incomplete penetrance," that is, not all individuals with the genotype will manifest the disease. It is estimated that about 20 per cent of males and 70 per cent of females with the mutation express no symptoms, making the designation of "at risk" extremely problematic. Moreover, the severity of symptoms varies enormously and cannot be predicted.

The first testing program, developed by an industry-university consortium, was organized in 1993 in the Colorado public school system as a prototype for developing a national program. The project was funded by Oncor, a private biotechnology company, and explicitly designed to save later public expenditure on children with behavioral problems. The research team developed a check list of "abnormal" behavioral and physical characteristics associated with the disease, including hyperactivity, learning problems, double-jointed fingers, prominent ears, and so on, and tested selected children. After two years, the anticipated number of cases had not come to light, the program was deemed uneconomical and suspended (Nelkin 1996: 538). Testing was not done in a clinical setting and, Nelkin notes, was driven by economic and entrepreneurial interests. Further, there are no known therapies for the condition once identified. The impact on the lives of those children who tested positive was significant, not the least of which was discrimination against them by health insurance companies. Nelkin points out that many parents actively supported testing for the Fragile X gene and that a significant number of them, particularly mothers, initially experienced relief once their child's so-called behavioral problem was identified as genetic; parents could no longer be found wanting for the condition of their child.

Even though extreme caution would seem to be in order in connection with the new genetics, we forge ahead rapidly toward making genetic testing and screening routine (Beeson and Doksum 2001). In support of an expansion of these technologies is the argument that people will be able to make rational choices about their marriage partners and about abortion, thus avoiding bringing diseased children into the world. There is no doubt that screening programs in connection with, for example, thallasaemia and Tay-Sachs disease, have brought enormous relief to some families (Angastiniotis et al. 1986; Kuliev 1986; Mitchell et al. 1996) and the Cuban government reports success with a screening program for sickle cell disease (Granda et al. 1991). Counseling of young people who are screened and found to be carriers of these genes is offered in all these programs, and success is measured in terms of the reduction in the incidence of the disease, that is in terms of the number of abortions carried out once the unwanted gene has been detected. One program based in New York that has tested more than 50,000 orthodox Jews in many parts of the world handles things a little differently. This program does not inform teenagers who are tested about their own status as carriers for Tay-Sachs disease because of the stigma associated with this disease. When a couple who have been tested plans to get married they may contact the Rabbi in charge of the program, and he will inform them confidentially if their match is at risk for producing diseased offspring. Such couples are then given counseling. Couples designated as not at risk, on the other hand, are not informed whether either one of them is a carrier, and the program has been criticized as a result of this policy as paternalistic (Ekstein: 1995).

Willis (1998) reminds us that abortion politics will effect the implementation and spread of screening technologies, with those countries and organizations where "right to life" campaigners are the most vocal having a direct influence on policy making. Certain advocates of gene therapy and germline engineering claim that with these technologies abortions can be avoided and, moreover, that "bad genes" will be disposed of entirely. Clearly this is self-promoting hype, because genetic manipulation will not be available for by far the majority of the people in the world for the foreseeable future.

When human germline engineering is brought up for discussion, as it increasingly is, people get agitated, but not usually, as one might predict, about inequalities of access to the technology, or about an inappropriate use of scarce resources. Just about everyone who participates in discussions relevant to germline engineering realizes that what has up until now been thought of as an unassailable boundary between nature and culture could be permanently transformed by such interventions. For this reason many individuals, involved geneticists among them, believe that germline engineering is an insidious threat to the social order, although others believe that we are on the verge of making scientific progress to an extent we have never before witnessed. It is pertinent to consider, while implementation of this particular technology continues to be banned, how arguments for and against its incorporation into the armoury of the new genetics are constructed.

Germline engineering involves the manipulation of germinal cells – eggs and sperm. In practice this means tinkering with fertilized eggs shortly after their formation while cells are at the "totipotent," or undifferentiated, stage. When an embryo is genetically manipulated in this way the modification will be copied into every single cell of the adult, including the sexual cells. Unless we learn how to reverse-engineer the ensuing generation of fertilized eggs, this transformation will be passed along to all future generations. Germline engineering in effect produces a eugenics, not of individuals, but of entire genealogies – a eugenics of normalcy that implicates future generations.

Animated discussion in connection with such engineering reveals two points about which virtually all involved scientists appear to be in agreement: first, that the technology, once off the ground, will be simpler and more manageable than the much more demanding sister technology of gene therapy. Before germline manipulation can be carried out, a safe, reliable way of delivering genes to a human embryo still has to be found, but the majority of scientists believe this to be a not too distant possibility and, once accomplished, will be replicable without much difficulty. Several hundred experiments have already been made with gene therapy, that is, with somatic cell as opposed to germline modifications, but so far with little success and with the untimely death of at least one subject. Virus vectors are used to deliver new genes to every cell of the human body and they must do so without causing untoward side effects if the therapy is to be successful. It is assumed that this delivery of replacement genes can be much more easily handled in embryos at a very early stage of development.

Second, there is general agreement that germline engineering is better characterized as an enhancement technology rather than as a therapy or even as genetic modification. In other words, germline engineering is not primarily about the elimination of specific diseases in living individuals, or even the abortion of embryos deemed as "undesirable." Germline engineering will constitute in effect not a "negative," but a "positive" eugenics, one expressly devoted to the improvement of the "race." Children, enhanced as embryos, will be in possession of genotypes that they ordinarily would not have possessed.

Aside from these points of agreement, those scientists currently arguing most vociferously for and against germline engineering sit in two firmly opposed camps. This opposition is characteristic, I suggest, of a stark divide readily apparent during the past two hundred years, throughout modernity, with respect to the relationship of science to ethics.

Arguments in favor of germline engineering

In June 1998 a one-day symposium was held at the University of California at Los Angeles (UCLA) as part of the Science, Technology, and Society program in the Center for the Study of Evolution and the Origin of Life. This symposium, entitled *Engineering the Human Germline*, was subsequently published as a book of the same name (2000) and involved nine scientists in addition to the two organizers, Gregory Stock and John Campbell, both of whom work in what can broadly be described as scientific philosophy. A small amount of superficial disagreement emerged among participants as to the potential dangers associated with manipulation of the germline, but no disputes of an epistemological kind erupted during the event. This group was overwhelmingly in favor of germline engineering (with one notable exception, French Anderson, the physician who has carried out more somatic gene therapy protocols than has anyone else to date) and declared that once the technology was available it would rapidly become "compelling" to "large numbers of parents" who would want to ensure that their offspring had the best of all possibilities for their future lives.

The symposium organizers made clear the dramatic nature of what was being discussed: "Germline engineering touches at the very core of what it means to be human. It palpably extends human power into a sacred realm, once mysterious and beyond reach ... it makes us look at how far we wish to intrude in the genetic flow from one generation to the next (Stock and Campbell 2000: 3–4). Perhaps the most outspoken participants were Daniel Koshland, Jr., past editor of *Science* and a professor of molecular and cell biology, and James Watson, Nobel Prize winner and past director of the National Center for Human Genome research at the National Institute for Health.

In discussing germline manipulations Koshland commented: "The demand for gene enhancement therapy will probably be very large, to give your children a better chance of success in the world" (2000: 27). Earlier he had noted that, "if the criterion [we make] is that children should turn out to be at least as good as their parents, my guess is that germline engineering will compete very well with those conceived the natural way. And if we make this criterion that the children should be up to their parent's expectations, then I think that the engineered child may have a good edge over the child conceived in the normal way" (2000: 26). When considering possible danger associated with this technology, Koshland argued that "there is no such thing as absolute safety in the world," and noted that the normal birth process is risky. He added, "if germline engineering is designed to be no more risky than 'normal' birth then the benefits will clearly outweigh the risks" (2000: 26).

French Anderson stated in 1998 that "none of us want to pass on to our children lethal genes if we can prevent it and that's what is going to drive germline gene therapy . . . you are not going to pass on a lethal gene to your child if you can have a simple, safe treatment that prevents it" (Engineering the Human Germline 1998). This statement, made at the symposium, does not appear in the book based on the symposium proceedings, where Anderson is much more cautious: "We know so little about the human body and so little about living processes, we would be unwise to attempt genetic engineering to try to treat, much less 'improve,' the human zygote or embryo" (2000: 48). Between the upbeat time of 1998 and the publication of the book on germline engineering two years later, 18-year-old Jesse Gelsinger had died as a result of gene therapy. French Anderson was not his physician (*New York Times* 1999).

When participants at the symposium turned to the issue of informed consent and possible harm to future generations, they were, for the most part, in agreement with the argument put forward by John Campbell that technology could be designed to solve this problem: "I think that if people are really concerned about consent we could take a human chromosome or a segment of it and put on a lock. None of those genes would have any effect until a person took an artificial hormone pill to unlock the cassettes and give him or herself the new engineered phenotype" (Engineering the Human Germline 1999: 13). Germline engineering will not, it seems, override individual choice. But who will judge whether the interests of society should override individual choice? Questions such as this were not raised at this gathering but in the book French Anderson (2000: 47) once again sounds a cautious note:

> . . . there needs to be societal approval prior to the first attempt at germline gene transfer. Almost all medical decisions are made between the patient and his or her physician. . . . Our rationalization for this is that "my body belongs to me." But our genes do not belong just to ourselves. The gene pool belongs to all of society.

Symposium participants briefly took up the question of the "sanctity of the gene pool." James Watson commented: "if we could make better human beings by knowing how to add genes, why shouldn't we do it?" (2000: 79). This was followed by a superficial examination of "what *really* is normal?" An ensuing discussion about "seizing control of our own evolution" culminated in comments about how it is difficult to sustain an argument for the "sanctity" of the human gene pool. Watson interjected with the comment:

I can't indicate how silly I think it is [the sanctity of the human gene pool]. I mean, we have great respect for the human species ... but . .. [e]volution is just damn cruel [a similar comment had been made by Francis Galton 100 years earlier] ... we should treat other people in a way that maximizes the common good of the human species.

(Watson 2000: 85)

Koshland was equally indignant at criticism of germline engineering:

We should start, perhaps, with the question raised by some who say we shouldn't tamper with the germline. I frankly don't understand these people. Where are they living? We are already altering the germline right and left. When we give insulin to a diabetic who then goes on to have children, we are increasing the number of defective genes in the population [the point made by Rene DuBos years ago in an entirely different context]. No one is seriously suggesting that we refuse to give life-saving drugs to genetically disadvantaged people.

(Koshland 2000: 26)

Arguments against germline engineering

The other side of the debate is succinctly set out in a 1992 paper published by scientists, all of whom participate in the Council for Responsible Genetics (CRG), located in Boston. They start out by criticizing the genetic reductionism present in the assertions of those in support of germline engineering, and then go on to outline the technical pitfalls and dangers associated with this particular technology. These authors argue that we may in fact already be modifying the germline inadvertently while doing experiments with somatic gene therapy.

The CRG confronts unexamined ethical assumptions built into the discussions in favor of germline engineering, including the likelihood that such technologies will go only to the economically privileged. But the Council is also concerned about the assumptions that "the value of a human being is dependent on the degree to which he or she approximates some *ideal* of biological perfection" together with the unexamined ideology that "all limitations imposed by nature can and should be overcome by technology" (Council for Responsible Genetics 1992: 1). The Council's position is that, "To make intentional changes in the genes that people will pass on to their descendents would require that we, as a society, agree on how to identify "good" and "bad" genes ... Any formulation of such criteria would necessarily reflect current social biases" (Council for Responsible Genetics 1992: 1).

The CRG is unconditionally opposed to germline engineering for three reasons:

1   because its target is "future" people rather than relieving the suffering
    of those of us already alive, in other words, there is no clinical justi-
    fication for germline engineering;
2   because people will increasingly be seen as "damaged goods" if they
    fall short of a technologically achievable ideal; *and*
3   no accountability toward future generations is taken into consideration.
        However, the Council is not opposed to further discussion of this
    technology and does not declare that it is categorically opposed to it
    for all time.

The ghost in the machine

The division between these protagonists reflects the divide already visible
200 years ago for which history has made Denis Diderot primarily responsible on the one hand, with Jean-Jacques Rousseau situated on the other
side. For the followers of Diderot, the encyclopedists as they came to be
known, science in effect usurps ethics and is charged with formulating and
implementing the goals of mankind and society. Human "nature" belongs
entirely to the realm of biology, and science will deliver what is needed.
This is the Standard View of technology, the position taken by those individuals currently in favor of germline engineering.

    Rousseau, in contrast, argued that ethics were autonomous and were
not only irreducible to science, but exercised tutelage over it. Rousseau
believed in perfectibility, but above all that humans have the freedom to
make choices. He came to represent the position that there are in effect
two cultures, one of humanism, distinct and in some ways superior to the
other of the scientific endeavor. Participants in the CRG fall for the most
part into the Rousseaian camp. In a paper published in the medical journal
The Lancet, three members go further and make it clear that in their
opinion discussion limited to existing values and conditions is not sufficient, nor are the usual parameters of bioethics. We must search, they
argue, for new ways to debate and monitor these technologies because
they will affect the lives not only of individuals, but of entire communities and future generations (Billings et al. 1999).

    But the perceived threat posed by several biomedical technologies whose
use is at present banned or carefully circumscribed – cloning, clinical use
of fetal tissue, the introduction of animal genes and organs into humans,
and germline engineering, among others – is felt not only because of their
potential effect on future generations. These technologies represent for
many the possibility of a radical break with our "natural" evolved selves
and with that which sets us apart from the rest of nature, our very "humanness." It is salient to observe how two well-known geneticists have chosen
to deal with this criticism.

    French Anderson, for example, in an article in *Human Gene Therapy,*
sets out by defining what for him is a "normal human being." He divides

humans into two unequal component parts: those characteristics and features that are measurable and that part which "all of our quantitative measurements will fail to define: perhaps it could be called a soul." A soul cannot be examined under a microscope, declares Anderson, nor can it be assigned a quantity. He believes that this is the "subjective, non-measurable, spiritual aspect ... of a human being," that which makes the whole greater than the sum of the parts. Anderson then argues that "if what is uniquely important about humanness (not about individual humans but about humankind as a whole) is *not* defined by the physical hardware of our body, and since we can only alter the physical hardware, it follows that we cannot alter that which is uniquely human by genetic engineering" (1994: 758). Anderson takes comfort from this conclusion, and believes that he should be free to go ahead with genetic manipulations, although it is possible that he has now modified this position in light of the poor track record of gene therapy.

Steve Jones, professor of genetics at University College, London, in a self-declared effort to show the extent to which we can tinker with nature without worry, insists that to speculate about mind and its origin is largely futile. He makes this argument in a recent book even though in the same publication he writes that "genes make brains and brains make behavior" (1999). Jones, like Anderson, resorts to the equivalent of Gilbert Ryle's Ghost in the Machine to justify his line of argument: "The birth of Adam," he writes, "whether real or metaphorical, marked the insertion into an animal body of a post-biological soul that leaves no fossils and needs no genes." As a reviewer of Jones's book notes, "this is almost identical to a line in the recent encyclical about evolution written by the Pope" (Evans 1999).

What is disturbing about these commentaries is that geneticists who embrace this type of thinking, by off-setting mind, soul, humanness, or spirituality as distinct from the physical hardware of our bodies, are able to rationalize a determinism that justifies genetic manipulations of all kinds. Our souls will emerge unscathed but our genomes will be suitably enhanced. One intransigent continuity from early modernity has survived intact, it seems: the idea of a stable, internalized, authentic subjectivity; a subjectivity that constitutes our uniquely human heritage, while our material bodies, along with the rest of the animal world, are constituted entirely from nature.

The philosopher Eric Parens, criticizing the Anderson paper, argues forcefully for keeping body and soul together; for recognition that our "humanness is within – not beyond – the reach of genetics, and for recognition of complexity." In contrast to both Diderot and Rousseau, and to those scientists for and against germline engineering, ethics should not be compartmentalized from science, Parens (1995) insists, nor should it be privileged. In another paper, Parens (1998) makes it clear that he is concerned that we may impoverish ourselves through enhancement and inadvertently reduce the diversity upon which we as humans have always flourished. I would add that we appear to be intent on creating not a "brave" new world, but a bland new world of sameness; the heritage of Galton lives on.

It has been pointed out by several commentators that critical discussion about genetic engineering is filled with inflammatory declamations about "playing God," "interfering with nature," and so on and that this type of language usurps any possibility of conducting useful discussion (Bonnicksen 1994; Boone 1988). Even when the debate is moderated, participants in symposia continue to talk past each other. On the one hand are those critics who insist that the scientific claims in favor of germline engineering are inaccurate and that the complexity of gene-gene and gene-environment interactions are grossly underestimated. It is also argued that even though the technology is feasible it is "medically irrelevant," because the same end result can be achieved for individual cases (but not for future generations) by using pre-implantation diagnosis with selective embryo transfer. We should therefore opt for the less grandiose intervention (Winston and Handyside 1993).

On the other hand, ethicists frequently black-box the technology itself and associated biological manipulations and set out in their argument the importance of creating an international ethical framework on the basis of which policy decisions will be made. It is recognized by these protagonists that an ethics of individual rights is no longer sufficient and there is discussion about communitarian ethics and "transnational harmonization" leading to an international "normative code" (Knoppers and LeBris 1991 361). These ethicists are concerned, rightly, that if no international standards exist then procreative tourism will become common, but they rarely take into consideration inequalities in access to health care or recognize divisions among scientists nor how problematic are some of the scientific claims made by them.

A third line of criticism points out that in an era of repeated cutbacks in health care systems, individuals are made increasingly responsible for their own health and for that of their offspring. The elderly, those with disabilities, and the mentally impaired are characterized at times in official documents as a "burden" on society. This rhetoric is not as far removed from Nazi Germany as we would like to think, argues Petersen (1998). The bioethical rhetoric of the "right to know," "informed choice," the assessment of risks and benefits associated with various medical interventions, and a focus on family health compound the problem, deflecting attention away from social and political factors implicated in disease incidence (Lippman 1998; Lock 1998, 1999c; Petersen 1998). Increasingly, under the simple-minded guise of utopian eugenics, pregnant women are required to undergo genetic testing in order that infants will be born with "healthy" genes. "Bad" genes will be systematically purged through abortion, IVF, and selective re-implantation of embryos, gene therapy, or germline engineering. Adolescents and adults targeted as carriers of "bad" genes are screened and, when found to be positive, are counseled about marriage partners and their reproductive lives.

The new genetics has enabled many families to avoid suffering, but there is plenty of evidence that it has increased anxiety for many more by furnishing people with information about their genes or those of their spouses, parents, siblings, or offspring about which they would rather not know. Uncovering the dilemmas and competing value systems associated with the new genetics that directly effect reproduction and family life is important. Rabinow (1999: 12) urges social scientists to focus on the larger picture, however, and argues that "values and opinions proliferate as a matter of course in democratic, consumer capitalist societies." Rather than focusing initially on competing value systems, he insists that we should pay attention to the new forms – the new assemblages – that precipitate these value conflicts.

Technology is central to this story, and it is well recognized that major changes are taking place constantly today in the scientific representation, intervention, and manipulation of life forms. Analysis of these new forms of thought and practices cannot be divorced from the social and political contexts in which they emerge, nor can a consideration of their effects on social life. Assessing the effects of the application of new biomedical technologies, including the new genetics, for individuals, families, communities, social relations, and for future generations, before the technologies are institutionalized, is a demanding task. The discursive practices, politics, rhetoric, undisclosed interests, and goals associated with these technologies need careful scrutiny. Such a critical perspective is made urgent now that the private sector is increasingly involved in funding and determining what technologies will be developed and marketed.

The pervasive idea of perfectability of the body through human intervention – a utopia of health based on the management of individual genomes – motivates some researchers associated with the new genetics, but not all of them, as we have seen. A rhetoric used to justify enhancement of the human genome by several of the geneticists who believe in perfectability makes use of fossilized assumptions about souls and spirits in order to deflect criticisms that they are playing God. Several of the genetic engineers of today have more in common with Francis Bacon than they realize, particularly when they posit body and soul as ontologically distinct, and when they are explicit that their task is to overcome nature's deficiencies and its cruelty. Meantime these same geneticists appear to have forgotten René DuBos's warning about the ever-changing environment – a process speeded up by the activities of humankind. There *is* talk of gene-environment interactions, but in the parlance of geneticists this often points to the way in which genes interact with the "milieu interior" of the body (as Claude Bernard put it); the environment exterior to the body is beyond the pale largely because it has proved resistant to reductionistic forms of manipulation. But it must be remembered that geneticists do not agree among themselves; most avoid archaic language, and many call for caution.

Highlighting the plurality of forms and practices at local sites that the new genetics and other technologies take, both at home and around the world, despite widely shared scientific premises, is an important task for social scientists (see, for example, Lock 1998b; 2001; Handwerker 1998). This activity has continuities with the classical anthropological task of making the strange familiar and lays bare the pervasiveness of pluralism and diversity of thinking. But equal emphasis should be given to making the familiar strange – to asking why, for example, particularly in North America, flying in the face of all that we know about molecular biology and population genetics, so many people are apparently captivated by a genetic reductionism as the best means to bring dignity to humankind and to ease all the pain and suffering in the world. We must also ask why the implementation of the new genetics is apparently widely supported and why a regime of *laissez-faire* eugenics, one grounded in individual interest, is acceptable when there has been rather little discussion of what might be best for society at large or the world as a whole. Of course, critical public discussion takes place today, as was not the case in the time of Francis Bacon or, much later, of Francis Galton. Such discussion cannot be productive without rapid widespread dissemination of the relevant debates and controversies – social scientists have a crucial role to play in ensuring that their particular interpretations of germline engineering and other new biomedical technologies are made available for public consumption.

References

Anderson, F. (1994). Genetic Engineering and our Humanness. *Human Gene Therapy* 5: 755–760.

—— (2000). A New Front in the Battle against Disease. In *Engineering the Human Germline*, edited by Gregory Stock and John Campbell. Oxford: Oxford University, pp. 43–48.

Angastiniotis, M., Kyriakidou, S. and Hadjiminas, M. (1986). How Thalassaemia was Controlled in Cyprus. *World Health Forum* 7: 291–297.

Bacon, F. (1942). *Essays and the New Atlantis*. Roslyn, NY: Walter J. Black, Inc.

Beeson, D. and Doksum, T. (2001). Family Values and Resistance to Genetic Testing. In *Bioethics in Social Context*, edited by Barry Hoffmaster. Philadelphia: Temple University Press, pp. 153–179.

Billings, P.R., Hubbard, R. and Newman, S.A. (1999). Human Germline Gene Modification: A Dissent. *The Lancet* 353: 1873–1875.

Bonnicksen, A. (1994). Demystifying Germ-Line Genetics. *Politics and the Life Sciences* 13(1): 246–248.

Boone, C.K. (1988). *Bad Axioms in Genetic Engineering*. Hastings Center Report 18(4): 9–13.

Callon, M. (1992). Techno-Economic Networks and Irreversibility. In *A Sociology of Monsters: Essays on Power, Technology and Domination*, edited by John Law. London: Routledge, pp. 132–164.

Campanella, T. (1981). *The City of the Sun: A Poetical Dialogue*, trans. Daniel J. Donno. Berkeley: University of California Press.

Caplan, A.L. (1993). Neutrality is not Morality: The Ethics of Genetic Counseling. In *Prescribing our Future: Ethical Challenges in Genetic Counselling*, edited by Dianne M. Bartels, Bonnie S. LeRoy, and Arthur L. Caplan. Hawthorne, NY: Aldine de Gruyter, pp. 149–165.

Council for Responsible Genetics Human Genetics Committee (1992). *Position Paper on Human Germ Line Manipulation*. Massachusetts: The Council for Responsible Genetics.

Darlington, C.D. (1972). Introduction. In *Hereditary Genius: An Inquiry into its Laws and Consequences*, edited by Francis Galton. Gloucester, MA: Peter Smith, pp. 9–21.

DuBos, R. (1959). *Mirage of Health: Utopias, Progress and Biological Change*. New York: Doubleday.

Duster, T. (1990). *Back Door to Eugenics*. New York: Routledge.

Ekstein, J. (1995). *The Dor Yeshorim Experience: A Case Study in Genetic Testing, Halacha, Humanity*. Conference Preceedings, "The Ethical Implications of the New Genetics". Tufts University, School of Medicine, pps. 42–53.

Evans, D. (1999). Evolutionary Matter Over Mind. *Guardian Weekly*, September 30–October 6, p. 16.

Foucault, M. (1980). *The History of Sexuality Volume 1: An Introduction*. New York: Vintage.

Fox Keller, E. (1992). Nature, Nurture, and the Human Genome Project. In *The Code of Codes: Scientific and Social Issues in the Human Genome Project*, edited by Daniel J. Kevles and Leroy Hood. Cambridge: Harvard University Press, pp. 281–299.

Franklin, S. (1997). *Embodied Progress: A Cultural Account of Assisted Conception*. London: Routledge.

Gilbert, W. (1992). A Vision of the Grail. In *The Code of Codes: Scientific and Social Issues in the Human Genome Project*, edited by Daniel J. Kevles and Leroy Hood. Cambridge: Harvard University Press, pp. 83–97.

Granda, H., Gispert, S., Dorticos, A., Martin, M., Cuadras, Y., Calvo, M., Martinez, G., Zayas, M.A., Olivia, J.A. and Heredero, L. (1991). Cuban Programme for Prevention of Sickle Cell Disease. *The Lancet* 337: 152–153.

Guardian Weekly (1999). Sterilization Drive Alarms Peruvian Women. January 2nd, p. 18.

Handwerker, L. (1998). Consequences of Modernity for Childless Women in China: Medicalization and Resistance. In *Pragmatic Women and Body Politics*, Margaret Lock and Patricia A. Kaufert eds. Cambridge: Cambridge University Press pp. 178–205.

Hara, H. (1996). Translating the English Term "Reproductive Health-Rights" into Japanese: Images of Women and Mothers in Japan's Social Policy Today. In *Proceedings of the 1996 Asian Women's Conference*, "The Rise of Feminist Consciousness Against the Asian Patriarchy". Ewha Women's University, Korea: Asian Center for Women's Studies pp. 44–49.

Haraway, D. (1991). A Cyborg Manifesto: Science, Technology, and Socialist-Feminism in the Late Twentieth Century – Chapter 8. In *Simians, Cyborgs, and Women: The Reinvention of Nature*. New York: Routledge, pp. 149–181.

Heilbroner, R.L. (1967). Do Machines Make History? *Technology and Culture* 8: 335–345.

Hill, S.A. (1994). *Managing Sickle Cell Disease in Low-Income Families*. Philadelphia: Temple University Press.

International Huntington Association (1990). Ethical Issues Policy Statement on Huntington's Disease Molecular Genetics Predictive Test. *Journal of Medical Genetics* 27: 34–38.

Jones, S. (1999). *Almost Like a Whale: The Origin of Species Updated*. London: Doubleday.

Kevles, D.J. (1984a). Annals of Eugenics: A Secular Faith I. *The New Yorker*, October 8th pp. 51–115.

—— (1984b). Annals of Eugenics: A Secular Faith II. *The New Yorker*, October 15th pp. 52–125.

—— (1984c). Annals of Eugenics: A Secular Faith III. *The New Yorker*, October 29th pp 92–151.

—— (1992). Controlling the Genetic Arsenal. *Wilson Quarterly* 16: 68–76.

—— (1995). *In the Name of Eugenics*. Harvard: Harvard University Press.

Kitcher, P. (1996). *The Lives to Come: The Genetic Revolution and Human Possibilities*. New York: Simon & Schuster.

Knoppers, B.M. and LeBris, S. (1991). Recent Advances in Medically Assisted Conception: Legal, Ethical and Social Issues. *American Journal of Law and Medicine* 27(4): 329–361.

Koshland, Jr., D. (2000). Ethics and Safety. In *Engineering the Human Germline*, edited by Gregory Stock and John Campbell. Oxford: Oxford University, pp. 25–30.

Kuliev, A.M. (1986). Thalassaemia can be prevented. *World Health Forum*. 7: 286–290.

Latour, B. (1993). *We Have Never Been Modern*. Cambridge: Harvard University Press.

Leslie, C. (1980). Medical Pluralism in World Perspective. *Social Science and Medicine* 14B: 191–196.

(1990). Scientific Racism: Reflections on Peer Review, Science and Ideology. *Social Science and Medicine* 31: 891–912.

Lewontin, R. (1992). The Dream of the Human Genome. *The New York Review of Books*, May 28th. pp. 31–40.

Leys Stepan, N. (1982). *The Idea of Racism in Science: Great Britain 1800–1960* Hamden, CT: Archon Books.

—— (1986). Race and Gender: The Role of Analogy in Science. *Isis* 77: 261–77.

Lippman, A. (1998). The Politics of Health: Geneticization Versus Health Promotion. In *The Politics of Women's Health: Exploring Agency and Autonomy*, edited by Susan Sherwin. Philadelphia: Temple University Press, pp. 64–82.

Lock, M. (1998a). Breast Cancer: Reading the Omens. *Anthropology Today* 14(4): 7–16.

—— (1998b). Perfecting Society: Reproductive Technologies, Genetic Testing, and the Planned Family in Japan. In *Pragmatic Women and Body Politics*, edited by Margaret Lock and Patricia A. Kaufert. Cambridge: Cambridge University Press pp. 206–239.

—— (1998c). Situating Women in the Politics of Health. In *The Politics of Women's Health: Exploring Agency and Autonomy*, edited by Susan Sherwin. Philadelphia: Temple University Press, pp. 48–63.

—— (2000). On Dying Twice: Culture, Technology and the Determination of Death. In *Living and Working with the New Biomedical Technologies: Intersections of Inquiry*, edited by M.Lock, A.Young, and A. Cambrosio eds Cambridge: Cambridge University Press, pp 233–262.

—— (2002). *Twice Dead: Organ Transplants and the Reinvention of Death.* Berkeley: University of California Press.

Manuel, F. and Manuel, F. (1979). *Utopian Thought in the Western World.* Cambridge: Harvard University Press.

Mitchell, J.J., Capua, A., Clow, C. and Scriver, C.R. (1996). Twenty-Year Outcome Analysis of Genetic Screening Programs for Tay-Sachs and β-Thalassemia Disease Carriers in High Schools. *American Journal of Human Genetics* 59: 793–798.

Mumford, L. (1934). *Technics and Civilization.* New York: Harcourt Brace.

Nelkin, D. (1996). The Social Dynamics of Genetic Testing: The Case of Fragile-X. *Medical Anthropology Quarterly* 10(4): 537–550.

New York Times (1999). Day for the Human Side of Gene Therapy. Friday Dec. 10th p. A19.

Office of Technology Assessment (1988). *Mapping our Genes.* Washington: Government Printing Office.

Otsubo, S. and Bartholomew, J.R. (1998). Eugenics in Japan: Some Ironies of Modernity, *1883–1945. Science in Context* 11(3–4): 133–146.

Pareus, E. (1995). The Goodness of Fragility: On the Prospect of Genetic Technologies Aimed at the Enhancement of Human Capacities. *Kennedy Institute of Ethics Journal* 5: 141–151.

—— (1998). Is Better Always Good? The Enhancement Project. *Hastings Center Report* Jan-Feb Special Supplement, pp. 51–515.

Paul, D.B. and Spencer, H.G. (1995). The Hidden Science of Eugenics. Nature 374: 302–304.

Petersen, A. (1998). The New Genetics and the Politics of Public Health. *Critical Public Health* 8(1): 59–71.

Pfaffenberger, B. (1992). Social Anthropology of Technology. *Annual Review of Anthropology* 21: 91–516.

Quaid, K.A. and Morris, M. (1993). Reluctance to Undergo Predictive Testing: The Case of Huntington Disease. *American Journal of Medical Genetics* 45: 1–45.

Rabinow, P. (1999). *French DNA: Trouble in Purgatory.* Chicago: University of Chicago Press.

Rapp, R. (1998). *Testing Women, Testing the Fetus: The Social Impact of Amniocentesis in America.* London: Routledge.

Rushton, J.P. and Bogaert, A.F. (1989). Population Differences in Susceptibility to Aids: an Evolutionary Analaysis. *Social Science and Medicine* 28: 211–1220.

Sanger, M. (1922). *The Pivot of Civilization*. Washington: Scott-Townsend Publishers.

Smith, J.M. (1988). Eugenics and Utopia. *Deadalus* 117(3): 3–92.

Stock, G. and Campbell, J. (editors) (1998). *Engineering the Human Germline Symposium Report: Summary Report*. http://www.ess.ucla.edu/huge/report.html

—— (2000). *Engineering the Human Germline: An Exploration of the Science and Ethics of Altering the Genes We Pass on to our Children*. Oxford: Oxford University Press.

—— (2000). A Vision for Practical Human Germline Engineering. In *Engineering the Human Germline*, Gregory Stock and John Campbell eds. Oxford: Oxford University Press, pp. 9–16.

Strathern, M. (1992). *Reproducing the Future: Anthropology, Kinship and the New Reproductive Technologies*. Manchester: Manchester University Press.

Stump, D.A. and Galison, P. (editors) (1996). *The Disunity of Science: Boundaries, Contexts, and Power*. Stanford: Stanford University Press.

Watson, J. (2000). The Road Ahead. In *Engineering the Human Germline*, edited by Gregory Stock and John Campbell. Oxford: Oxford University Press, pp. 73–95.

Willis, E. (1998). Public Health, Private Genes: The Social Context of Genetic Biotechnologies. *Critical Public Health* 8(2): 31–139.

Winston, R.M.L. and Handyside, A.H. (1993). New Challenges in Human in Vitro Fertilization. *Science* 260: 932–936.

Winner, L. (1977). *Autonomous Technology: Technics-out-of-Control as a Theme in Political Thought*. Cambridge, MA: The MIT Press.

Yoxen, E. (1984). Constructing Genetic Diseases. In *Cultural Perspectives on Biological Knowledge*, edited by Troy Duster and Karen Garett. Norwood, NJ: Ablex, pp. 41–62.

Chapter 11

Killing and healing revisited

On cultural difference, warfare, and sacrifice

Margaret Trawick

Preliminary thoughts

In an essay I wrote twenty years ago for Charles Leslie, entitled "Death and Nurturance in Indian Systems of Healing" (1983), I made an effort to show how seemingly very discrepant systems of healing in southern India complemented one another and fit together into an overall pattern. I was attempting to build on Charles Leslie's theories about medical pluralism in India. One of the thoughts I expressed in that essay was that (in the healing systems I was examining) powerful medicines, beings, and acts were ones that had both killing and healing potencies. A pervasive mythology underpinning these medical systems linked suffering with power, and life with death. These conclusions were not original, but they were expressed in an elegant fashion. In fact, the means of expression would be considered too elegant today. Everything fitted together a bit too nicely.

Historically the discussion among medical anthropologists about the relationship between warfare and healing has centered upon the question of how to heal the damage caused by warfare and on the larger question of how, if at all, to comprehend the deep suffering that human beings inflict upon one another in war. The experience of suffering – whether of the lone individual or of vast numbers of victims together, or both – has been a focal concern (Kleinman et al. 1997; Das et al. 2001). This essay takes a somewhat different approach, but the topic here also is cultural pluralism – or more precisely, plurality – about how different "systems" juxtaposed and intermingling in time and space get sorted into mutually complementary niches. But the fit here is not so nice, and the complementarity of which I speak is not benign. As a first approximation of an appropriate metaphor, I thought of a poisonous compound, made of two distinct, more-or-less benign-in-themselves ingredients. This poisonous compound is lethal almost beyond imagining: it is warfare.

For ordinarily peaceful human beings to support such a horrible enterprise as warfare, they must, in the words of one embattled school child, "change their minds to fit the circumstances." The circumstances are the realities of war, and the minds of people who normally deplore violence must change radically to adapt to war, to become fit for it.[1] To effect such a radical change of people's minds, some powerful tool or mechanism must be already in place in those minds. That powerful tool may be a combination of reason and experience, a carefully thought-out descriptive model that explains changed circumstances and offers a plan of action to address them effectively.

That powerful tool may be a myth, a story that defies all reason and direct experience, all the unpleasant facts of day-to-day life, and offers a dream of transcendence, out of the dreary world of fact, and into the glorious world of the holy. For a myth to compel a people to war, it cannot be new or unfamiliar, because if it were, they would see its obvious falsehood and reject it. To be effective in mobilizing a people to acts of extreme, gratuitous violence, a myth must be old and familiar, deeply ingrained in habitus, in religious practice, in all the ways that the people in question are accustomed to stitching together the epistemological holes in their world and fantasizing a reason for existence.

A descriptive model and a plan of action are sufficient for people already trapped inside a war to bring them to come to terms with it, because they will already be seeking such a model and such a plan. Immediately and desperately endangered, considering that if they do nothing they and their loved ones will certainly die, people offered a single, risky chance of escape, an all-or-nothing gamble, may take the gamble, and not be judged irrational for doing it. But for unimperiled people to enter the peril of warfare, for ordinary kind people to applaud and even directly engage in the massacre of innocents, something stronger than reason is needed, something strong enough to disable reason altogether. For this, only myth will do.

I describe here a situation in which warfare is constructed as, and thus becomes, an act of sacrifice on the part of the two parties at war with each other. Sacrifice, in turn, is constructed by the warring parties as an act of healing on the part of the sacrificer. Therefore each party wages war against the other as a healing act, even as the war itself, with all the affliction it causes, is perceived by both sides as the main affliction to be healed. The irony of a war waged for healing purposes, a war to end war, is, as liberal Westerners perceive it, an antique folly. What is the liberal anthropologist to make, then, of the intelligent young rebel combatant who tells him or her in fullest sincerity, "We are fighting so the next generation will not have to fight"?

The war of which I write is the war currently raging between the Government of Sri Lanka and the Liberation Tigers of Tamil Eelam (LTTE). This war is confounding in its complexity, as many wars must be, but the complexity of this one is rendered all the more confounding by the fact that it is waged in a very small area, by the militant sectors of two small ethnic groups (the Sinhalese people, who constitute the great majority of the Sri Lankan populace, and Lankan Tamils who constitute the largest ethnic minority in the country), while larger powers have little interest in getting involved. In this essay, I must of necessity oversimplify the situation, which otherwise would defy description altogether.

This essay discusses sacrificial sentiments in relation to warfare, and the paradox of war that is waged for healing purposes. Certain aspects of the current war in Sri Lanka are examined in this light. Viewed from one angle, this war is an "ethnic" war, waged between two different ethnic groups with two different and mutually incompatible worldviews. The problems of such an essentialist position are clear, and I must immediately declare that I do not adopt this position. I propose instead that essentialist definitions of ethnicity are part of the mythology of warfare. The polarization of two previously commingled intermarrying groups, their definition of themselves in opposition to one another, and their failure (or deliberate refusal) to "understand" one another, inhere in the war mythology itself.

Different meanings of sacrifice, with the deep-seated emotions infusing these meanings, come into play in the war mythology. My claim here is *not* that people use myth to *make sense* of the chaos and suffering of war, but rather that myth is invoked (sometimes deliberately, sometimes not) to *motivate* people to join in war in the first place, and to keep them fighting long after the fighting has surpassed the bounds of reason, if there were any bounds in the first place.

The Sri Lankan conflict contains rational elements, and people act according to rational motives, but these rational motives are not sufficient to explain the ferocity and destructiveness of the conflict. Tamils and Sinhalese in Sri Lanka have defined themselves against one another, and fundamental to the self-definition of each is the peculiar sacrificial sentiment nurtured by each. Tamil and Sinhalese sacrificial sentiments are not the same, except insofar as each considers sacrifice to be a healing act. Sinhalese militants (most notably, the Sinhala Buddhist clergy and its followers) consider the war to be a sacrificial destruction of something utterly evil, which they name "terrorism." They wage war for the sake of healing the Sinhala people and their homeland of this evil affliction. Tamil militants (most notably the LTTE) consider the war to be an act of supreme *self-sacrifice*, for the sake of redeeming (*miiLa*) Tamil Eelam from subjugation.

The joining of these two mythologies, neither of which acknowledges the validity of the other, has led to the tolerance of massive bloodshed and atrocities in the conduct of the war. Murder, torture, and slaughter of civilians are commonplace. National and local resources are thrown into the "war effort," as though the war were a sacred purpose surpassing in importance the present and future well-being of the island's human population.

Through this essay I am trying to show that this particular war is characterized by an additional irony, on top of all the ironies inherent in destruction of life for the sake of improving life. It is not just that the affliction of warfare is created for the purpose of healing the affliction which is the war itself. It is also that, in this particular war, the parties attempting to defeat each other and heal themselves in the process are engaged in a single *cooperative* act of sacrifice. I will try to show that, for the Sri Lankan Government, which ostensibly represents and acts in accordance with the views of the Sinhala people, the supreme act of healing consists of purifying the patient by sacrificing the malign *other* that has invaded the patient's life. This interpretation of SL Government ideology has been made by other scholars (notably Kapferer 1997) and countless newspaper stories substantiate this view. The LTTE is literally demonized (in a Western evangelical sense – see below) by the Sri Lankan Government, and sometimes all Tamils are demonized, and when captured they are all too often tortured as demons would be tortured. Not only their bodies, but their very souls, their self-respect, their will to live, their minds, their memories, their monuments, their libraries, and all the rest must be rendered irretrievably nonexistent. The aim of Sinhala militants is to destroy every trace of Tamil resistance, as a man-eating monster would be destroyed, to obliterate it violently and completely.[2] But this is only half of the sacrificial picture.

The other half of the picture is the sacrificial ideology of the LTTE. For the Liberation Tigers, and arguably for civilian Tamils of both the Saiva and Christian religions, the supreme act of healing consists of *self-sacrifice*. Thus the most highly honored members of the LTTE are Black Tigers, people who go on missions in which their death is assured, by explosions in vehicles or boats they are driving at targets they aim to destroy, or by detonation of explosives strapped to their bodies. The target can be anything from a politician to a bank to a naval vessel. Often the target is missed, and the only harm done is to the Black Tiger himself or herself, whose body is always blown to pieces – obliterated like a flower *pandal* (a temporary structure covered with flowers) at the end of a Sinhala *yaktovil* (a demon exorcism ceremony described below). But even when the target is missed, the memory of the Black Tiger is deeply honored.[3]

Not only Black Tigers, but everyone who joins the LTTE is considered to have chosen a path of self-sacrifice. They renounce family and home (though in practice, not absolutely) and in general they lead spartan lives. There are material rewards to joining the LTTE – a continuous supply of good nourishing food is probably the most important, but all members are expected to be ready to give their lives in combat if need be, and most of them do in fact die in combat within a few years of joining the movement. As of this writing, over sixteen thousand LTTE members have died in service to the movement.

In short, both Tamil and Sinhala militants are engaged in the project of sacrificing Tamils, although they join in this project with different aims in mind. This is the penultimate conclusion I reach in this essay. The final conclusion is one I reached as I was writing the essay, and was trying to articulate my ideas. In the process of putting my thoughts into words, I found there was something more that needed to be said.

Colonial and neocolonial contributions

Obviously, Sri Lanka does not exist in a vacuum, and neither do Tamil and Sinhala cultures. The island formerly known as Ceylon was colonized for about 150 years by the British, and before that for the same length of time by the Dutch, and before that for the same length of time by the Portuguese. Since independence, the Sri Lankan Government has been a friend and ally of the US (as opposed, for instance, to India, which was a "nonaligned" nation and therefore was sometimes treated by the US as an antagonist). The influence of these "outsiders" (assorted western countries, to say nothing of India) upon the ways of life and thought of Lankan peoples has been manifold and immense. One cannot even imagine what modern and ancient Lankan history would have been like without these others, these outsiders. Forgetting India and thinking just of the West, one can say that certain aspects of Lankan social and cultural order have been magnified in importance by the West, others diminished, others rewritten. Some new things have been introduced and have been integrated into the whole. Some old things have disappeared. I cannot recite all the influences and changes wrought by colonial and postcolonial powers upon Ceylon/SriLanka, but certain ones are important to note for the sake of this essay.

First, the class hierarchy of the island was reinforced by British colonial practices and prejudices. The modern upper class in Sri Lanka is more British in its markers of distinction than it is Sinhala or Tamil or anything else. This class prides itself on its Britishness – perhaps more than anything else, on its command of the Queen's English. Prince Charles was the guest of honor at the Golden Jubilee Celebration of the 50th Anniversary of Sri Lankan Independence. In the mid-1990s, Princess Diana was an icon of Sri Lankan middle-class youth, both Tamil and Sinhala. Class is a more important factor in such matters as marital and political alliances than is ethnicity or religion. The old ruling-class families still remain in control of the Sri Lankan Government. The current President, for example, is the daughter of two former Prime Ministers (when her father was assassinated, her mother became PM). Her brother is in the opposition party in Parliament. When she was elected, she appointed her elderly mother Prime

Minister (again), and she made her mother's brother Deputy Minister of Defense, and de facto commander of the Sri Lankan Armed Forces.

The British may have thought that only the upper classes were made of the proper "stuff" to rule. It would have been a matter of blood and breeding. Certainly the Ceylonese upper classes were happy to share and propagate this view. Those who migrated to England saw themselves as superior to the common South Asian riff-raff (Daniel 1997: 312–313). The Tamils among them saw (and still see) themselves as "the best of the Tamils." All of them saw themselves as better than the poor. The consequence of this rigid(ified) class hierarchy has been terrible corruption and incompetence in government, a large number of educated but unemployed young people among the working classes, and a bloody Marxist insurrection, among numerous other problems. Tamils were resented and subjected to violent pogroms because they were "over-represented" in the Government and in the professions (i.e., in the culturally and educationally Anglicized upper class). Tamil-owned economic establishments in Colombo were burnt to the ground during the pogroms of 1983.

Second, the alliance between the Buddhist clergy and the state, whereby one lent authority and power to the other, was made law by British colonials, effectively making Buddhism the state religion. In the Kandyan Convention of 1815, the Kingdom of Kandy was ceded to the British in exchange for a promise that "the religion of the Boodhoo professed by the Chiefs and inhabitants of these Provinces is declared inviolable, its Rites, Ministers, and Places of Worship are to be maintained and protected" (Scott 1994: 155, 269n).

The concession to Buddhism was a trade-off; when England got control of Kandy, it consolidated its control over the entire island. Only the missionaries were unhappy. In signing a treaty which mandated protection of Buddhism in "these Provinces" (eventually, all of Ceylon), the colonial administrators must have thought they were doing something not only politically expedient, but also liberal and benign: writing into law the protection of a religion that was what the majority of the natives adhered to, and that was in its philosophical versions high-minded by European standards. But it was contrary to England's own hard-learned principle concerning separation of Church and State, and it contributed to trouble in modern Ceylon.

In 1946, two years before Ceylon was granted independence, a constitution came into law that scrupulously protected minority rights. A key passage was article 29, in which it was stated that "No law [made by Parliament] shall prohibit or restrict the free exercise of any religion; or make persons of any religion or community liable to disabilities or restrictions to which persons of other communities or religions are not made liable; or confer on persons of any community or religion any privilege or advantage which is not conferred on persons of other communities or religions. . . ."

Modern Tamil nationalists point to this 1946 constitution as a good one, made by good administrators, and consider that this is the way things should have stayed. But Sinhala nationalists were not happy with it. For one thing, they thought it was too heavily influenced by Christian missionaries. They considered that it had been written *for* the Lankan people and not *by* them. They considered that it had been written by a group appointed by foreign dominators (with whom they considered the Tamils to be in league). In 1972, a new constitution was passed by a two-thirds majority of Parliament, in which a key clause stated, "The Republic of Sri Lanka shall give to Buddhism the foremost place and accordingly it shall be the duty of the State to protect and foster Buddhism while assuring to all religions the rights granted by Section 18(1)(d)."

This tie between religion and state, combined with a religious belief that the island is the sanctuary of Buddhism, and combined in addition with a modern belief in the sanctity of the sovereign, territorially bounded nation-state, has made it very difficult for anyone in Government to oppose the clergy and keep their positions (or indeed their lives) intact. The assassination of Prime Minister S.W.R.D. Bandaranaike by a Buddhist monk seems to have gotten this message across.[4]

The constitution of Sri Lanka has been subject to many debates and quarrels, but the clause protecting Buddhism is not likely to be repealed by the required two-thirds majority of Parliament.

Overthrow, or even major revision, of the existing sociopolitical order is unthinkable for right-wing Sinhala Buddhists because the hierarchical order of the state is mandated by the hierarchical order of the cosmos. The British did not invent this idea, although they seemed to have helped it along in Sri Lanka. The close link between Theravada Buddhism and early ideals of kingship is well documented. It is not surprising to find that in early Lankan Buddhist mythology, the Buddha is portrayed not as an exemplar of human virtue and wisdom, but as the very embodiment of supernatural power and authority. The ideal of divine kingship that finds expression in this myth was propagated in numerous variants throughout South and East Asia some thousand or two thousand years ago, and in West Asia long before that. In the Lanka of myth, the Buddha *is* King. Like many a mortal ruler, he subdues by force and terror those beings who question his authority (Scott 1994: 193–199). The Buddha controls all creatures; his word is law. In this mythological order, defiance of the Buddha is not possible. Everyone must bow to him in the end. I think it probable that this worldview, if one can call it that, would eventually have faded away many years ago from Sri Lanka, had it not been revived by Sinhala nationalists and given the stamp of authority by a British treaty.

A third contribution of westerners to modern Sri Lankan culture consisted of Christian missionaries' insistence that there is only one "true" religion. Buddhist revivalists of the nineteenth and twentieth centuries decided that Buddhism was it. The Buddha dhamma was/is equivalent to the truth, and everything contradicting it was/is a lie. I think it would not be incorrect to refer to this view as Buddhist fundamentalism and to suggest that it has been inspired, in a way, by Christian fundamentalism. Religious intolerance thus becomes part of the modern picture. Old texts (*Mahavamsa, Dipavamsa*) have been exhumed and special passages under-lined to justify this picture, the portrait of modern Sinhala nationalist identity.

In addition, Evangelical missionaries imbued Sri Lankan religion with a sharp kind of Manicheanism that was not present before. Sinhala *yakku* were regarded as "demons," as representations of the very Devil himself, and were seen by Evangelical missionaries as totally evil; Sinhala people were said to "worship" these "demons" by committing "various abom-inable evils" (Scott 1994: 161). It is no wonder that Sinhala people did not like these missionaries.

From a modern western point of view, the Sinhala *yakku* are great psychic medicine, complex personalities whose horrific early childhood experiences made them into monsters, tortured torturers with deliciously gruesome histories steeped in forbidden fantasies. They are as scary and funny, hungry and horny, as Michael Keaton's Beetlejuice. Their faces, if one is to judge by the masks sold in tourist shops, are beautiful and appealing in their weirdness. Their ears are explosions of flowers, their hair is a profusion of pretty snakes with angry faces. Their expression is that of a lonely psychopath. "Love me or I'll eat you," it says. The "devil dancers" have thus become an insignia of Sinhala culture, brought out for parades and displays, featured in National Geographic articles, and celebrated by anthropologists. Sinhala people are *proud* of them and of the ceremonies that take place around them. To host such a ceremony enhances a person's prestige within the local community. If "demon-worship" is perceived as the "heart" of Sinhala "religion" and philosophical Buddhism is relegated by Western observers to the status of façade, this is no doubt because the Buddhist monks are so boring compared to the *yakku*.

Nineteenth-century Evangelical missionaries complained that Sinhala people "have no fixed principles" and that these people would irritatingly agree to call themselves Buddhists or Christians or both at the same time (Scott 1994 165–167). Modern observers might praise such flexibility, such tolerance. There is room in modern Christendom for the idea that much lies between absolute good and absolute evil. But the harshly judgmental, damned-or-saved view introduced by those missionaries has been born again, one might say, in the intransigence of the present-day Sinhala Buddhist clergy, who assert with absolute certainty that the island "belongs" to the Sinhalese, that no "concessions" must be made to the Tamil inhabitants of the island, that the LTTE must be defeated militarily, and that everyone who fails to acknowledge this fact is simply deluded, if not downright evil. Sinhala Buddhist clergy view the LTTE as the Evangelicals viewed the Sinhala "demons" of yore – as absolutely evil and at the same time as senseless monsters who must be destroyed. It would be better if the LTTE were treated as actual yakku are treated (more on this topic later), although better yet would be to treat them as fellow human beings.

A fourth contribution of western civilization to Sri Lankan culture is the introduction by Americans into Sri Lanka of a new (to Sri Lanka) war mythology. It is important to point this out, because otherwise it is dangerously easy to accept culturalist explanations of the Sri Lankan war among others. To do so is to blame "a culture" for a war (along the lines of "national character" studies of Germans and Japanese) or, what is just as bad, to blame cultural difference for ethnic conflict. Worst of all, is to suggest that quaint native "beliefs" are what give rise to such wars and to promote an attitude of superiority of us over them, an attitude to which we are not entitled. For, if culture and mythology are undoubtedly aspects of why and how war is waged, then it must be acknowledged that Americans are subject to the same kinds of "irrational" influences – that is, Americans of the recent past have been motivated by culture-specific mythology to engage in war. I give evidence below that American war-mythology has gotten into the Sri Lankan military, and the result has been to make a bad situation worse.

The American people's response to the Gulf War has already become a classic example of the mobilization of myth to support embarkation on warfare. The myth used by the (former) Bush administration to support America's attack on Iraq has been termed by Lakoff, "The Fairy Tale of the Just War" (1992: 446). Lakoff characterized this fairy tale thus:

> Cast of characters: A villain, a victim, and a hero. The victim and the hero may be the same person. The scenario: A crime is committed by the villain against an innocent victim (typically an assault, theft, or kidnapping). The offense occurs due to an imbalance of power and creates a moral imbalance. The hero either gathers helpers or decides to go it alone. The hero makes sacrifices; he undergoes difficulties, typically making an arduous heroic journey, sometimes across the sea to a treacherous terrain. The villain is inherently evil, perhaps even a monster, and thus reasoning with him is out of the question. The hero is left with no choice but to engage the villain in battle. The hero defeats the villain and rescues the victim. The moral balance is restored. Victory is achieved. The hero, who always acts honorably, has proved his manhood and achieved glory. The sacrifice was worthwhile. The hero receives acclaim, along with the gratitude of the victim and the community.

In the Gulf War version of this fairy tale, Saddam Hussein is the villain, Kuwait is the innocent victim, American soldiers are the heroes. The heroes leave family and friends to journey across the seas into the hostile terrain of the Arabian Desert. Their sacrifice is separation from family and endurance of the heat of the desert. They defeat the villain, rescue the victim, and return home to the acclaim and gratitude of all. In the whole process no good guys (or hardly any) have come to harm, nor have the good guys ever departed from their role as good guys, they have never behaved ignobly, they have never victimized innocents. They remain wholly good, and wholly triumphant as well.

The mythic depictions of what happened in the Gulf War were quite at odds with reality, as many scholars and members of the press were at pains to point out. But the American people, by and large, believed the story anyway. The popularity of President Bush soared to an all-time high.

In Sri Lanka, the current Government has attempted to invoke a similar myth. Perhaps the Sri Lankan commanders were even tutored in this myth – as a lesson in psy-ops – by their American advisors. One SL Army incursion into the (dry) north of the island was called "Desert Attack," although the area in question is not exactly a desert. The name for this operation, if not its content, was surely inspired by the US Operation "Desert Storm."

In the Sri Lankan version of the American war-hero fairy tale, Velupillai Prabhakaran (head of the LTTE) is the villain, Jaffna (the peninsula in which the LTTE first came to power and which it controlled for some time) is the victim, and the Sri Lankan soldiers (sent by the Government to wrest control of Jaffna from the hands of the LTTE) are the heroes, leaving behind family and friends (in southern Sri Lanka) and journeying at risk of their lives into the hostile terrain of Tiger territory (the northernmost part of Sri Lanka, where the Jaffna Peninsula is). This offensive was called Operation Riviresa ("Operation Sunshine") presumably because it was supposed to bring light into the lives of the Jaffna people. Prabhakaran, like Hussein, was called a "monster," a "psychopath," a "megalomaniac" and such. He was, and is, almost accused of eating little children – the horrific image of the suicide bomber being merged with the pathetic image of the child soldier in descriptions of what Prabhakaran does.[5]

Such was the story from December 1995 through January 1996. The Sri Lankan Army (comprised entirely of Sinhalese soldiers) marched into the northern peninsula of Jaffna (inhabited entirely by Tamil people) and took it over, while the LTTE withdrew to the jungles south of the peninsula, encouraging civilians to flee the invading army and come with the LTTE into the jungles, which many civilians did.

With the "rescue" of Jaffna, that should have been the end of the story. The monster/villain, if he wasn't killed, was at least driven off to the jungle. The Sinhalese soldiers should have returned home as heroes, the popularity of the President should have risen, and everyone but the villainous Tigers should have been happy.

But the story did not work out as planned. I will suggest two reasons for failure – one obvious, the other perhaps not quite so obvious but equally significant. The obvious reason for the failure is that the Sri Lankan invasion of Jaffna differed in a thousand ways from the American bombardment of Baghdad and the return of Kuwait to her throne. (During "Operation Desert Attack" some expatriate Jaffna Tamils bitterly joked, "If the Vanni is such a desert, why does the Army bother with it? It doesn't even have oil.")

In the American fairy story outlined by Lakoff, a clear separation of good and evil is presupposed at the outset. The triumph of good over evil is expected. Human suffering exists, but is easily manageable, and is incorporated into the moral victory of the strong and good. This black-and-white mythology, which I have called Manicheanism, was sufficient to mobilize American support for a quick and brutal bombing raid overseas.

But Manicheanism in Sri Lanka, as I have suggested above, leads into serious quagmires. In short, Western myths do not always work well in Sri Lanka. They can and do contribute to violent conflict, and to a general breakdown of social order, such as we see in Sri Lanka at this time. Equally important, however, is that Sri Lanka has myths of its own, quite different from the western myths.

Enactments of sacrifice

In Sri Lanka there are four major, institutionalized religions: Buddhism, Saivism, Christianity (primarily Catholic), and Islam. Militant monks notwithstanding, on the popular level in Sri Lanka, these four religions have no quarrel with one another. If an alliance of religious sympathies exists, then it takes the form of a close alliance between Saivism and Christianity and a looser alliance between Buddhism and Islam. Triumphalism and its opposite, sacrificialism, pervade all four religions. But Saivism and Christianity are (in modern Sri Lanka) more sacrificialist, Buddhism is more triumphalist, and Islam takes a kind of live-and-let-live, kill-or-be-killed position, as the situation mandates. Most Buddhists are speakers of the Sinhala language, most Saivas are speakers of the Tamil language, most Muslims are Tamil speakers but profess no attachment to the Tamil language. Christians include both Sinhala speakers and Tamil speakers, but more of the latter than the former. Sinhala Christians and Tamil Christians are divided by their ethnicities, not their faith. Sinhala Buddhism and Tamil Saivism are both founded upon and deeply pervaded by pre-nominalist faiths and beliefs. Sinhala Buddhists and Tamil Saivas still attend and enjoy each other's ceremonies, even as the war goes on.[6]

Popular Tamil Saivism consists of an elaborate set of ritual addresses to deities who are not wholly benign. Popular Sinhala Buddhism involves (but is not confined to) an elaborate set of ritual addresses to *yakku* ("demons") who are not wholly malign.[7] Sinhala rituals addressing troublesome *yakku* often entail clear efforts to get the reluctant *yakku* to bow to the will of the Buddha; these same rituals also entail clear efforts to drive the *yakku* far away ("back" to the land of the *yakkus*, wherever that is), to sever the bond between the yakku and the afflicted person, and to symbolically "kill" the *yakku* (by means of mock funerals, cutting of lemons, pumpkins and such, and destruction of the central pandal where much of the ritual drama takes place). Scott considers that the ritual specialist's relationship with the *yakku* is like the relationship of someone at war with an enemy (see note 7). In this respect, the "mission" of Sinhala Buddhism is analogous to an Islamic *jihad* (only with less historical, cultural, and religious depth and complexity). Right wing extreme Sinhala Buddhist nationalists think of Tamils as infidels who like yakka must submit to the will of Buddha, leave the island, or be killed.

Tamil Saivism, on the other hand, easily embraces the image of Christ crucified. The death of Christ under torture to redeem the sins of all humankind, the spiritual comfort and nourishment of his good blood, and the sharing of his suffering are all understood by Tamils. There has even been some arcane debate over whether Tamil Saivas got this idea from early Christians, or the reverse. For the purposes of this essay, it does not matter who got what idea from whom, but only that these four religions mix in numerous ways on the island they all inhabit. The nature of the mix affects and is affected by wartime alliances and ideologies.

In the present war in Sri Lanka, LTTE members who die in battle are honored by the movement as Maaveerarkal, "Great Heroes." Their cemeteries are called "sacred" (*punniyam*). The coffin of a fallen LTTE combatant is covered with an LTTE flag. Their blood is said to redeem and nourish the homeland. So far, we are fully in line with the treatment of fallen soldiers in western countries.

The death of one Tiger in combat is said to cause others to come forward and take the place of the one who has fallen. In actual fact, many young people do follow their elder brothers or sisters into the field of combat, presumably out of love for those brothers or sisters. Whole families of siblings have joined the rebels in this way, despite the policy of the LTTE that only one member of each family should join, and whole families of siblings have been killed (other whole families resist joining, or send their sons abroad if they can). Each year, throughout the world, in the month of November, a commemorative ceremony is held, called Maaveerar Dinam, or "Great Heroes Day." Every fallen LTTE combatant is honored. Their reward is just this – to be remembered. To the families of those who were killed, the memorial ceremony is also a comfort. We remain on familiar territory.

The most highly esteemed of Sinhala Army personnel, conversely, are not those who have died. They are not among the countless, unacknowledged dead – the foot soldiers who, we are told, "gave their lives for their country." Who were they? How did they die? Did they die at all, and if so, where are they buried? The families of many Sinhala soldiers missing-in-action will tell you they do not know. (We are still in familiar territory, here). The most esteemed people in the Sinhala military are the men of high rank under whose command the largest number of lives, resisting and unrepentant, have perished. The top brass of the Sri Lankan Army consider that their mandate is to destroy the terrorists. Their reward for wreaking destruction upon large numbers of terrorists (or presumed terrorists) is promotion. By comparison, the rank of an LTTE member is not known until his or her death, and at his or her death, he or she is usually promoted.

While the LTTE venerates its dead, records every name of each fallen hero, and maintains sacred cemeteries for them, the Sri Lankan military hides its dead, their numbers, and their names. For the Sri Lankan military, each fallen combatant is a source of shame, a sign of defeat. The LTTE will tell anyone who asks the precise number of LTTE members who have died. But it keeps as a very close secret the number of LTTE members who are living. The Sri Lankan military does exactly the opposite.

To return to the original basic point, war is an affliction, and this war is no different. It causes suffering to the good and innocent, it kills the people and ravages the soil, it has decimated the economy and exacerbated poverty. Few would openly admit that they want the war to continue because they like warfare, or because they profit from it. We hear little if anything from either side about the necessity of eternal struggle, or ongoing revolution.

And yet, as I have stated above, for both parties to the conflict, including many who hate the war, the war is an act of healing – the only possible act. To understand this view, it is necessary to tap into pre-existing views.

For the LTTE and its supporters, the purpose of their fighting is to drive the Sinhalese Army off of Tamil soil. This in itself, however, is only a means to the ultimate end of creating a healthy Tamil Eelam. The LTTE considers that Tamil society, even before the current conflict, was not healthy. It was riven with caste inequalities, gender oppression, and exploitation of the poor by the rich. Tamil society will never be strong and healthy until such inequalities have been completely abolished.

None of these ideas was created from scratch by the LTTE. Modern and pre-modern Tamil history are replete with stories of the oppressed overcoming their oppressors by means of extreme suffering, self-discipline, and sacrifice. The oppressed as a rule does not kill the oppressor, but shames him into seeing the error of his ways. Often, the oppressed dies violently, only to return as a powerful immortal deity (or memory) demanding justice for the living oppressed. In this Mariamman, Kannakiyamman, Nandanar, Kannappan, Ciruttondan, Nallatangal, countless village deities, cinema heroes and heroines enact this story in one way or another.[8]

Living oracles heal as mediums for deities such as Mariamman and Kaliyamman. The oracle also must suffer throughout his or her life in order to continue healing others. Lawrence (1997) describes the dramatic suffering taken on by one oracle in the eastern war zone, purely for the purpose of ascertaining what has become of one "disappeared" young man. In this case, the healing act did not even entail a demand for justice; it only entailed answering the question, "Where is he?" The suffering of the supplicants was just barely lessened.[9]

Anti-caste movements in southern India can be traced back at least a thousand years. Though caste was never abolished, it came to be ignored in many ritual and secular contexts. The modern Dravidian Renaissance, as it has been called, adopted a number of the values expressed in the early myths and strengthened the anti-Brahminical sentiments that had been expressed in folklore from long before then. The aim was not to kill Brahmans, or even to drive them from the south, but simply to deprive them of their privileges. Brahmans came to be seen as exogenous "Aryan invaders" and a general mistrust of Brahmans is expressed by some Tamil nationalists even to this day.

Among some Tamil nationalists favoring the establishment of an independent Tamil Eelam, the Sinhalese people, who claim original descent from the north, have been assimilated to the "Aryan invader" image. The composers of the Rig Veda called themselves "Aryas" and downgraded the indigenous peoples they conquered as dark-skinned and inferior. The fact that Sinhalese consider themselves to be lighter-skinned than Tamils (a perception that escapes most western observers) adds another log to the fire of Sinhala-Tamil discord. Finally, the fact that Sinhala soldiers are sent into Tamil areas to fight Tamil-speaking Tigers apparently does give them a sense of being in a foreign land surrounded by people whose speech they cannot understand, and vice versa.

The LTTE consider themselves to belong to the earth – and indeed, probably most of the combatants come from farming families. Though they have taken an animal name, the vegetative imagery pervading their verbal art is striking. I will offer as an example one of many poems that have been published in the pro-Eelam Tamil newspaper *Kalattil*. This appeared in the issue of 16 July 1997, on page 9. The editors wrote this preface:

In the battle of Elephant Pass, Captain Kasturi embraced heroic death. These are the lines of poetry she wrote at the end but was unable to finish.

My translation from the Tamil is as precise as I can make it:

Deathless

Severed hands
grow back fast.
The more they're cut,
the more they sprout.

Like stubborn plants,
sliced hands
bear buds
and mangled ones
burst red.

Strangled throats
in streaks of flame
oppose a ripe death,
screaming.

Burnt lungs
scald the occupier,
and sear him
with their breath
forced free.

"He's dead and gone,"
the enemy mocks,
and in that place,
corpses take life.

You enemies cause trembling agony.
Torture. Kill. What of it?
Severed, amputated,
cut down, warriors sprout.

Our warriors
will not die until
your armies flee
beyond our bounds.

Hands raised for rights
submit to no invasion.

Not only members of the LTTE compose such poetry. The poem below
was written by a young man who chose not to join the LTTE, but fled
abroad instead. Again, this is my translation. The poet is Tamil. The poem
is addressed to an imaginary Sinhalese person:

Neighbor,
your mouth says you don't understand,
but I understand the grin on your mouth.
your timeless hypocrisy
is nothing new.

Nevertheless,
firm in my gentleness, I will not kill my words,
but will keep telling you to the end,

"The severed palmyrah tree may die,
but deep in the earth, its root will send forth new sprouts."

At least this much you will see,
on my earth that you burnt, from every ash-pile,
a palmyrah will spring like a phoenix.

Wind, animals, birds, rivers, travelling out,
will all carry bits of my rich soil
to plant its living seeds to grow again
thick green in their ripeness,
while blood-red flowers will pour
from the sharp-thorned drumstick tree,
showing its anger.

On that day,
do not stand at my threshold,
knocking at my door,
asking flowers for your daughter's wedding garland.

Today my people's corpses are falling,
Crumbling like rich manure, they will rise
and laugh like destiny's faces,
their scattered blood smiling
from all the red flowers.

But no matter how much time passes,
tomorrow's howling wind will proclaim
today's stench of death in my land.

The battle cry of Sinhala militants is, "Destroy the Tigers." Popular Sinhala rhetoric stresses and amplifies the evil of the Tigers. It also stresses and amplifies the power of the Tiger forces, representing them as a world-threatening affliction, a dangerous perpetrator of global terrorism, a spreading infection that all right-thinking people will strive to eradicate. As a kind of virus, the LTTE has no moral status of its own. Its sole, unthinking aim, in the eyes of Sinhala militants, is self-replication. When the LTTE achieves a military victory, kills so many soldiers and takes so many weapons and so much territory, Sinhala militants, as though they were doctors, blame other doctors. The ruling party blames the opposition party, and the opposition party blames the ruling party. The free press is blamed for reporting what is happening on the warfront, and weakening the morale of the Sinhala people in their struggle against this deadly disease. Foreign governments are blamed for allowing supporters of the LTTE to subsist and act within their shores, thereby providing pockets for the disease to develop and grow. Humanitarian organizations (NGOs) are blamed for treating the LTTE as human and showing compassion for this disease that is wholly evil and inhuman and must be destroyed for the sake of the wholeness of the world. Young people who join the LTTE are characterized as victims-turned-into-monsters by the bite of the werewolf, or as humans turned into zombie slaves ("drugged" and "brainwashed") by the growing zombie army. Once zombified, they lose their humanity and their natural fear of death, and are "thrown into the front as suicide bombers." They are no longer real people.

The original intent of this essay was to show that the sacrifice of Tamil lives constitutes a moral and spiritual victory both for the LTTE and for the Sri Lankan military. The aim of the Sri Lankan military is to "eradicate terrorism" by killing Tamil people. The aim of the LTTE is to achieve liberation of Tamils through Tamil self-sacrifice. One would guess that the inevitable end of this war would be sacrifice and obliteration of Tamils on the island.

And yet, since 1983, the LTTE has just become stronger and stronger. It has achieved victory after victory in its confrontations with the Sri Lankan Army. Part of the reason for this – and here is another irony – is that Sinhala soldiers fighting for the Sri Lankan Army do not want to die. For them, personal death at the hands of an enemy is the ultimate defeat. If they are threatened with death, they retreat (run away if they can) instead of holding their ground to the end. Like most "normal" soldiers, few want to go to the front. Therefore, the Sri Lankan Army suffers problems with desertion. About 20,000 deserters are said to be still at large. These deserters are not necessarily cowards. Indeed, it takes some bravery to flee the army, given the consequences if one is caught by either side. But those who desert consider that it is better to take their chances than to live what turns out to be the miserable life, and possibly die the miserable death, of a soldier. The point here is simply that Sinhala soldiers have a healthy and strong will to live and be free, whatever else one might say of them.

People who join the LTTE have already decided to die fighting. Recent recruits that I met, teenaged girls who had run away from home only that day, told me that they *wanted* to die. They had left their parents' homes because life there held no hope for them. They decide to die, and *then* they join the LTTE. It is not so much that they are sacrificing their lives for a greater cause, as that the greater cause gives them an honorable way of leaving civilian life, or indeed of leaving life altogether. Faced with the grim reality of combat, even combat-training, some of them subsequently change their minds, just as a person who has swallowed a bottle of pills in a suicide attempt may change her mind and look for a doctor. Others, however, just become more hardened in their resolve. For more experienced members who have been in the movement for years and who are committed to it for ideological reasons and because it is their *only* family, death in combat is the ultimate victory.[10] They lose their fear, and this absence of fear protects them, to a certain extent. They say that they do not panic. Those who do probably do not last long. But some, who joined young, have been in scores of battles. Jungle combat is their whole life. They are accustomed to death. They say, convincingly, that they are quite happy with this life. More sentimental ones say they know that their names will be written in history, and they have faith that each single death will yield multiple new lives, as a seed fallen on the ground will grow and yield a plant with multiple new seeds. This agrarian metaphor has deep meaning for them.

Sinhala people grow up in an equally agrarian environment. But indigenous agrarian views have not been incorporated for them into a fighting ideology. The poorest of Sinhala people, those from whom the Sri Lankan military forces are recruited, seek salvation through revenge.

O Kali *maniyo*. You are the most powerful of the seven mothers. I have heard of your great power and how you stopped the storm which flooded the land. I have heard how you protected your husband from the Asura. Punish my enemy who brought the *vina* against me. I cannot feed my children. I cannot send them to school. I know a *kodivina* has been made. My husband's relatives have brought this sorrow.

O Bhadrakali, break the legs of my enemies. I want to see the pig who has caused my suffering hobbling lame. O Fire Kali, burn their lives. Never let them sleep. O Kali, look at me. Help me. O Kali, heal my husband's legs. Make him well to work again. These people are jealous because we are sending our children to school. O *maniyo*, punish these cruel people.

(Kapferer 1997: 232)

This is the prayer of an impoverished woman whose husband had been injured in a traffic accident. She suspects the cause of this misfortune to be someone close at hand – her husband's relatives. The larger causes, such as failure of traffic law enforcement and failure of the vehicle driver or anyone else to provide compensation or relief, are subsumed under the powers of the divine. We do not know the prayers of the kin of soldiers wounded or killed in battle against the LTTE, but perhaps they are much the same. For most Sinhalese, the LTTE is a vast and distant demonic force far beyond their prayers. This force can be mobilized by closer individuals for destructive purposes – hapless soldiers can by sent by higher commanders, supposedly on the same side, into the jaws of death. Evil and its attendant suffering are always out there waiting. No human force and no divine force can make the evil cease to be. Each human being alone must seek deliverance.

In popular Sinhala Buddhist practice, the most powerful earthly forces are demonic. Sinhala Buddhist mythology represents Tamils as invaders of the island, constantly threatening to fragment it and thus destroy it, in much the same way that a demon will threaten the integrity of a human life. Demons are not stupid. They are cunning and deceptive. Therefore, to defeat a threatening demon, the services of a wise specialist in the form of a demon exorcist are required, and spectacular expensive ceremonies must be performed. Finally the demon-or more precisely the power that sent the demon-is obliterated in a cataclysmic act of destruction of an elaborate "palace" (a decorated structure made for the purpose of the ceremony) into which the afflicted has entered, step-by-step, to come to terms with his or her being.[11] The ceremonies are said to be frightening, but hugely entertaining.

It is easy to find an analogy between Sinhala nationalists' views of the LTTE and popular Sinhalese Buddhist views of the demonic. In fact, it is too easy. Buddhist clergy and members of government who unequivocally advocate the continuation of the "war against terrorism" at any cost intentionally provoke and seek to mobilize terrible fears among the Sinhalese-the fear of sudden death, the fear of being taken by surprise, the fear of being cheated, the fear of losing everything, the fear of being left with nothing to hold onto. The LTTE embodies all these fears. The clergy and the military encourage the projection of all fears upon the LTTE, and so, for that matter, does the LTTE itself.[12] The clergy and the military insist that no negotiation with the LTTE should ever take place. No compromise whatsoever is possible. "Terrorism" must be destroyed, and that is that.

However, their equation of terrorism with the demonic is shallow and simplistic, not only from the viewpoint of an external observer who does not believe in demons, but also from the viewpoint of an internal observer who understands some of the complexities of popular Sinhala religion. In rural exorcism ceremonies, negotiation with the afflicting demon does in fact take place. The demon is offered food and so forth, and long dialogues occur between demons and exorcists in which the attempt of the exorcist is to get the demon to submit to the will of the Buddha and leave the afflicted patient alone, in exchange for certain concessions. If the demon does not submit to the will of the Buddha, it is not annihilated. Something is annihilated, and that is the bond between the demon and the afflicted. Imagery of conception and parturition or even abortion is common. The demon "enters" the victim by casting the light of its eyes upon the victim. The light of the eyes is, in Sinhala myth, a sexual substance than can lead to fertilization. A pumpkin on the belly of the patient may be sliced. Vines and cords will be cut. The demon has to be gotten out of the body of the afflicted, because the demon drinks the blood and eats the flesh of his host, as a fetus is said to drink the blood and eat the flesh of its mother. Several of the great Sinhala demons originated in this way. The demon was conceived in an evil fashion, his mother died under torture as punishment for her sin, the demon-baby was born as she died and subsisted by eating the body of his dead mother before going out in the world and becoming a major force (Wirz 1954). It is not the demon's fault that he is a demon. All he wants is to be fed and housed inside someone else's body. Many scholars consider that these "demons" are really in some way a part of the afflicted person, a demanding part, but a part from which the afflicted does not entirely wish to be separated. Exorcism ceremonies are addressed both to the afflicted person and to the part of the afflicted person that is causing trouble. The ceremonies literally work out a negotiated settlement between the warring parts of the afflicted self. Thus Scott's metaphor (see note 5 above) is supremely apt.[13]

Sinhala Buddhist exorcism ceremonies have in common with exorcism ceremonies everywhere, including South Indian Tamil ceremonies, an acknowledgment that the afflicting ghost or demon attacks not out of malice but out of desire. A demon (or ghost) becomes one through no serious fault of its own. The Tamil exorcist asks the afflicting demon, "Who are you and what do you want?" The demon gradually and elliptically spells out its identity and its needs. Then it is induced to go away by means of certain offerings. However, the demon is not thereby destroyed. It will come back again to afflict someone else some other day. Possessing demons can turn into deities if they are lucky. There is no sharp line between one category of being and the other.

Sinhala demons also are not destroyed. Indeed, the pantheon of demons is an intrinsic part of the Sinhala cosmos. The pantheon of demons has been represented as a near-perfect mirror-reflection of the pantheon of deities (Yalman 1964). Both demons and deities are immortal but flawed. They have in common their great power over human lives. Human beings seek to manipulate these powers to improve their own earthly well-being and to destroy *human* enemies.

Thus, if one were to fully equate terrorism with Tamil and the demonic in Sri Lanka, one would have to acknowledge that both Tamils and terrorism are part of the overall Sinhala world and will never be destroyed.

The equation of terrorism with Tamil and the demonic also fails in that there has also been Sinhala terrorism, in the form of the JVP youth uprising between 1987 and 1989, during which period some sixty thousand Sinhala youths, "suspected terrorists," were massacred by Government forces. Tamil extremists as well as Sinhala extremists refuse to acknowledge the significance of this event and the obvious similarities between Government brutalization of Sinhala youth during the JVP uprising and Tamil youth thereafter. But non-extremists on both sides are well aware of the parallels.

Kapferer (1997) discusses the rise of the demon-deity Suniyam in popular Sinhala Buddhism during the twentieth century. The name Suniyam means "sorcery" and Suniyam is the master of the power of sorcery. Sorcery is destructive human agency, turned against other human beings.

Whether Suniyam as an agent in his own right is good or evil is beside the point. He embodies Sinhala people's view that destructive human agency is an enormous power in their world. Suniyam is a master not only of destructive human agency, but of authority, judgement, and punishment. His body is "covered in snakes, representations of the world-destroying, body-enveloping poisons of sorcery that Suniyam both sends and controls." (Kapferer 1997: 27) Kapferer proposes that in post-independence Sri Lanka, the rise of a series of dictatorial prime ministers and presidents, who increasingly accrued individual powers and exercised these powers in violent and destructive ways, all the while promoting Sinhala nationalism and allowing their personal images to be assimilated with the divine, was the context in which Suniyam came to prominence in popular Sinhala Buddhism (Kapferer 1997: 29). In other words, Suniyam, master of human malevolence, is none other than the head of the Sri Lankan Government, reflected in the shining eyes of popular Sinhala Buddhism.

Kapferer records the prayer of a Sinhala woman who came to a Suniyam shrine in October 1989, when the Government was in the process of putting down the JVP uprising by massacring tens of thousands of Sinhala youth. This woman's son had disappeared and she feared he had been killed by Government forces:

> O God who fought and conquered the Asuras,
> Listen to my plea! My son has not come home for
> seven days. O God, we have tried our best
> to find out what has happened. I have been told that
> he has been killed by the special forces. O God, use
> your powerful heat (*tejas*) to destroy them!
> I still hope that my son is alive. O God, can you
> find some way that I can meet him? O God, destroy
> those who have killed my son. O God, who carries

the pot of fire, burn them, tear them
into pieces, kill them with your sword!
May you live ten thousand years!

This prayer was uttered eleven years ago. The JVP uprising was utterly crushed, and direct massacres of Sinhala boys by Government forces ceased. Today, Sinhala boys are recruited into the Government army, and generally if they are killed, they are killed by the LTTE. In recent years, the LTTE has overrun a series of large Government military installations – most notably at Mullaitivu in 1996, at Kilinocchi in 1998, and at Elephant Pass (Anai Iravu) in 2000. During these operations, and in smaller raids against smaller bases, some thousands of Sinhala soldiers have been killed. Often the families of soldiers who have been killed or gone missing in action are not notified as to what has happened, and the families are left to wonder, hope and pray in agony.

What kinds of prayers are uttered by mothers of Sinhala boys killed or missing in action during conflicts with the LTTE? Perhaps they pray for the destruction of the LTTE. Or perhaps they pray for something else. Some have formed organizations seeking to make the Government account for the soldiers killed in battle or missing in action.

Among Tamils in Sri Lanka and elsewhere, demon-exorcism rituals are common, but they are small and specialists in exorcism are not held in especially high esteem. They cannot match the magnificent and elaborate Sinhala exorcism ceremonies. Similarly among Tamils, sorcery is acknowledged as a reality, and counter-sorcery rituals take place for the purpose of neutralizing the spell. But Tamil people do not openly engage in sorcery for the sake of destroying or damaging another person, because sorcery is considered an evil activity engaged in by evil people.

The most spectacular Tamil religious ceremonies are temple festivals in which people participate to gain merit and absolution of their sins. Personal acts of *tavam* (or *tapas*) for the purpose of self-purification and incurring the grace of a deity range from making donations to the temple, to providing religious service (such as preparing food for pilgrims), to fasting, to the piercing of tongue or cheek with knives, through to fire-walking and hook-swinging. Participants in these last acts insist that they are not painful. Sometimes the person engaging in such an act is clearly in deep trance. Other times he or she appears to be in a normal, if concentrated, state of mind. Sometimes the person engaging in such an act does it for a particular purpose, such as to fulfill a vow to a deity who has healed him or her of sickness or to protect a loved one in danger from harm. Other times, a person who engages in fire-walking (for instance) does so not for any particular purpose, but as a regular act, to maintain personal purity and the grace of the deity. In the Batticaloa District of eastern Sri Lanka, which has always been famous for its many fine old temples and the ceremonies surrounding them, intensification of the war has been accompanied by magnification of the temple ceremonies (Lawrence 1997). No deity can be said to reflect a recent political development.

Both the Sinhala Buddhist ceremonies and the Tamil Saiva ceremonies are performed for the general purpose of healing and renewal of self and world. Both sets of ceremonies have been deployed in recent times to address the afflictions of violence and warfare. Both sets of ceremonies contain an element of violence, and for this reason alone, both sets of ceremonies may be called sacrificial in nature. But the nature of the sacrifice is quite different on the two sides. On the Sinhala side, violent and destructive sentiments are directed outward. On the Tamil side, such sentiments – or at least their overt expressions – are forbidden, and self-sacrifice is perceived as the means to grace and power.

In Tamil Saivism, the god himself bleeds. The great god Siva, represented in the form of a lingam, very often suffers injury in the stories told about him and endures this injury for the sake of love.

An exemplary tale of Siva is the origin story of the Sri Taantondriswaran Koil ("The Temple of the Lord Who Made Himself Appear") in the town of Kokkaddichcholai, which is the very heart and showpiece of LTTE territory in the east, although it is at the same time dangerously close to the edge of Army-controlled territory. The massacres, the shellings, the strafings, the round-ups, the tortures, and the disappearances that have afflicted the people of this town and its environs are too many to list here. The number of young people who have left their homes in this town and its environs to join the LTTE, and the number of those who have died in the conflict are countless. Their cemeteries are maintained as holy ground, and from time to time the army razes these cemeteries, and then they are reconstructed and reconsecrated as means allow.

The origin story of the temple in Kokkaddichcholai is this. Once the area was all forest. Some hunters came and saw some honey in the top of a Kokkaddi tree. They took an axe to the tree in order to fell it and get the honey. Blood then flowed from the wound in the tree. The hunters then realized that God was in the tree, and they fled. A woman came and out of compassion, bound the wound in the tree. From the wound in the tree, a small sivalingam budded forth. It grew and was discovered by a holy man, who sat by the tree and did *tavam* there. As time went on, a great temple grew around the spot.

One may conclude from this and similar evidence that the LTTE ethos of self-sacrifice and regeneration emerged from the already existing local Tamil religious ethos. A similar religious ethos is stressed by Tamil Christians. In discussing with me the question of whether suicide-bombing by Black Tigers was a sin, a Catholic clergyman from Batticaloa said, "In defying the authorities of the time, Christ knew he was going to die. He knowingly walked into his death. He could be said, therefore, to have committed suicide. But giving your life for the sake of others is not suicide. It is the supreme sacrifice." In the view of this person, those who went to their deaths for the sake of others were martyrs in the truest sense.

One may also conclude that the Sinhala chauvinist ethos of saving Sri Lanka by killing the Tamils is not an indigenous ethos. It is a construct, appropriating parts of some old mythic texts, the reverence of Sinhalese for their monks as upholders of Buddhism and transformation of deep fear and injury into rage and desire for vengeance. This construct fails to take into account Sinhalese understandings of power and suffering. It would seem that for Sinhalese, to suffer is to be disempowered, whereas for Tamils, suffering is the very source of power. This is not to say that the average Tamil person likes or wants to suffer. But suffering in itself is not a source of shame; it may even be a cause for pride.

When I first thought of this essay, I was planning to write that Tamil and Sinhalese cultures are caught in a kind of complementary schizmo-genesis, following Bateson. The Sinhalese try to heal their own suffering by pushing it onto Tamils, while Tamils gobble this suffering up and turn it into triumph, thus causing the Sinhalese to fear the Tamils even more and to inflict more suffering upon them, and so it goes on and on. But obviously the situation is much more complicated than this. A whole set of vicious circles is in operation here, and not only one. The big vicious circle to which they all contribute is the increasing militarization of both sides and the consequent increase in impoverishment, suffering, and death on both sides. In this way, warfare is perceived by the people as the cause of suffering, and more warfare is offered by the government (and to a lesser extent by the LTTE) as the only cure for this suffering.

Not really a conclusion

As I write, however, I come to the view that this circle itself is a construct, equally if not more a product of deliberate design than the prescription of destroying Tigers (the demonic "other") for the sake of preserving Sri Lanka (the whole and healthy "self"). The cycle of destruction and defeat, followed by increased militarization, followed by more destruction and defeat, followed by further increased militarization, and so forth, did not happen accidentally, and was certainly not the inevitable consequence of a certain kind of cultural difference.

The events of the year just past (2000) tell an instructive story. In April, the LTTE succeeded in capturing Elephant Pass, a large Army base that guarded the entrance to the Jaffna Peninsula, the former stronghold of the LTTE, which the LTTE is seeking to recapture from the Government. During this battle, the LTTE, as is their habit, captured what they called a "huge cache" of weaponry. They made things easier for themselves by allowing many soldiers to escape onto the peninsula, where these soldiers are now trapped. The Government immediately responded by putting itself on a "war-footing" and demanding that all resources being used for "non-essential" civilian services, such as development projects, be made available for military use. It insisted that it needed more and bigger military equipment, including destroyers and minesweepers that the Navy had been coveting. The Government said that it needed more weaponry because the LTTE had weapons the Government did not have, in the form of multibarreled rocket-launchers (MBRLs) and therefore the LTTE was better armed than the Government, and this was why it was able to take the base. (It turns out that these MBRLs are antiquated but still usable items leftover from the former Soviet Union.)

Meanwhile, supporters of the LTTE in overseas countries were celebrating the latest victory and were promising expatriate Jaffna Tamils that very shortly all of Jaffna peninsula would be again in control of the Tigers. They said that now was the time to contribute, to assist the LTTE in its final push to re-take Jaffna.

The taking of Elephant Pass was thus a win-win proposition for both the Sri Lankan arms procurement people and for the LTTE. The LTTE obtained more weaponry in the form of all the materiel it got from Elephant Pass, and the Sri Lankan Government arms procurement people also were allowed to buy new weaponry and other war-making equipment as a kind of compensation for the losses the Security Forces suffered at the hands of the LTTE. None of these military acquisitions will help the civilian population at all. Taxes on goods such as petrol have been raised to enable the Government to pay for the military equipment it says it needs to fight the Tigers.

By the end of the year 2000, it was clear that the LTTE would not be able to take control of Jaffna. It was not that the Tigers lacked armaments or personnel, but rather that they could not attack the Army because the soldiers were living so closely among the civilian population. It would have been easy to evacuate the soldiers from the peninsula – India even offered to help do it after the storming of Elephant Pass by the Tigers – but the Government refused. Thus the soldiers are stuck in a place they do not want to be, among people who do not want them to be there.

Around mid-December, the LTTE declared a unilateral month-long truce (reserving the right to engage in defensive military activity, however), which was to begin December 26, and asked the Government to reciprocate, which the Government did not do. Then the LTTE said that if the Government undertook a military offensive toward Elephant Pass, the war would get very nasty. In response, the Government undertook a military offensive toward Elephant Pass.

It is like a dance, but a dance of death. Or like two powerful male animals of the same species perhaps, engaged in ritual combat. The two dance partners have been together long enough to know each other well. They anticipate each other's moves and respond with perfect grace, as though their nervous systems were attached. They could go on like this forever. They will go on for a while, I think. While they are dancing – one might even say, while they are playing games with each other – many more people will certainly die. The damage will be permanent and irreparable. There will be no redemption. There will be no purification. There will probably not even be any lessons learned.[14]

Thus I have come to a different conclusion from the one that I first intended. There is a third kind of sacrifice – not ethnic fratricide at all, but a kind of intranational and international filicide, in which the young and the poor are the first to die, while the rich and the old get richer and older, and pass their riches on to their spoiled and stupid children.

This is a scene we have seen many times before, hardly just in this century and hardly just in Sri Lanka. To heal it will take not a new kind of medicine, nor a new kind of cultural understanding, but a new kind of government, and enforcement of responsibility upon the demons of power.

Notes

1 This essay is based in part upon field research conducted in the Batticaloa District of Sri Lanka from November 1997 through June 1998, under a grant from the American Institute of Sri Lankan Studies for research on children's agency in Sri Lanka. I was most interested in the way that children exercised agency with respect to the war. The embattled school child mentioned above was one of those I interviewed during this time. She lived in an "uncleared" (LTTE-controlled) area of Eastern Sri Lanka. The war was going on all around her.

Daniel (1997) refers to something he calls "the agentive moment." As I understand him, he means by this term a moment when a person or group of people together discover that their habitual way of living and being does not work anymore, and therefore they must change their habits. To break out of habitual patterns (which, because they are habitual, are largely below the threshold of awareness) is to exercise agency, according to this model. Daniel considers that some unexpected, hard reality ("secondness") has to break into people's lives, demonstrating to them that their old habits are inadequate, in order for them to exercise agency (i.e. conscious control over their lives and selves) and change their habits. Such a process is exactly what the child quoted above was referring to, I believe. This child was not alone in using the phrase I have quoted. Several children used it to explain to me how they transformed themselves to adapt to what Daniel would call the "bruteness" of the war. Sometimes this change of mind involved radically reducing expectations for the future – most of the children I interviewed "doubted" that the war would ever end, and therefore doubted that they would ever be able to live in peace. They felt that they simply had to come to terms with this fact, and be prepared for violent disruptions in their lives at any time. Other times the change of mind involved transforming oneself from a peaceful, non-violent person into an LTTE combatant.

2 A recent example of the destruction of Tamil resistance has been the arrest
of student peace demonstrators by the Sri Lankan Army (Reuters 2001; AFP
2001). Numerous other examples of such events can be gleaned from news
reports of international news agencies. Amnesty International, among other
agencies, provides reports of torture.

3 See Roberts (1996) for an argument that this self-sacrifice is religiously motivated. LTTE supporters were unhappy with Roberts's article, in part because
of the derogatory implications of the word "cult." In general, Tamil nationalists are ecumenical, secularists, or even atheists. A Tamil nationalist may
have his or her religion, but religious intolerance is deeply shunned. The question of whether certain nationalisms (such as American flag-worship) constitute
religions in themselves is another issue.

4 This murder happened in 1959. The motives for it are not clear, but some
speculate that Bandaranaike was killed by the monk because he had made
too many compromises with the Tamils. A more recent incident happened in
1999, when M.H.M. Ashraff, the Minister of Transport and powerful head of
the Sri Lanka Muslim League (the largest Muslim party) published a poem
entitled "Lord Buddha and the Poet." The gist of the poem is that the Buddha
laments the strife and corruption in Sri Lanka and says that he will come soon
to teach the Dhamma in the Tamil language, and he hopes that "these people"
will learn Tamil in order to receive the message. The character of the Buddha
himself is not impugned in the poem, but Sinhala Buddhists were outraged.
One Major General Ananda Weerasekera was quoted in the Sunday Times
(Colombo) as saying, "The fact that Minister Ashraff is still alive inspite of
his attitude toward the Sinhala Buddhists is the clearest evidence that the
Dhamma is still very much alive in this land, for in any other land he would
have been stoned to death." (*Sunday Times* [Colombo] 28 November 1999).
On 16 September 2000, Ashraff died in a helicopter crash, a day after resigning
from the ruling coalition, the People's Alliance. The cause of the crash remains
unknown.

5 Many LTTE members are in their teens. The Sri Lankan Government makes
good propaganda use of the younger ones it is able to capture alive. See for
instance Dugger 2000. When I presented an earlier version of this paper to a
Stockholm audience that included Sinhalese, and used the term "filicide" as I
do at the end of this one, Sinhala members of the audience thought that I
meant "child-killing" or "child-sacrifice" of the kind they consider the LTTE
to engage in. It is probably worth mentioning here that most present-day guer-
rilla organizations, such as FARC and the Chechnyan rebels, include fighters
under the age of fifteen. The existence and prevalence of lightweight but high-
powered combat weaponry enables small-bodied people to be effective
combatants.

6 To give just one example, a young Tamil woman I knew, nominally Methodist,
who had been shot in both knees and crippled by a Sinhala soldier, still attended
both Saiva temple festivals to which the LTTE contributed *and* Buddhist festivals sponsored by the Army, even when these festivals were held at the same
time in competition with one another. My friend simply enjoyed the festivals.
She said she was not the only one who attended both.

7 Different social scientists have put forward different ideas as to "the meaning"
of these ceremonies and their assorted components. Amarasingam (1973)
stresses the healing effects of the humor and laughter characterizing the
ceremonies; Kapferer (1997) writes about the recreation of self through violent
sacrifice of malign beings who have taken control of the victim's life;

Obeyesekere (1969) and Yalman (1964) discuss psychosexual, structural, and functional aspects of the ceremonies; Scott (1994: 208) citing Asad (1987: 197n) citing Clausewitz, considers the ceremonies to be a special kind of "strategy" "of antagonistic wills struggling for supremacy over a terrain that may not always be delimited, with forces that are not always constant, in conditions whose changing significance cannot always be anticipated. Such an aim *does* require some theoretical understanding and knowledge of rules, although that is not all it requires."

8 The principle of self-sacrifice is intrinsic to Tamil religious practices, not only in Sri Lanka but also in India. For a detailed ethnographic discussion of this matter, see Nabokov (2000.)

9 Lawrence also noted that Sinhala soldiers seemed to respect the power of this oracle, at least to the point of getting out of the way when she (an unarmed old woman) fiercely charged them. They might just as easily have arrested her or shot her. Lawrence's observation is a powerful comment in itself. Combined with my observation, in note 6, that even a Tamil woman who had been shot by a Sinhala soldier had no problem enjoying Sinhala Buddhist ceremonies, it points to a level of shared belief that has not been changed even by the atrocities of the war.

10 Quite a few, however, decide after a few years that they want to leave the LTTE, marry and start a new family. If their reasons for leaving the movement are strong enough, or if they have been in the movement for more than five years, they are allowed to "retire" to civilian life.

11 This is my brief summary of Kapferer's (1997) densely detailed description and analysis of an anti-sorcery ceremony. One obvious point that needs to be stressed is that the ceremonies described by different analysts happened at different times in different places, were performed by different people, and therefore should be expected to have different "meanings." Kapferer considers (as I understand him) that the ceremony he observed involved a sacrifice on the cosmic level – the whole world, or at least the whole self of the afflicted, was being destroyed so that the afflicted could emerge whole. Scott considers that nothing is being symbolically destroyed in the ceremony he describes, that it is not even properly speaking an exorcism, and the "sacrifice" spoken of is nothing more than the small offerings given to the *yakku*, to make them go away. In descriptions of *yaktovil* by other authors (Wirz 1954, Yalman 1964, Obeyesekere 1969) the violent destruction of the focal decorated structure played an important part. In the ceremony viewed by Scott, the structures were simply dismantled as the ceremony was ending. Even when it is obvious in a ceremony that *something* is being symbolically destroyed, when for instance the central ceremonial structure is dramatically destroyed, or when a mock corpse is carried away, it does not seem to be at all obvious *what* the thing is that the celebrants are symbolically destroying or killing. Whatever it is, it is the source of affliction, it is *not* intrinsic to the afflicted himself or herself, and it is something that has to be gotten rid of so that the suffering of the afflicted will be alleviated. In other words, it is *other*; it is *not self.*

12 The Tigers do try to frighten their enemies and their potential enemies. The idea (so one member of the LTTE told me) is to teach the Sinhalese not to harass the Tamils. Also, frightened soldiers do not make good fighters.

13 I say this even though Scott dismisses the functionalist-psychoanalytic way of explaining spirit possession, which in its latest version is a variant of the theory of multiple personality disorder (Castillo 1998). In my view, Scott's own data supports the theory that Scott rejects.

14 Langer (1997) observes that the Holocaust of World War II was not about redemption. It had no silver lining, no healing of it was or ever will be possible. We might extend his idea to other mass atrocities, other wars.

References

Anonymous (2001). January 15. Sri Lanka arrests students over truce pressure. 123 India.com & AFP.

Amarasingam, L.R. (1973). Laughter as Cure: Joking and Exorcism in a Sinhalese Curing Ritual. Unpublished doctoral dissertation, Cornell University.

Asad, T. (1987). On Ritual and Discipline in Medieval Christian Monasticism. *Economy and Society* 16(2): 159–203.

Castillo, R.J. (1998) *Meanings of Madness*. Pacific Grove, California: Brooks/Cole.

Daniel, E.V. (1997). Suffering Nation and Alienation. In *Social Suffering*, edited by Arthur Kleinman, Veena Das, and Margaret Lock, pp. 261–283. Berkeley, Los Angeles and London: University of California Press.

Das, V., Kleinman, A. and Ramphele, M. (eds) (2001). *Violence and Subjectivity*. Berkeley and Los Angeles: University of California Press.

Dugger, C.W. (2000). September 11. Rebels Without a Childhood in Sri Lanka War. *New York Times*.

Kapferer, B. (1997). *The Feast of the Sorcerer: Practices of Consciousness and Power*. Chicago: University of Chicago Press.

Kleinman, A., Das, V. and Lock, M. (editors) (1997). *Social Suffering*. Berkeley, Los Angeles and London: University of California Press.

Lakoff, G. (1992). Metaphor and war: the metaphor system used to justify war in the Gulf. In *Thirty Years of Linguistic Evolution: Studies in honour of Rene Dirven on the occasion of his sixtieth birthday*, edited by Martin Putz, pp. 463–481. Philadelphia and Amsterdam: Benjamins.

Langer, L.L. (1997). The Alarmed Vision: Social Suffering and Holocaust Atrocity. In *Social Suffering*, edited by Arthur Kleinman, Veena Das, and Margaret Lock, pp. 47–66. Berkeley, Los Angeles and London: University of California Press.

Lawrence, P. (1997). Work of oracles, silence of terror: Notes on the injury of war in eastern Sri Lanka. Doctoral dissertation, University of Colorado, Boulder.

McDonald, S. (2001). January 15. Sri Lanka students detained ahead of peace protest. London: Reuters Limited.

Nabokov, I. (2000). *Religion Against the Self: An Ethnography of Tamil Rituals*. Oxford: Oxford University Press.

Obeyesekere, G. (1969). The Ritual Drama of the *Sanni* Demons: Collective Representations of Disease in Ceylon. *Comparative Studies in Society and History* 11(2): 174–216.

Roberts, M. (1996). Filial Devotion and the Tiger Cult of Suicide. *Contributions to Indian Sociology* 30: 245–272.

Scott, D. (1992). Anthropology and Colonial Discourse: Aspects of the Demonological Construction of Sinhala Cultural Practice. *Cultural Anthropology* 7(3): 301–326.

—— (1994). *Formations of ritual: colonial and anthropological discourses on the Sinhala yaktovil*. Minneapolis: University of Minnesota Press.

[Trawick] Egnor, M. (1983). Death and Nurturance in Indian Systems of Healing. *Social Science and Medicine* 17: 935–945.

Yalman, N. (1964). The Structure of Sinhalese Healing Rituals. *Journal of Asian Studies* 27: 115–150.

Wirz, P. (1954). *Exorcism and the Art of Healing in Ceylon*. Leiden: E.J. Brill.

Charles Leslie's Publications

Books

1960   *Now We Are Civilized: A study of the world view of the Zapotec Indians of Mitla, Oaxaca.* Detroit, MI: Wayne State University Press.

1960   *Anthropology of Folk Religion.* New York: Vintage Books.

1965   *Uomo a mito nelle culture primitive.* Sansoni: Florence (Italian edition of *Anthropology of Folk Religion*)

1976   *Asian Medical Systems: A comparative study.* Berkeley: University of California Press.

1980   Reprint of *Now We Are Civilized.* Westport, CT: Greenwood.

1992   *Paths to Asian Medical Knowledge,* co-edited with Allan Young. Berkeley: University of California Press.

1993   Indian edition of *Paths to Asian Medical Knowledge.* New Delhi: Munshiram Manoharlal Publishers.

1998   Indian edition of *Asian Medical Systems: A comparative study.* New Delhi: Motilal Banarsidas Publishers.

Articles and Reviews

1952   "Style tradition and change: An analysis of the earliest painted pottery from North Iraq." In *Journal of Near Eastern Studies.* 11(1): 57–66.

1956   Review in Man, Culture and Society, H.L. Shapiro, ed. In *American Sociological Review.* 21: 802–3.

1958   Review of *Cuentos Mixes* by Walter Miller. In *Journal of American Folklore.* 71(383): 584–5.

1960   "From the Guest Editor," Special Issue, *The Social Anthropology of Middle America. Alpha Kappa Deltan,* XXX, winter issue.

1960   "Fox Impressions." In *Documentary History of the Fox Project,* edited by Fred Gearing, R. McNetting and Lisa Redfield Peattie. University of Chicago Press, pp. 87–92.

1963   Comment on "Magic and Religion" by Rosalie and Murray Wax. In *Current Anthropology.* 4: 509–10.

1963   "The Rhetoric of the Ayurvedic Revival in Modern India." In *MAN.* LXII(82): 72–73.

1965   Review *of Talea and Juquila: A comparison of Zapotec Social Organization* by Laura Nader. In *American Anthropologist.* 67: 1320–5.

1966   Review *of Folk Practices in North Mexico* by Isabel Kelley. In *Western Folklore.* XXV(4): 264–65.

1967   Review of Social Change In Modern India by M.N. Srinivas. In *American Anthropologist.* 69(3–4): 420–21.

1967   "Professional and, Popular Health Cultures in South Asia." In *Understanding Science and Technology in India and Pakistan,* edited by Ward Morehouse, University of the State of New York Press, pp. 27–42.

1968   Robert Redfeld. In *International Encyclopedia of the Social Sciences,* 13, Macmillan, pp. 350–53.

1968   "The Professionalization of Ayurvedic and Unani Medicine." In *Transactions of the New York Academy of Sciences.* 30(4): 559–72. (Reprinted in *Medical Men and Their Work,* edited by Eliot Freidson, J. Lorber, Aldine, 1972).

1969   "Modern India's Ancient Medicine." In *Trans-Action.* June, 46–55. (Reprinted in Sociological Realities, edited by I. L. Horowitz and M.S. Strong, Harper & Row, 1970.)

1970   Review of *Humanity and Modern Sociological Thought* by R.P. Cuzzort. In *American Anthropologist.* 72: 718.

1970   "Symbolic Behavior" (Review of *The Ritual Process* by Victor Turner). In *Science.* 168: 702–4.

1971   Review *of The Zinantecos* of Mexico by E.Z. Vogt. In *MAN.* 6 (new series): 513–14.

1972   "Research Needs to Develop the Comparative Study of Asian Medical Systems." In *Asian Studies Professional Review.* 1(2): 12–17.

1972   "Burg Wartenstein Symposium." In *Medical Anthropology Newsletter.* 3(2): 9–11.

1972   "Asian Medicine." In *Medical Anthropology Newsletter.* Vii: 13–14; and 3(4): 10–11.

1973   "The Professionalizing Ideology of Medical Revivalism." In *Entrepreneurship and Modernization of Occupational Cultures in South Asia.* Edited by Milton Singer, Duke University Press, pp. 16–42.

1973   "Asian Medical Systems: A Symposium on the Role of Comparative Sociology in Improving Health Care", with co-author, Carl E. Tylor. In *Social Science & Medicine.* 7(4): 307–18.

1973   Review of Edwin H. Ackernecht, *Medicine in Ethnology Selected Essays.* In *Contemporary Sociology.*

1974   "Scientific Medicine in a Secular Society." In *Religion and Medicine,* edited by K.N. Udupa and Germohan Singh. Banaras Hindu University Press, pp. 17–29.

1974   "The Modernization of Asian Medical Systems." In *Rethinking Modernization: Anthropological Approaches,* edited by John Poggie and R. Lynch. Greenwood Press, pp. 69–108.

1975   "The Role of Indigenous Health Practitioners in Family Health." In *Health of the Family: Proceedings of the* 1974 *International Health', Conference.* National Council for International Health, pp. 155–181. (Introduction by C. Leslie, Chair, and papers by Chang Wei-hsun, Arthur Kleinman and K.N. Udupa.)

1976 "Pluralism and Integration in the Indian and Chinese Medical Systems."
In *Medicine in Chinese Cultures: Comparative cross cultural studies of health
care in Chinese and other societies* (John E. Fogarty International Center
for Advanced Study in the Health Sciences). Reprinted in *Culture, Disease
and Healing* edited by David Landy. New York: Macmillan, 1977.

1976 "The Hedgehog and the Fox in Robert Redfield's Work and, Career." In
American Anthropology: The Early Years, edited by John Murra,
Proceedings of the American Ethnological Society, West Publishing Co.

1977 "Foreword" to *Ayurveda: The Knowledge of Life by* Kumar Alagoppan.
Madras Association of Medicine Press.

1978 "Foreword" to *The Quest for Therapy in Lower Zaire* by John Janzen,
University of California Press.

1978 Review of Joe Loudon, ed., Social Anthropology and Medicine. In *American
Ethnologist.* 386–389.

1978 "Introduction" to *Theoretical Foundations for the Comparative Study of
Medical Systems,* edited by Charles Leslie. Special issue of *Social Science
& Medicine.* 12(2B): 65–69.

1980 "Medical pluralism in world perspective." In *Medical Pluralism,* edited by
Charles Leslie. Special issue of *Social Science Medicine.* 14B(4): 190–96.

1981 Review of The Future of Academic Community Medicine in Developing
Countries edited by Willoughby Lathem. In *Medical Anthropology
Newsletter.* 12(4): 25.

1982 Review of Judith Farquhar and D. Carlton Gajdusek, Kurul, Early Letters
and Field Notes, and of Shirley Lindenbaum, Kuru Sorcery. In *Bulletin of
the History of Medicine.* 56(2): 144–147.

1982 Review of George Murdock, "Theories of Illness: A World Survey". In
Bulletin of the History of Medicine. 56(2): 305–b.

1983 "Policy options in regulating the practice of traditional medicine." In
Traditional Medicine and Health Care Coverage edited by Robert
Bannerman, John Burton, Ch'en Wen-Chieh. Geneva: World Health
Organization.

1985 "What caused India's massive community health workers scheme: A sociology of knowledge." In *The Chinese Model in Health Care Planning,*
edited by Charles Leslie. Special issue of Social *Science & Medicine.* 21(8):
923–930.

1987 "Interpretations of illness: syncretism in modem Ayurveda." In the 9th
International Symposium on the Comparative History of Medicine, East
and West, *The History of Diagnoses,* pp. 7–42, The Taniguchi Foundation,
Japan.

1987 "Medicine in Asia." In *Encyclopedia of Asian History,* The Asia Society,
New York: Charles Scribner Sons.

1988 Review of Stephen Frankel, *The Huli Response to Illness.* In *Bulletin of the
History of Medicine.* 62: 339–40.

1988 "Social research and health care planning in South Asia." In *Ancient Science
of Life, Journal of the International Institute of Ayurveda.* Vlll(I): 1–12; and
Vill(2): 75–91. Coimbatore.

1988 "Foreword" to D.N. Kakar, *Primary Health Care and Traditional Medical
Practitioners.* New Delhi: Munshiram Manoharlal Publishers.

1988   "Foreword" to *The Context of Medicines in Developing Countries Studies in Pharmaceutical Anthropology* edited by Sjaak van der Geest. Kluwer Academic Publishers.

1989   "Magic and Curing in Thailand." In *Reviews in Anthropology*. 14(4) back issue 1987.

1989   "Indigenous Pharmaceuticals, the Capitalist World System and Civilization." In *Kroeber Anthropology Society Papers*. 1, 69–70: 23–32.

1989   "India's Community Health Workers Scheme: A Sociological Analysis," *Ancient Science of Life*. IX(2): 40–53.

1990   "Scientific Racism: Reflections on peer review, science and ideology," *Social Science & Medicine*. 31(8): 801–912.

1995   "The Blind Anthropologist and the Elephant of Traditional Asian Medicine." In *Proceedings, Part 9, The 4th International Congress on Traditional Asian Medicine,* published by Department of the History of Medicine, Juntendo University, Tokyo.

1996   Review of Priya Vrat Sharma, (editor), "History of Medicine in India." In *Bulletin of the History of Medicine*. 70: 308–9.

1998   Review of George Foster, *Hippocrates' Latin American Legacy: Humoral Medicine in the New World,* in *Transcultural Psychiatry*. 35(1): 140–43.

Forthcoming:

"Robert Redfield." In the *Oxford Encyclopedia of Mesoamoican Cultures,* Oxford University Press.

Comment on "Heaps of health, metaphysical fitness, Ayurveda and the ontology of good health in medical anthropology" by Joseph Alter. In *Current Anthropology*.

Index

Printed and bound by CPI Group (UK) Ltd, Croydon, CR0 4YY

01/11/2024

01782635-0009